Vital Pulp Treatment

Vital Pulp Treatment

Edited by

Henry F. Duncan
Professor and Consultant in Endodontics
Division of Restorative Dentistry and Periodontology, Dublin Dental University Hospital
Trinity College Dublin, Lincoln Place, Dublin 2, Ireland

Ikhlas A. El-Karim
Clinical Professor and Consultant in Restorative Dentistry
School of Medicine, Dentistry and Biomedical Sciences, Queen's University
Belfast, Northern Ireland, UK

WILEY Blackwell

This edition first published 2024

Registered Offices
John Wiley & Sons, Inc., 111 River Street, Hoboken, NJ 07030, USA
John Wiley & Sons Ltd, The Atrium, Southern Gate, Chichester, West Sussex, PO19 8SQ, UK

For details of our global editorial offices, customer services, and more information about Wiley products visit us at www.wiley.com.

Wiley also publishes its books in a variety of electronic formats and by print-on-demand. Some content that appears in standard print versions of this book may not be available in other formats.

Library of Congress Cataloging-in-Publication Data
Names: Duncan, Henry, 1971- editor. | El-Karim, Ikhlas A., editor.
Title: Vital pulp treatment / edited by Henry F. Duncan, Ikhlas A. El-Karim.
Description: Hoboken, NJ : Wiley-Blackwell, 2024. | Includes index.
Identifiers: LCCN 2023043780 (print) | LCCN 2023043781 (ebook) | ISBN 9781119930389 (hardback) | ISBN 9781119930396 (adobe pdf) | ISBN 9781119930402 (epub)
Subjects: MESH: Dental Pulp Diseases–therapy
Classification: LCC RK351 (print) | LCC RK351 (ebook) | NLM WU 230 | DDC 617.6/342–dc23/eng/20231107
LC record available at https://lccn.loc.gov/2023043780
LC ebook record available at https://lccn.loc.gov/2023043781

Cover Design: Wiley
Cover Images: © Henry Duncan

Set in 9.5/12.5pt STIXTwoText by Straive, Pondicherry, India

Printed and bound by CPI Group (UK) Ltd, Croydon, CR0 4YY

C9781119930389_020224

Contents

List of Contributors

Isaac J. de Souza Araújo
Department of Cariology, Restorative Sciences, and Endodontics
University of Michigan School of Dentistry
Ann Arbor, MI, USA

Department of Bioscience Research, College of Dentistry
University of Tennessee Health Science Center
Memphis, TN, USA

Lars Bjørndal
Cariology and Endodontics, Section of Clinical Oral Microbiology, Department of Odontology, Faculty of Health and Medical Sciences
University of Copenhagen
Copenhagen, Denmark

Marco C. Bottino
Department of Cariology, Restorative Sciences, and Endodontics
University of Michigan School of Dentistry
Ann Arbor, MI, USA

Department of Biomedical Engineering, College of Engineering
University of Michigan
Ann Arbor, MI, USA

Roberto Careddu
Division of Restorative Dentistry and Periodontology
Dublin Dental University Hospital, Trinity College Dublin
Dublin, Ireland

Bruno Cavalcanti
Department of Cariology, Restorative Sciences and Endodontics
University of Michigan School of Dentistry
Ann Arbor, MI, USA

Daniel Chiego, Jr.
Department of Cariology, Restorative Sciences and Endodontics
University of Michigan School of Dentistry
Ann Arbor, MI, USA

Paul R. Cooper
Faculty of Dentistry, Sir John Walsh Research Institute
University of Otago
Dunedin, New Zealand

Siobhan Cushley
Centre for Dentistry, School of Medicine Dentistry and Biomedical Sciences
Queen's University Belfast
Belfast, Northern Ireland, UK

Renan Dal-Fabbro
Department of Cariology, Restorative Sciences, and Endodontics
University of Michigan School of Dentistry
Ann Arbor, MI, USA

Till Dammaschke
Department of Periodontology and Operative Dentistry
University of Münster
Münster, Germany

Henry F. Duncan
Division of Restorative Dentistry and Periodontology
Dublin Dental University Hospital, Trinity College Dublin
Dublin, Ireland

Ikhlas A. El-Karim
Department of Restorative Dentistry, School of Medicine, Dentistry and Biomedical Sciences
Queen's University Belfast
Belfast, Northern Ireland, UK

Helena Fransson
Department of Endodontics, Faculty of Odontology
Malmö University
Malmö, Sweden

Lara T. Friedlander
Faculty of Dentistry, Sir John Walsh Research Institute
University of Otago
Dunedin, New Zealand

Johnah C. Galicia
College of Dentistry, Manila Central University
EDSA-Monumento
Caloocan City, Philippines

Kerstin M. Galler
Department of Operative Dentistry and Periodontology
Friedrich-Alexander-University
Erlangen, Germany

Bill Kahler
Faculty of Medicine and Health, Department of Restorative and Reconstructive Dentistry, Sydney Dental School
The University of Sydney
Surry Hills, NSW, Australia

Asma A. Khan
Department of Endodontics, School of Dentistry
UT Health San Antonio
San Antonio, TX, USA

Yoshifumi Kobayashi
Department of Oral Biology
Rutgers School of Dental Medicine
Newark, NJ, USA

Mark Lappin
Department of Restorative Dentistry, School of Medicine, Dentistry and Biomedical Sciences
Queen's University Belfast
Belfast, Northern Ireland, UK

Fionnuala T. Lundy
The Wellcome-Wolfson Institute for Experimental Medicine
School of Medicine, Dentistry and Biomedical Sciences
Queen's University Belfast
Belfast, Northern Ireland, UK

Venkateshbabu Nagendrababu
Department of Preventive and Restorative Dentistry
College of Dental Medicine, University of Sharjah
Sharjah, UAE

Giampiero Rossi-Fedele
Adelaide Dental School, The University of Adelaide
Adelaide, SA, Australia

Emi Shimizu
Department of Oral Biology, Rutgers School of Dental Medicine
Newark, NJ, USA

Matthias Widbiller
Department of Conservative Dentistry and Periodontology
University Hospital Regensburg
Regensburg, Germany

Foreword

In this era of sustainability, the need for minimally invasive, conservative and biologically based treatment approaches has never been more compelling. The patient-centred benefits of such strategies have been clearly illustrated in the success of selective removal of deep caries in operative dentistry, and this approach is now attracting significant interest in the field of vital pulp treatment (VPT). VPT offers a suite of minimally invasive therapies that have the potential to make treatment less invasive, simpler and biologically based while replacing more complex and invasive traditional root canal therapies.

Although not a new concept, the last two decades witnessed a remarkable interest in VPT. Advances in pulp biology research and an improved understanding of the nature of the reparative and regenerative processes in dental pulp, coupled with the continued development of biomaterials, have contributed to the trend. Many published clinical studies have recently demonstrated success for VPT over conventional root canal treatment. It is evident that there are advantages in preserving pulp vitality, highlighted by the simplicity of the techniques and potential cost savings and to that end, VPT has now been endorsed by major professional bodies including the European Society of Endodontology and the American Association of Endodontists. However, many dentists point out that they do not feel well-trained in the area. As the area evolves and the quality of the research supporting VPT continues to improve, it is important that current evidence is summarized and explained systematically in order to improve the understanding of the dental practitioner interested in carrying out VPT. To date, VPT techniques are usually reduced to one chapter in an operative dentistry or endodontic textbook, so we thought it imperative that the breath of VPT, from reasons to keep the pulp, through diagnosis, to management and outcome, were detailed in one user-friendly text.

Furthermore, at present, controversial practices and lack of consensus among clinicians on the best approach to manage deep caries and exposed pulp remain, and there is a need for more education and training to increase awareness and improve the clinical decision-making process and appropriate case selection for VPT. The aim of this book is to provide contemporary, evidence-based and scientific reference to the clinical development and application of VPT in permanent teeth. For this, an international group of experts in pulp biology, cariology, dental trauma, VPT, dental materials and regenerative endodontics contributed chapters highlighting their state-of-the-art skills and knowledge in their respective fields. The result is a book that provides an in-depth knowledge and understanding of the scientific basis for pulp preservation therapies and the importance of maintaining pulp vitality. Secondly, clear clinical guidance with evidence-based clinical protocols is provided for all VPT procedures such as direct pulp capping and partial and complete pulpotomy for both the cariously and traumatically exposed pulps. Accurate diagnosis is a prerequisite for successful VPT; therefore, pulpal diagnosis is considered as a standalone chapter, but the subject is covered throughout the book, reflecting the importance and also the limitations of our current practice in this area. The development in applied biomaterials, revitalization and regenerative endodontic treatment as well as expected outcomes and follow-up, are covered in the later chapters of the book.

The book combines cutting-edge information with protocols and an array of illustrations, making it suitable for a wide range of clinicians including undergraduate students, postgraduate clinical trainees and researchers, endodontists and general dental practitioners. The book aims to provide a contemporary evidence-based reference in the first book dedicated to VPT, providing answers to existing controversies and considering future perfectives and development in the field. VPT is no doubt evolving, and the hope is that future editions of this book will keep with the momentum. We hope you enjoy the text.

Ikhlas A. El-Karim, Belfast, Northern Ireland, UK
Henry F. Duncan, Dublin, Ireland

Preface

Vital pulp treatment in its various forms has been a subject discussed in dentistry courses for decades. However, it is only recently, in the last five years or so, that converging developments in dental material science, pulp biology and dental have made this treatment a valid, predictable and evidence-based strategy.

It is not even 25 years ago that the long-term success rate of direct pulp capping was estimated as well below 50%, or a flip of coin; this poor outcome understandably has led many clinicians to view vital pulp treatment as somewhat of a second-class treatment, more like an attempt rather than as a bone fide definitive treatment. This perception is changing due to clear and compelling evidence from clinical trials supporting vital pulp therapy and it is rather exciting to see a case made for its application made in this book.

Reasons to maintain a functional pulp-dentine complex are numerous and can be summarized broadly into categories: adding positive features and avoiding potentially negative elements inherent to the main comparator, i.e. root canal treatment (RCT). Vital pulp treatment or VPT retains immunocompetent tissues that effectively provide microbial clearance and protection from apical periodontitis. Moreover, in teeth with incomplete root formation, VPT promotes further dentine apposition and apical maturation. Conversely, RCT is associated with a larger damage to structural integrity, higher cost and specifically for molars with significantly higher clinical complexity.

Indeed, many patients may benefit from VPT in their desire to retain the natural dentition for the long term. It is therefore very fitting and timely that Ikhlas El-Karim and Henry (Hal) Duncan, two clinicians with a strong biomedical understanding, have edited this book; it offers a compelling and comprehensive update on all aspects of VPT, from the case for the selection of the procedure, over material choices to related biology and outcomes.

A balanced group of international authors has contributed to this volume, providing a broad and well-reasoned approach. First the case for treating, rather than removing, the pulp is made by Daniel Chiego and Bruno Cavalcanti succinctly from a functional and a biologic approach. The next chapter authored Paul Cooper, Lara Friedlander and Fionnuala Lundy draws from the vast experience of these authors in pulp biology to strengthen the rationale even more.

This book is directed towards clinicians with a scientific mindset and the following chapters provide contemporary viewpoints on practical aspects of vital pulp therapy. First Asma Khan and Johnah Galicia describe various aspects of pulp diagnostics, an essential step in predicable VPT. With the understanding that VPT is often prescribed in treatment of deep caries, Lars Bjørndal and Helena Fransson provide relevant information from the viewpoint of caries removal strategies.

Moving forward to VPT procedures that are more extensive Till Dammaschke in his chapter looks at direct pulp capping, a procedure that has received much attention with the development of silicate-based biomaterials. Pulpotomy, an approach that aims to physically remove all coronal pulp with little or no capacity to heal is then discussed by the editors themselves, supported by Roberto Careddu and Mark Lapin.

Chapters 7–10 provide important information for other areas that are critical to the current understanding, including materials (Renan Dal Fabbro, Isaac De Souza Araujo and Marco Bottino), treatment of traumatic injuries (Giampiero Rossi Fedele and Bill Kahler) and regenerative procedures (Matthias Widbiller and Kerstin Galler).

The last chapter on epidemiology and outcomes (Siobhan Cushley, Venkatesh Nagendrababu and Emi Shimizu), again written by authorities in the field, completes this volume.

The enthusiasm of the editors and authors for the topic is palpable and fits where the field is moving internationally, that is towards a much broader acceptance of vital pulp therapy. Providing current and directly applicable information that underpins this therapy is a crucial step in this direction. I am convinced that this book will enjoy a wide readership, equally for seasoned clinicians those at the beginning of their careers.

Ove A. Peters, Professor of Endodontics,
School of Dentistry, The University of Queensland,
Brisbane, QLD, Australia

1

The Importance of Maintaining Pulp Vitality

Bruno Cavalcanti and Daniel Chiego, Jr.

Department of Cariology, Restorative Sciences and Endodontics, University of Michigan School of Dentistry, Ann Arbor, MI, USA

Introduction

When the pulp is inflamed, either reversibly or irreversibly, it is important for clinicians to question the success rates, possible outcomes and patient satisfaction associated with each treatment option. This is also true when considering using more conservative options like vital pulp treatment (VPT) or traditional therapies such as root canal treatment. As highlighted elsewhere in this book, both have a good success rate and can be used as reliable options for the management of pulpal disease.

In this context, one question commonly asked by clinicians is 'what are the real benefits of maintaining the pulp?' It is well-known that immature teeth benefit considerably from VPT. However, clinicians may not see the importance of keeping the pulp tissue for other cases, as the only perceived benefit would be the maintenance of tooth sensitivity. While this benefit is correct, the pulp plays other important roles within the tooth, most notably with the molecular mechanisms to defend the body from bacterial challenge. Furthermore, with the fast development of regenerative therapies, the pulp will be essential to rebuild lost tooth structures and improve the tooth's prognosis. This book chapter will show a number of molecular mechanisms that are involved in this regenerative process, how the pulp physiology contributes to clinical practice and, most important, show the importance of the pulp tissue in the maintenance of tooth homeostasis.

Dental Pulp Development

To appreciate the importance that the pulp plays on tooth homeostasis, it is necessary to appreciate how the dentine-pulp complex develops. The developmental stages bring a number of insights into the participation of different cell types and the subsequent organization of dental tissues, which can also be recapitulated into the desired repair and regeneration processes after dental procedures.

Tooth development is a process that involves a well-coordinated effort between cells from different origins, leading to the formation of a complex organ (detailed in Chapter 2). Unfortunately, when analysing pulp repair/regeneration processes, the clinician is not able to mimic whole tooth formation. This is complicated further by the cells present in the pulp tissue that may not have the

Vital Pulp Treatment, First Edition. Edited by Henry F. Duncan and Ikhlas A. El-Karim.

same potential as the original cells during tooth development. Nonetheless, the translation of the process at the molecular level to the clinical activity can be of great importance to direct future studies and biomaterial development.

In this context, the participation of stem cells in the development process is important. It is now well established that the pulp tissue has its own reserve of multipotent cells, capable of differentiating into the necessary tissues and/or replacing cells that were damaged or simply completed their function and enter into senescence (1). In fact, most dental tissues have their own mesenchymal stem cells; the enamel, for obvious reasons, is deprived of any cells after tooth eruption and, thus, does not have the same regenerative potential as other tissues. The discovery of dental pulp stem cells (DPSCs) brought many possibilities, more specifically in the understanding of the success of VPT and regenerative endodontics. DPSCs are capable of differentiation into a myriad of cells and tissues, including odontoblasts, fibroblasts, endothelial cells and neurons (2–4), being capable of regenerating all cell types necessary to form a new pulp tissue. This potential appears superior to responses observed with other stem cell populations (3). In addition, the literature shows, in animal models, that the neoformed pulp tissue in complete root models is very similar to the original pulp tissue (5, 6) (Figure 1.1). Moreover, these new pulp tissues were induced only in the presence of the host vasculature and DPSCs, suggesting that the potential is there for complete regeneration or at least functional repair.

Cell Signalling and Dental Pulp Development

Most studies using DPSCs have focused on the potential of these cells to differentiate into odontoblasts (7–9). This is understandable as, in the reparative process, clinicians want the neoformed pulp tissue to produce dentine in order for this barrier to serve as protection to the tissue. Understanding odontoblast differentiation is a difficult process: some studies have shown that the reparative dentine, particularly when induced by certain materials, can be tubular (10–12); other studies have shown that, most of the time, the barrier does not have the tubular aspect, meaning that the formed tissue is more akin to 'osteodentine' than to actual dentine (13, 14). This brings uncertainty, as there is no specific odontoblast marker(s) to confirm that the differentiated stem cell is a real odontoblast. Studies have looked into dentin-matrix-acidic-phoshoprotein 1 (DMP-1), dentin-sialophosphoprotein (DSPP), matrix extracellular phosphoglycoprotein (MEPE), nestin and others, generally trying to observe their presence in combination with each other (2, 7, 15–17). However, it is important to emphasize that some of these genes can be expressed by osteoblasts and other cell types, meaning that the differentiated cells observed in molecular analysis may not be a typical odontoblast cell.

With this, it is possible to separate the two concepts of regeneration and repair: from a clinical standpoint, having an adequate regeneration/repair with a solid dentine (or osteodentine) barrier, pulp vitality and functional tooth is good enough for patient satisfaction. On the other hand, from a research standpoint, it can be frustrating that with all the potential observed from the stem cells, we are still not able to regenerate the tissues as they are, complete with an odontoblast pseudostratified layer, cell junctions and tubular dentine.

Some answers for this dichotomy may be due to a shortage of information on molecular signalling. As discussed above, during tooth development, there is a very well-coordinated effort and interaction between different cell types and layers to induce tissue formation and even tooth shape (18, 19). For example, it is known that the signalling between the ameloblasts and mesenchymal cells in the dental papilla induces the initial cell differentiation towards odontoblasts, which consequently directs the deposition of an initially 'disorganized' layer (the mantle dentine) and then starts the construction of the typical tubular pattern of orthodentine, by a centripetal

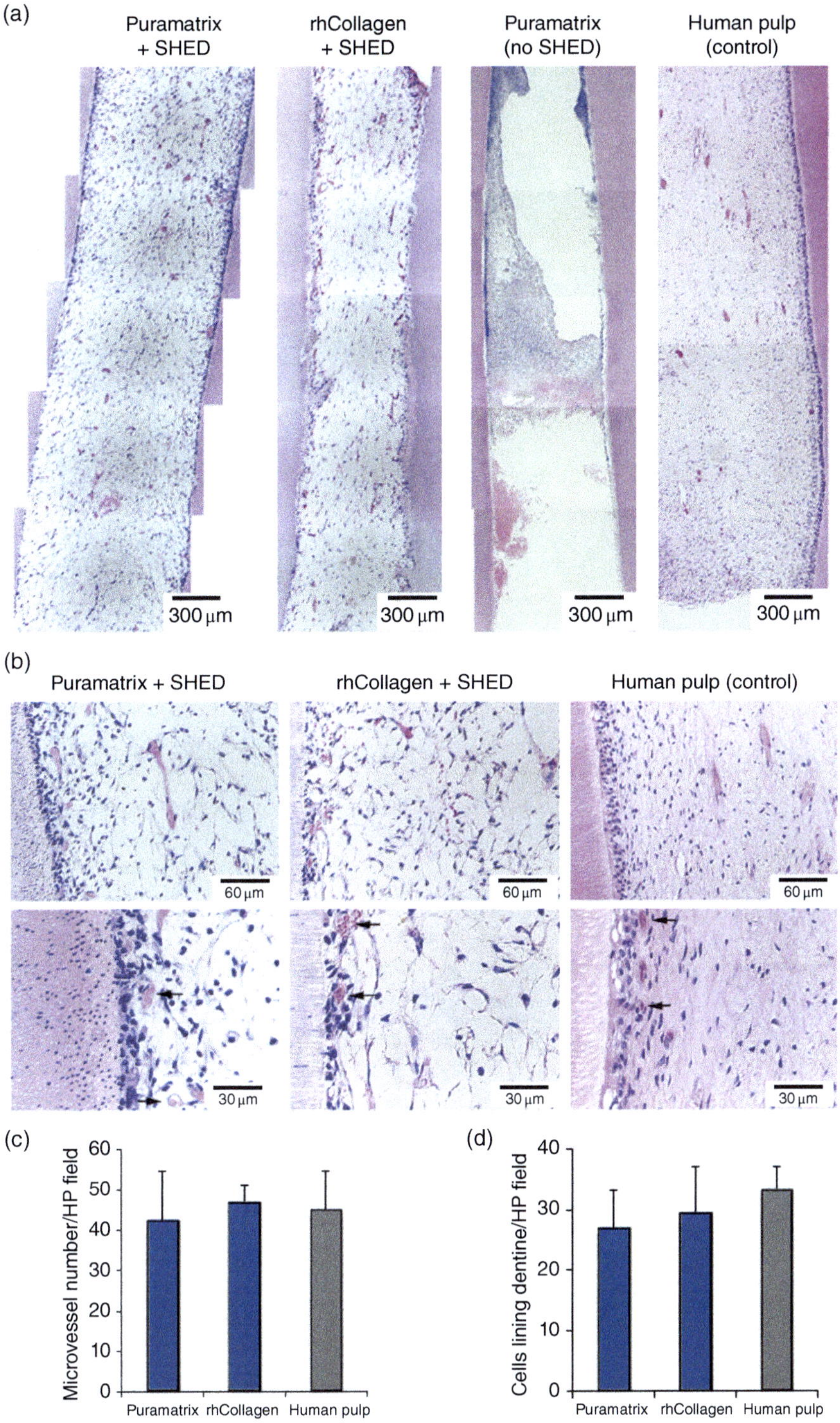

Figure 1.1 Dental pulp tissue engineering with SHED injected into human root canals and transplanted into immunodeficient mice. (a) Low-magnification and (b) high-magnification images of tissues formed when SHED mixed with scaffolds (Puramatrix™, rhCollagen type I groups) were injected into full-length root canals of human premolars. A vascularized connective tissue occupied the full extension of the root canal. Cell densification and many blood vessels were observed along dentin walls. Scaffolds (Puramatrix™) injected into the root canals without cells were used as controls for SHED. Freshly extracted human premolars were used as tissue controls. Black arrows point to blood vessels close to the odontoblastic layer. (c) Graph depicting microvessel density and (d) cellular density of dental pulp tissues engineered with SHED injected into full human root canals. Microvessel density and cellular density were similar in both experimental conditions and the control group (human pulp), as determined by one-way ANOVA (5). Reproduced with permission from International & American Associations for Dental Research.

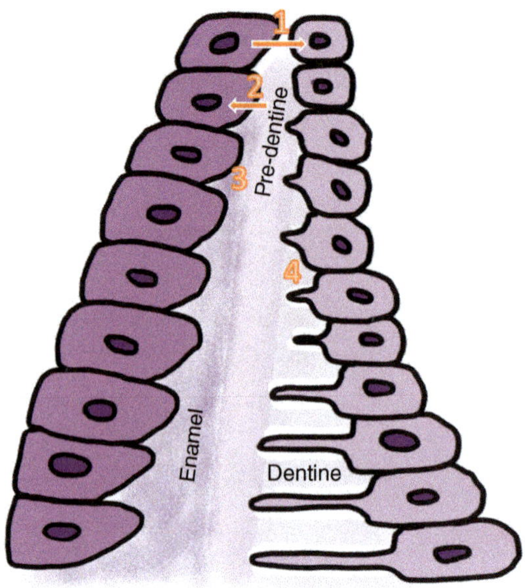

Figure 1.2 Sequence of dentine formation – (1) signalling from pre-ameloblasts to pre-odontoblasts (DSPP, enamelysin and ameloblastin) and deposition of a baseline collagen matrix; (2) deposition of pre-dentine by the immature odontoblasts, leading to signalling to ameloblasts; (3) enamel deposition; (4) dentin (tubular deposition). Both ameloblasts and odontoblasts mature throughout the process.

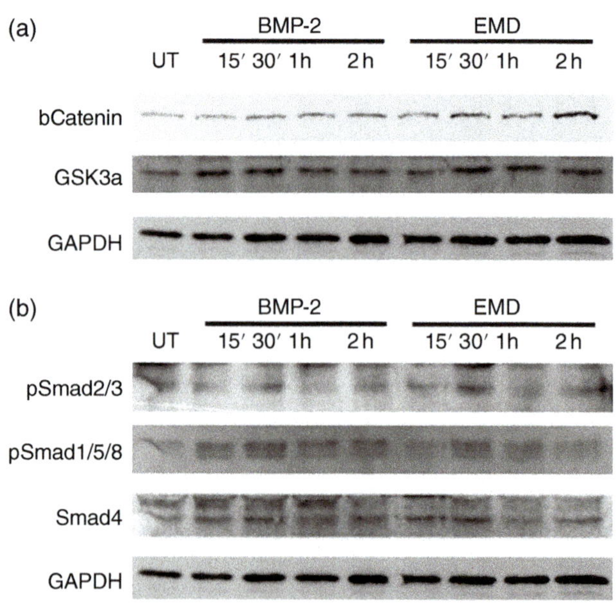

Figure 1.3 Western blotting analysis of pathways affected by BMP-2 (a known dentine inducer) and EMD (enamel matrix derivatives) on dental pulp stem cells. Differences can be seen by the increase of expressed Wnt pathway proteins for EMD (a) and the increase of Smad 4 for BMP-2 in the canonical BMP pathway (b). Unpublished data.

direction of movement of the odontoblast layer (Figure 1.2). This signalling is comprised principally of DSPP, enamelysin and ameloblastin (20). However, it is evident that the Wnt and Sonic hedgehog (SHH) pathways and the deposition of a baseline collagen matrix are also essential for the correct cell lining (18, 21). With this, attempts were made to use enamel derivative proteins to induce pulp repair. However, there are differences between the differentiation induced by enamel matrix derivatives (EMD) and mineral trioxide aggregate (MTA), for example, even if the gene expression changes are similar (Figure 1.3). Clinically, none of the materials used for pulp capping and/or regenerative procedures is capable of synthesizing and secreting the original signalling molecules layered by ameloblasts. This does not mean that the regeneration process is impossible. The literature has shown examples that the dentine itself is a major reservoir of multiple growth factors that can activate multiple signalling pathways into DPSCs (22). More importantly, these growth factors can be mobilized by current materials used for pulp capping (e.g. calcium hydroxide and MTA), which can be of great importance in chemotaxis prior to inducing cell differentiation and production of the dentine barrier (23–25).

The Role of the Apical Papilla

Last, but not least in tooth development, is the role of the apical papilla. While considered an embryonic tissue, the apical papilla is a mesenchymal tissue that remains active until the complete maturation of the tooth (Figure 1.4). After the deposition of the first layers of dentine at the crown level and subsequent formation of the primitive pulp tissue, the remnants of the dental papilla continue to work with the Hertwig's epithelial root sheath in order to guide the development of the cementum, alveolar bone, radicular dentine and periodontal ligament (26, 27). As with the crown, the signalling between epithelial and mesenchymal cells is responsible for tissue differentiation of the stem cells present in this tissue and consequent dentinogenesis. Even after the tooth eruption, the root(s) will continue to develop and, until the development is complete, the apical papilla will remain. As the original dental papilla, the apical papilla is rich in undifferentiated cells with multipotent capacity, which makes it a great source of stem cells for revitalization or revascularization procedures (28).

This understanding of the tooth development process brings insight into the repair process induced by VPTs. The first associated with the presence of undifferentiated cells and its potential to differentiate into odontoblasts and other cell types necessary for repair and regeneration. Second, it is expected that an effective material will closely mimic the interactions between these mesenchymal stem cells and the epithelial cells that formerly underlined the primitive pulp tissue. Third, molecules that participate not only in the differentiation process but also in the cell recruiting events may be of interest for using dental materials. This can happen directly or indirectly as dentine serves as a reservoir for many of these factors, and materials can be affected by extracting them from the tissue and mobilizing them for cell intake.

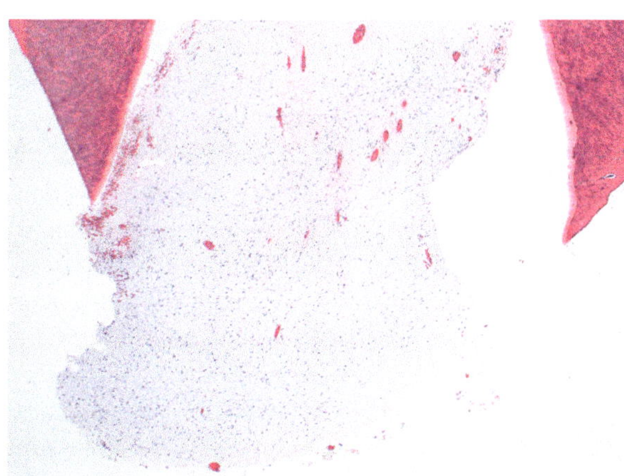

Figure 1.4 Histologic image from the apical papilla, detaching from the root apex of an immature third molar. Observe the high cellularity and vascularization of the tissue, which can be preserved partially and used for endodontic regenerative purposes (HE, 40×).

Stem Cell Reserve and Healing/Regeneration Potential of the Dental Pulp

Current concepts on pulp regeneration rely on stem cells, either by transplantation or by attracting stem cells present in the body to the area, also known as cell homing. The same can be said about the repair process: it is known that the pulp has a reparative potential, and most of this potential comes from the cellularity of the tissue. Notably, previous research has shown that older patients present lower healing potential in the pulp, and that conservative pulp procedures should be mostly reserved for young patients. This comes from the fact that older connective tissues will have their cell turnover and cellularity negatively affected, and the constant production of secondary dentine determines that cells in this 'older' pulp tissue may enter senescence (29, 30). The aged pulp tissue will appear radiographically to have smaller pulp chambers and clinically have less profuse bleeding and higher levels of fibrosis. This means that a tooth that has been previously decayed with tertiary dentine production and then restored is pathologically 'older' than a completely sound tooth. It is important to differentiate this pulp age from the patient's age. With this, the literature has shown that the patient's age has little effect on the success of VPT procedures (31).

Of course, a clinical evaluation of the cellularity of the pulp tissue is not possible currently; in fact, dentistry, despite all the evolution in the last century, still does not have a reliable way to determine an exact pulp diagnosis (see Chapter 3). Thus, the professional opting for a conservative or radical procedure needs to take other factors into account besides the patient's age. Indeed, the patient's age still plays a role as the fibre: cell ratio changes over time. But other factors such as clinical diagnosis, dental history and presence of tertiary dentine and/or internal calcifications are also signs that the pulp tissue in question has already been irritated and responded. Having a clinical understanding that an aged tissue can respond less ideally in a young patient and vice versa is essential to explain both success and failure in VPT.

Pulp Vascularization and its Clinical Implications

As with most connective tissues, the dental pulp can be seen as comprised of structural fibres, cells, nerves, blood vessels and lymphatic vessels. However, when looking closely, it is clear that the pulp is more complex; it is made up of different anatomical zones and is encircled by a hard tissue secreted by odontoblasts (Figure 1.5). The impact of these anatomical attributes and other factors on the potential of the pulp to heal and/or on the determination of success in clinical procedures will be discussed further below.

Among these complexities, the internal anatomy of the pulp chamber and canals is one of the factors contributing to the evolution of inflammatory and reparative processes. As stated above, the pulp is surrounded by dentine, which is a hard tissue. This makes it impossible for the pulp tissue to swell and/or expand in case of inflammation. The apical foramen is the main point of entry for the neurovascular bundles, and the more immature the tooth is, meaning that the foramen is increased in size (open-apex), the better the tissue vascularization is. This happens even in inflammatory events and, thus, can result in better clinical outcomes when performing pulp capping and/or pulpotomy procedures. In addition, due to their small size and inconsistent numbers, lateral canals, for example, do not appear to contribute significantly to the presence of neurovascular bundles.

If clinical outcome and success of VPTs is considered, the presence of vascularization is important, as it is responsible for providing the immune cell response and the nutrients for a successful repair. It is known that angiogenesis can be induced by the presence of hypoxia, which

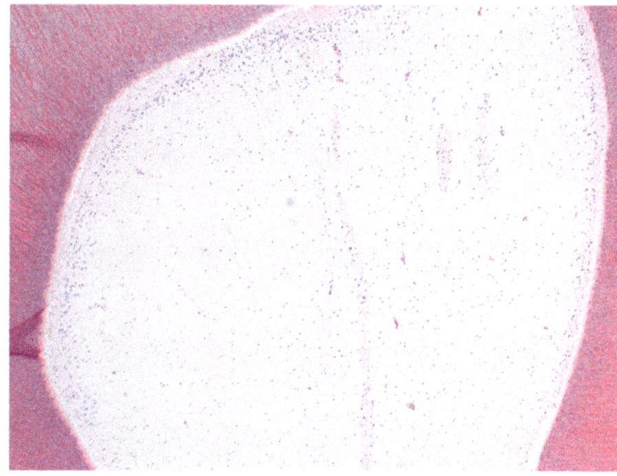

Figure 1.5 Histologic image from the pulp tissue encircled by dentine/enamel structure (HE, 40×).

is observed in a connective tissue that achieves 200 µm in size (32). The dental papilla does not have any blood vessels until it achieves this diameter, and cells start to suffer from the lack of oxygen. This lack of oxygen induces the production of hypoxia-inducible transcription factor 1–alpha (HIF1-alpha), which then induces the activation of vascular endothelial growth factor (VEGF), responsible for cell differentiation and formation of new blood vessels (33, 34). This factor is important and explains why the coronal pulp is much richer in microvessels per mm^3 than the radicular pulp, as its volume is larger. Moreover, HIF-1alpha has been connected to increased production of tertiary dentine in inflamed pulps, suggesting these factors can also contribute to the repair process (33, 35). It is essential to understand the role that hypoxia plays, not only in pulp development but also in other aspects of the homeostasis of the tissue. After any sort of damage and/or induced inflammatory process by the presence of bacterial lipopolysaccharides (LPS), it is possible that small areas of the pulp tissue will undergo different levels of hypoxia. The lack of oxygen in this tissue has the primary participation in the angiogenic process, particularly by the expression of HIF1-alpha and VEGF (Figure 1.6). Other molecules are also related to angiogenesis, more specifically the B-cell lymphoma 2 (Bcl-2) (36) and cytokines such as interleukin 1 beta (IL-1beta) and tumour necrosis factor-alpha (TNF-alpha) (37), which all have a clear effect on both the angiogenic and inflammatory processes. Moreover, the presence of hypoxia is known to activate DPSC differentiation and consequent mineralization (35, 38, 39), illustrating the close connection between the pulp damage and the repair process.

In addition to the simple presence of blood vessels, it is well-known that a vascularized tissue can also respond more effectively to harm from bacteria and materials in order that the tissue can be repaired or regenerated properly. Many studies on pulp regeneration have been focusing on the importance of vascularization and have specifically shown that, without proper angiogenesis, true regeneration cannot occur. In this context, the use of angiogenic factors such as the above-cited HIF1-alpha or the VEGF has been proven as a way to promote angiogenesis by the differentiation of DPSC into endothelial cells and by assisting with anastomosis with the host original blood vessels (2, 33). This process is essential to allow for the complete fill of the pulp space with functional tissue and, in the case of repair, VEGF, for example, could be used as an adjuvant to promote adequate oxygen levels for the pulp tissue during the initial inflammatory process and, consequently, allowing the cells to migrate and differentiate.

Besides blood vessels, lymphatic vessels appear to be of major importance in regulating inflammatory and repair processes. While the literature has opposing views on this subject, with

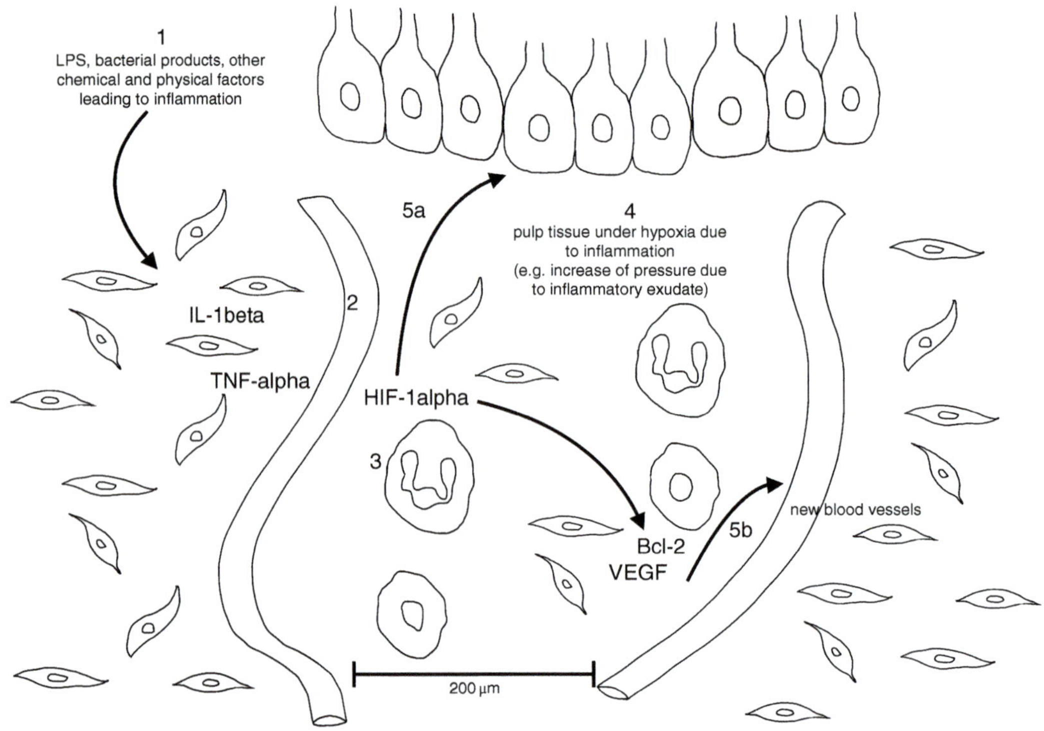

Figure 1.6 Mechanisms of hypoxia-induced dentinogenesis and angiogenesis. (1) Induction of cell response due to LPS, bacterial products and/or other irritants; (2) promotion of vasodilation by cytokines; (3) increase in inflammatory exudate on the affected tissue; (4) hypoxia; (5) as the hypoxia reaches 200 µm, affected cells release HIF-1alpha, which directly affects odontoblasts to induce tertiary dentine and/or induces the release of VEGF and Bcl-2 to form new blood vessels.

data showing the complete absence of this type of structure (40, 41) and others showing its presence (42–45), it is important to understand how lymphatic drainage can contribute to control inflammation. In this context, lymphatic vessels have the initial function of removing catabolites from the tissues, including inflammatory cells, cytokines and dead bacteria, amongst others, directing them to lymph nodes, which then will work on these drained fluids to eliminate harmful factors (46). When looking at this function in pulp tissue, the controversy regarding the presence or absence of lymphatic vessels continues: in theory, the absence of lymphatic vessels would be a confirmation that pulp does not recover from intense inflammatory processes, as the cytokines and other harmful factors will be chronically acting on the tissue without proper drainage. However, even the studies that show the lack of lymphatic capillaries in the dental pulp state that these studies were done under normal conditions (40, 41), while other studies have specifically shown the presence of these capillaries under inflammation (42, 45). All this conflicting information may, in fact, indicate that the pulp indeed lacks lymphatic circulation, although lymph angiogenesis appears to occur in the presence of pulp damage and inflammation. Additionally, the fact that the pulp tissue is only vascularized from the apical region can also be responsible for the lack of removal of these factors. As the pulp containment within hard tissue walls can contribute to that as blood vessels are dilated, there is an increase in intrapulpal pressure and, consequently, if lymphatic vessels are present, they would be less effective given this pressure. Among the studies that show the presence of lymphatic vessels, there are some observations that are also important, such as the fact that these types of vessels are more prevalent close to the apical region and not in the coronal pulp tissue (47). Clinically, this can also explain why pulpotomies tend to be successful, as the radicular pulp tissue can be more resilient to the inflammatory process because it has higher capability to modulate the inflammatory process due to the presence of lymphatic vessels. Again, these facts can be only observed if pulp vitality is preserved, since true regeneration is not yet achieved clinically, at least in any clinically available technique.

Pulp Innervation and its Contribution to Physiologic Changes

Maintaining pulp vitality also results in the presence of functional nerves in the tissue. The pulp is a highly innervated tissue, with many of the nerve bundles close to the odontoblast layer. The pulp possesses sympathetic nerves, which are associated with the blood vessels and their ability to respond with vasodilation or constriction and the ability to participate in the 'neurogenic inflammation' process (48, 49). Evidently, the normal physiology (homeostasis) of the tissue is only maintained in case the tissue is preserved properly. This is factually true for the pulp tissue; however, the physiology of the dentine itself is completely dependent on the maintenance of the pulp tissue, with an interrelationship so intertwined that these two tissues together have been called the dentine-pulp complex. This relationship starts during tooth development stages and goes on through the tooth's life, and some of the functions discussed here are very important in terms of the long-term prognosis of the tooth.

Much has been presented about pulp tissue physiology and how its structure affects treatment outcomes. When discussing pulp preservation, the first factor that comes to mind is the ability of the tooth to respond to pain, and it serves as an alert in case something is wrong. Many dentists have had the experience that a devitalized tooth (a root canal-treated tooth) became decayed, and the carious lesion evolved with no warning underneath a crown, resulting in extensive structure loss and an unrestorable tooth. One can then infer that the pulp tissue, when present, can 'detect' this carious lesion, leading the patient to seek dental work before such destruction occurs. Indeed, the pulp has this ability, and it all comes down to the presence of vitality in the tissue.

As stated previously, the pulp tissue is rich in nerves. The most important ones from the point of view of tooth response are the A-delta and C fibres (50), which include both afferent and post-ganglionic sympathetic fibres. A-delta fibres are myelinated which are bundled in a plexus that is mostly located between the core of the pulp tissue and the cell-free zone. These fibres lose their myelin layer (but not their Schwann cells) when penetrating the cell-rich and cell-free zones until reaching the odontoblast layer and, occasionally, the dentine tubules. The literature does not show any evidence of real synapses between these fibres and odontoblasts (51, 52). Independently of the presence or absence of these connections, the close relationship between these A-delta fibres and the dentine is of major importance in many aspects of pulp physiology, from dentine sensitivity (for example, the hydrodynamic theory) to inflammatory and repair responses (53, 54).

A-delta fibres conduct the stimuli very quickly, and this translates into a response that is sharp and of short duration. So, when cold is applied on the tooth surface, the dentinal fluid present in the tubules moves towards the pulp, and this movement stimulates the A-delta fibres present either in the tubules or close to the odontoblast layer. In healthy tissue, this response rapidly subsides as the body temperature stabilizes the fluid movement, eliminating the stimulus to the nerve fibres (53). Sometimes, patients present with hypersensitivity due to exposed dentine. The principle for the painful response is the same. However, the process known as neurogenic inflammation has been proven to happen in the pulp tissue also (55, 56). In this case, the stimulation of a sensory (afferent) nerve fibre can lead to the release of substance P, which is a neuropeptide with major role in the inflammation (55). Substance P has been detected as released from C fibre terminals and is associated with increased pulpal blood flow and, consequently, vasodilation (57). Other neuropeptides such as calcitonin gene-related peptide (CGRP) also work towards the neural immune response, with a dose-dependent effect on recruiting T-cells, for example (58). Understanding this process may bring therapeutic options, as it is clear that the nerves and all neuropeptides detected in the pulp tissue can impact pain control, immune response and inflammation (59) (Figure 1.7). Stimulating the pulp nerves due to tooth damage can lead to hyperalgesia and allodynia at the trigeminal ganglion level (60), so the sensitized tissue will respond to pain more easily. This response, either from a normal pulp or for a pulp with reversible pulpitis, is a good way to raise the patient's awareness and assist the provider with a pulp diagnosis that does not demand a more radical intervention. In the case of a carious tooth, this inflammatory process can continue to develop. With this and the presence of bacteria, areas of necrosis and anoxia can be observed in the pulp tissue and these fibres, due to the presence of their Schwann cells, start to lose their efficiency as these cells depend on oxygen to survive (54). This helps to explain why tissues with irreversible pulpitis have lingering pain when tissues are stimulated with cold. The speed at which the stimulus is conducted is not the same anymore, and the increase in intrapulpal pressure can lead to a more severe response. This intrapulpal pressure, on the other hand, will not be stimulating the A-delta fibres but, instead, will be stimulating the C fibres. These fibres, as stated above, are unmyelinated nerve fibres, generally located in the pulp core. In this context, these fibres do not respond to cold stimulus, for example, as they are not connected to the

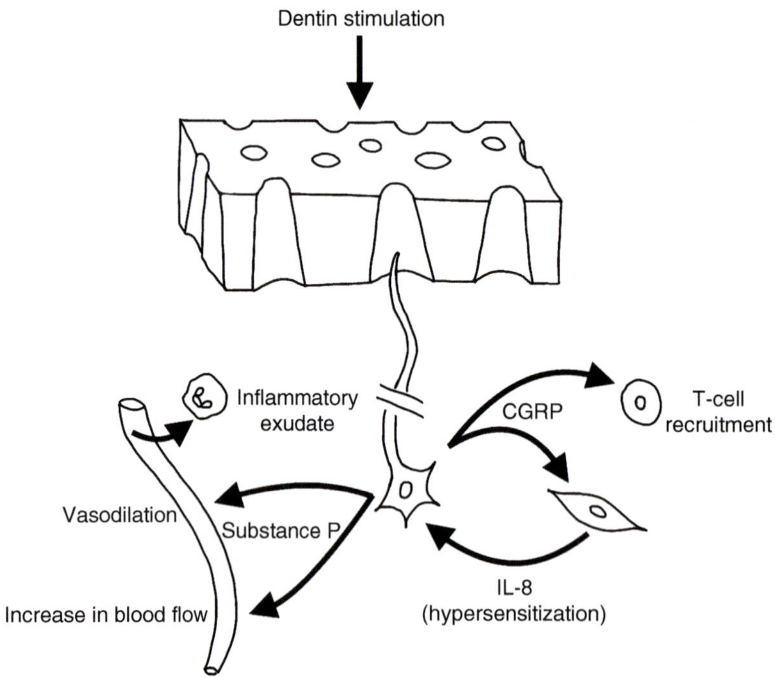

Figure 1.7 Mechanism of neurogenic inflammation. Dentine stimulation can lead to C fibres to express and release both substance P and CGRP. Substance P can induce an increase in blood flow and vasodilation, while CGRP can induce the recruitment of T-cells. CGRP also induces pulp cells to express IL-8, which can increase the sensitization of neural fibres and make the inflammatory cycle persistent.

tubular fluid movements. In a normal pulp tissue, these fibres would not be responsible for typical tooth pain; however, given the fact that they respond with a more dull, aching pain, they can assist in diagnosing referred pain, for example (61). In cases of pulpitis, they tend to lead to the most painful episodes, particularly due to their effectiveness in detecting changes in intrapulpal pressure (57). These fibres are also more resistant to hypoxia, meaning that they can be responsive even in cases where the pulp tissue is close to complete necrosis. Again, responses like this can only be used for diagnosis in vital pulps and losing these references can impair the awareness about harmful processes like caries.

Pulp Response to Restorative Processes

Preserving tooth vitality also has an impact on restorative processes. *In vitro* studies have shown that the presence of pulp tissue alone does not change dentine hydration and, consequently, does not make the tooth more brittle (62). On the other hand, there is evidence showing that the absence of dentinal fluid and consequent maintenance of the collagen structure of the dentine may affect the bonding process (63, 64). The hybridization process with adhesive and the etched dentine can be more effective if a certain level of moisture is present, particularly if the moisture comes from the dentinal tubules. The correlation between the use of dental materials and dentine permeability can also serve as a good reason for keeping pulp vitality, as it is well-known that the application of chemical, bacterial and thermal stimuli on the dentine surface can have an impact on how the pulp tissue responds (65). When applying dental material against dentine, even without pulpal exposure, one can expect a tissue reaction. Initially, the tissue reaction comes from the simple fact that dentine is being cut by a bur with heat (66). When that happens, some odontoblast extensions will be cut or overheated, leading those cells to their death and consequent release of cytokines that will initiate the inflammatory process. Most of the time, in healthy pulp tissue, this will not result in more damage as the stimulus is of short duration. As we are going to discuss later in this chapter, the inflammatory process is, in fact, necessary for adequate repair and even for regenerative procedures.

With respect to dental material application, studies have shown, for example, that eugenol can have a soothing effect on the pulp, even though it is very cytotoxic (67, 68), indicating that dosage and composition are significant when attempting pulp repair. In addition, when looking for repair, a vital pulp provides an environment where the factors released by the dentine due to the action of dental materials can be effective in promoting cell differentiation, control of inflammation, angiogenesis and other actions (23, 24). In this context, as obvious as it can be, preserving the pulp vitality is essential to promote adequate repair and dentinogenesis, all necessary for adequate healing of the tissue and reestablishment of the homeostasis of the dentine/pulp complex. The same can be said about the presence of bacteria: the vital pulp tissue, besides reporting tissue destruction with pain, can also be responsible for the initial line of defence against microorganisms. There is a lot of information on how bacteria affect odontoblasts and how, even in cases where the pulp is not exposed, bacterial byproducts are known to have an effect on the pulp tissue and, as explained for dental materials, this reaction can start an inflammatory reaction and consequently, the production of tertiary dentine in an attempt to recover tissue homeostasis. Recent studies show that even small amounts of LPS and lipotheicoic acid (LTA) can induce alkaline phosphatase, an indicator of mineralization, in DPSCs (69, 70). This information, associated with dentine permeability, shows the role played by the pulp tissue in the protection of the tooth when faced with microbial and chemical agents. The molecular aspects of this protective effect will be discussed in the next subsection.

Pulp Vitality and Inflammation

Much has been researched and discussed about the effects of inflammation on pulp repair. Currently, it is well established that the reparative process needs some level of inflammation to be effective. While we still cannot control the 'threshold' level of inflammation clinically, the knowledge of the participating molecules in both processes is essential to improve the odds of being able to do so in the future.

The molecules involved in the inflammatory process are numerous and have different specific functions. Among these, it is possible to name proinflammatory cytokines, for example. These include some of the already discussed molecules (e.g. HIF-1alpha) but also interleukin 1 beta (IL-1beta), interleukin 6 (IL-6), interleukin 8 (IL-8) and others. Most of them have been shown to be associated to pulp tissues with irreversible pulpitis, a fact that can also be reproduced with pulp cell cultures under stress (71–76). These studies have proven a direct correlation between levels of cytokines and inflammatory status. However, we have also shown that even a healthy pulp has basal levels of those cytokines, and, as we have demonstrated in previous work, they can be localized in the odontoblast layer of a non-inflamed tissue (74). This supports that proinflammatory cytokines may also be involved in the regular dentinogenesis process and that this process may be exacerbated in case of higher levels of these cytokines, leading them to induce more tertiary dentine and, consequently, collaborate in the tissue repair (71, 74, 77–80). These papers show that this process can occur on a number of different fronts, such as the activation of the Wnt pathway by the inflammatory cytokines, the activation of substance P by neural stimulus and even the direct release of cytokines by competent cells (e.g. odontoblasts, DPSCs and fibroblasts) when challenged by bacteria and their subproducts (Figure 1.8). As stated above, the repair process is dependent on some level of inflammation, and the expression of these cytokines opens opportunities in the translational research field. The first one can be associated with the qualification and quantification of these cytokines to facilitate pulpal diagnosis and increase treatment success rates (81). Although this is still not feasible clinically, the understanding of the development of pulpal inflammation, its stages, and the cytokines involved with success and repair is essential to keep pulp vitality. On another note, there are opportunities for using immunotherapy as a way to control and modulate these cytokines and, thus, direct the repair process (82).

Mechanisms of Pulp Repair

Other molecules involved in the pulp repair are transcription factors associated with cell differentiation and mineralization, which is essential to protect the pulp tissue from the external environment. Transcription factors are proteins that encode a number of genes and thus regulate a large number of functions in cell metabolism and response. The literature is rich in examples of transcription factors that participate in the dentinogenesis process, namely Runx2 (21, 35, 69, 83) and homeobox genes (Msx1, Msx2, Dlx3, Dlx5, Sox2), which can be expressed to direct the cell differentiation and consequently the proper tissue formation (83–87). It is important to emphasize that the pulp capping materials may have a role in this expression and that the sequence where these proteins are expressed also plays a role in determining the outcome towards an osteodentine or tubular dentine phenotype (16). Recently, some focus has been put on the role of microRNA in the inflammatory process. MicroRNA (miR) are small molecules, more specifically single-stranded RNA molecules, that regulate the expression of genes. They can be present in the blood and inside

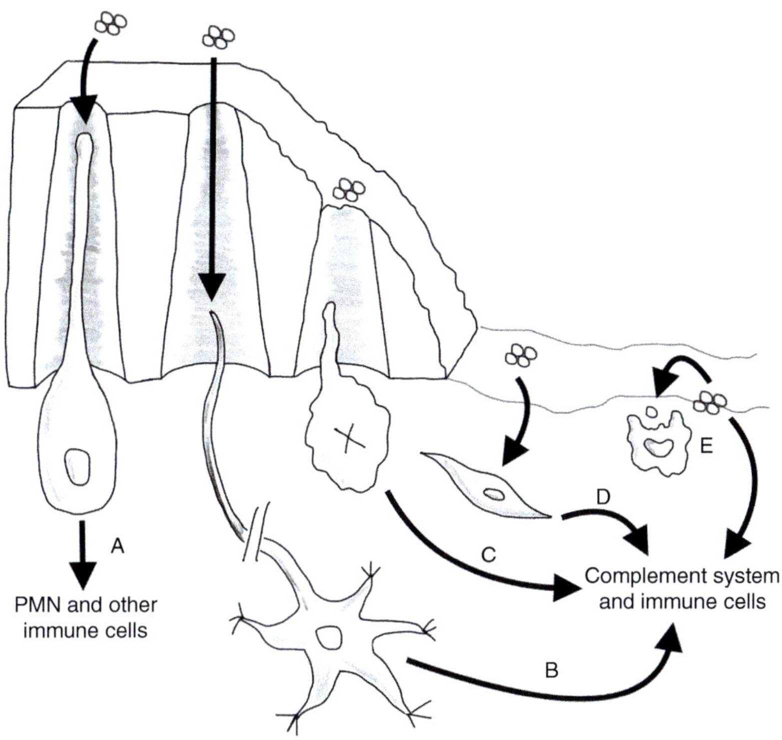

Figure 1.8 Molecular responses to activate pulp inflammation. The presence of bacteria in different levels of dentine and their products can activate odontoblasts, which will subsequently release cytokines such as IL-1beta and IL-8 (A). These same products can lead to the activation of nerve fibres and the release of substance P and CGRP (B). The complement and immune systems can also be activated by dead cells (C) and immunocompetent pulp cells (D), by the presence of necrosis (e.g. leading to release of HIF-1alpha) and also cytokines released from pulp cells (Il-6, IL-8 and others). When bacteria reach the pulp, they will face macrophages and activate the immune system themselves (E). The activation of the immune system is essential for pulp repair, as it will induce cell differentiation and activation of the existent and viable odontoblasts.

cells and are seen as an alternative for controlling diseases. This makes them candidates for epigenetic regulation in pulp repair as well. In the last few years, there has been a large amount of research being directed at identifying the miRNA in the inflamed pulp tissue. MicroRNAs were observed as playing a role in inflammation, opening the prospect that regulating them can assist as well in the control of tissue inflammation (88–90). Furthermore, another aspect of microRNA is that these molecules are not only responsible for the control of inflammation, but they also play a role in cell differentiation and tissue repair, with some of these molecules having action on both processes (89, 91). More specifically, pulp studies have identified many different microRNAs, and, unfortunately, this makes it difficult to discuss specifically which ones would be ideal targets. For example, there is data on miR-126 controlling the expression of IL-1beta in human pulps (88); that miR-21 can regulate many cytokines and factors in LPS-induced dental pulp cells (90); miR-let7c-5p is responsible for blocking inflammatory pathways and promoting osteogenic differentiation (91).

Thus, when looking at VPT and the maintenance of the pulp tissue, we focused more on the aspects that can lead to a successful pulp-induced regeneration. In a still unpublished study, our group identified the miR-200c as one of the targets based on the collection of healthy and inflamed

(a)

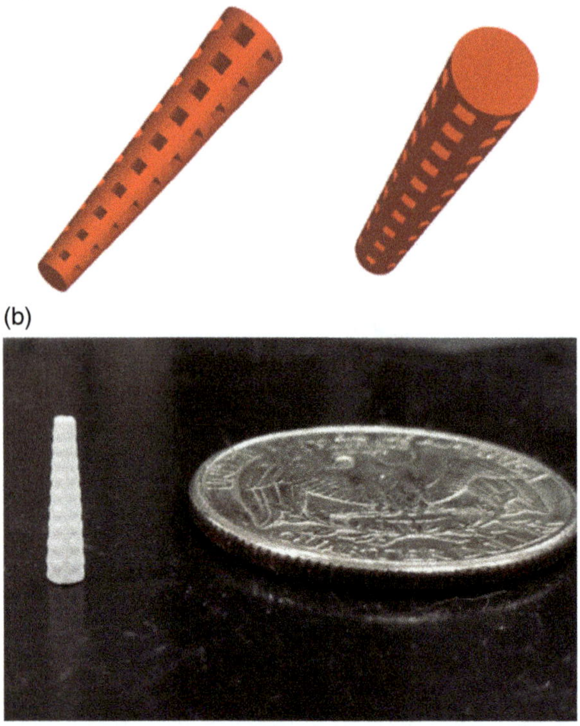

(b)

Figure 1.9 Design of a miRNA 'rich' scaffold encoding miRNAs to control inflammation and induce pulp regeneration. This particular shape was reproduced to allow for implantation in a standardized root canal. (a) Computer design for the standardized scaffold; (b) 3D printed scaffold compared to coin for perspective.

pulp tissues. This miR was closely associated with the levels of IL-6 in human pulp tissues and was also not expressed in normal pulps, while being directly correlated with cytokine expression in cell cultures; moreover, it has also shown the ability to induce pulp repair and control inflammation in a rat pulpitis model, when delivered directly as a 'pulp capping agent' in collagen sponges (unpublished data), plus the fact that it is possible to 3D print scaffolds in the desired shape to allow for pulp tissue regeneration using them (Figure 1.9). This mimics another study by our group, which also has shown the capacity of inducing pulp repair using gene-encoding plasmids on collagen sponges as an alternative to customize pulp repair (92). Fortunately, we may be moving towards more biomimetic and directed VPTs in the future and rely much more on the potential of the remaining tissue to induce pulp repair.

Conclusions

Based on the previous discussion, it is clear that the preservation of the pulp tissue has numerous benefits for clinical practice. First and foremost, maintaining pulp vitality will allow the tooth to perform its full function by responding to stimuli, completing tooth development and alerting the patient of something wrong. In addition, the pulp tissue can also contribute to its own repair, particularly to protect the tooth organ from external harmful factors. In this context, the comprehension of how the pulp tissue reacts against specific materials and promotes repair is also the basis for developing more efficient and biocompatible restorative options, which will, in the future, be more effective at the molecular level to control the inflammation and promote dentinogenesis.

References

1 Gronthos S, Mankani M, Brahim J, Robey PG, Shi S. Postnatal human dental pulp stem cells (DPSCs) in vitro and in vivo. *Proc Natl Acad Sci U S A.* 2000;97(25):13625–30.
2 Sakai VT, Zhang Z, Dong Z, Neiva KG, Machado MA, Shi S, et al. SHED differentiate into functional odontoblasts and endothelium. *J Dent Res.* 2010;89(8):791–6.
3 Karaoz E, Demircan PC, Saglam O, Aksoy A, Kaymaz F, Duruksu G. Human dental pulp stem cells demonstrate better neural and epithelial stem cell properties than bone marrow-derived mesenchymal stem cells. *Histochem Cell Biol.* 2011;136(4):455–73.
4 Sanen K, Martens W, Georgiou M, Ameloot M, Lambrichts I, Phillips J. Engineered neural tissue with Schwann cell differentiated human dental pulp stem cells: potential for peripheral nerve repair? *J Tissue Eng Regen Med.* 2017;11(12):3362–72.
5 Rosa V, Zhang Z, Grande RH, Nor JE. Dental pulp tissue engineering in full-length human root canals. *J Dent Res.* 2013;92(11):970–5.
6 Iohara K, Imabayashi K, Ishizaka R, Watanabe A, Nabekura J, Ito M, et al. Complete pulp regeneration after pulpectomy by transplantation of CD105+ stem cells with stromal cell-derived factor-1. *Tissue Eng Part A.* 2011;17(15–16):1911–20.
7 Cavalcanti BN, Zeitlin BD, Nor JE. A hydrogel scaffold that maintains viability and supports differentiation of dental pulp stem cells. *Dent Mater.* 2013;29(1):97–102.
8 Dong Q, Wang Y, Mohabatpour F, Zheng L, Papagerakis S, Chen D, et al. Dental pulp stem cells: isolation, characterization, expansion, and odontoblast differentiation for tissue engineering. *Methods Mol Biol.* 2019;1922:91–101.
9 Lim HM, Nam MH, Kim YM, Seo YK. Increasing odontoblast-like differentiation from dental pulp stem cells through increase of beta-catenin/p-GSK-3beta expression by low-frequency electromagnetic field. *Biomedicines.* 2021;9(8):1049.
10 Faraco IM Jr, Holland R. Response of the pulp of dogs to capping with mineral trioxide aggregate or a calcium hydroxide cement. *Dent Traumatol.* 2001;17(4):163–6.
11 Tziafas D, Pantelidou O, Alvanou A, Belibasakis G, Papadimitriou S. The dentinogenic effect of mineral trioxide aggregate (MTA) in short-term capping experiments. *Int Endod J.* 2002;35(3):245–54.
12 Zarrabi MH, Javidi M, Jafarian AH, Joushan B. Histologic assessment of human pulp response to capping with mineral trioxide aggregate and a novel endodontic cement. *J Endod.* 2010;36(11):1778–81.
13 Cuadros-Fernandez C, Lorente Rodriguez AI, Saez-Martinez S, Garcia-Binimelis J, About I, Mercade M. Short-term treatment outcome of pulpotomies in primary molars using mineral trioxide aggregate and biodentine: a randomized clinical trial. *Clin Oral Investig.* 2016;20(7):1639–45.
14 Tziafa C, Koliniotou-Koumpia E, Papadimitriou S, Tziafas D. Dentinogenic responses after direct pulp capping of miniature swine teeth with Biodentine. *J Endod.* 2014;40(12):1967–71.
15 Demarco FF, Casagrande L, Zhang Z, Dong Z, Tarquinio SB, Zeitlin BD, et al. Effects of morphogen and scaffold porogen on the differentiation of dental pulp stem cells. *J Endod.* 2010;36(11):1805–11.
16 Zanini M, Sautier JM, Berdal A, Simon S. Biodentine induces immortalized murine pulp cell differentiation into odontoblast-like cells and stimulates biomineralization. *J Endod.* 2012;38(9):1220–6.
17 Duncan HF, Kobayashi Y, Yamauchi Y, Quispe-Salcedo A, Chao Feng Z, Huang J, et al. The critical role of MMP13 in regulating tooth development and reactionary dentinogenesis repair through the Wnt signaling pathway. *Front Cell Dev Biol.* 2022;10:883266.
18 He P, Zhang Y, Kim SO, Radlanski RJ, Butcher K, Schneider RA, et al. Ameloblast differentiation in the human developing tooth: effects of extracellular matrices. *Matrix Biol.* 2010;29(5):411–9.
19 Sharpe PT. Neural crest and tooth morphogenesis. *Adv Dent Res.* 2001;15:4–7.

20 Bègue-Kirn C, Krebsbach PH, Bartlett JD, Butler WT. Dentin sialoprotein, dentin phosphoprotein, enamelysin and ameloblastin: tooth-specific molecules that are distinctively expressed during murine dental differentiation. *Eur J Oral Sci.* 1998;106(5):963–70.

21 Lim WH, Liu B, Cheng D, Hunter DJ, Zhong Z, Ramos DM, et al. Wnt signaling regulates pulp volume and dentin thickness. *J Bone Miner Res.* 2014;29(4):892–901.

22 Liu J, Jin T, Ritchie HH, Smith AJ, Clarkson BH. In vitro differentiation and mineralization of human dental pulp cells induced by dentin extract. *In Vitro Cell Dev Biol Anim.* 2005;41(7):232–8.

23 Graham L, Cooper PR, Cassidy N, Nor JE, Sloan AJ, Smith AJ. The effect of calcium hydroxide on solubilisation of bio-active dentine matrix components. *Biomaterials.* 2006;27(14):2865–73.

24 Tomson PL, Grover LM, Lumley PJ, Sloan AJ, Smith AJ, Cooper PR. Dissolution of bio-active dentine matrix components by mineral trioxide aggregate. *J Dent.* 2007;35(8):636–42.

25 Tomson PL, Lumley PJ, Smith AJ, Cooper PR. Growth factor release from dentine matrix by pulp-capping agents promotes pulp tissue repair-associated events. *Int Endod J.* 2017;50(3):281–92.

26 Zeichner-David M, Oishi K, Su Z, Zakartchenko V, Chen LS, Arzate H, et al. Role of Hertwig's epithelial root sheath cells in tooth root development. *Dev Dyn.* 2003;228(4):651–63.

27 Retana-Lobo C, Reyes-Carmona J. Immunohistochemical characterization of stem cell, vascular, neural, and differentiation markers in the apical papilla and dental pulp of human teeth at various stages of root development. *J Histotechnol.* 2022;46:1–11.

28 Ruparel NB, de Almeida JF, Henry MA, Diogenes A. Characterization of a stem cell of apical papilla cell line: effect of passage on cellular phenotype. *J Endod.* 2013;39(3):357–63.

29 Morse DR, Esposito JV, Schoor RS, Williams FL, Furst ML. A review of aging of dental components and a retrospective radiographic study of aging of the dental pulp and dentin in normal teeth. *Quintessence Int.* 1991;22(9):711–20.

30 Baker A, Karpagaselvi K, Kumaraswamy J, Ranjini MR, Gowher J. Role of dental pulp in age estimation: a quantitative and morphometric study. *J Forensic Dent Sci.* 2019;11(2):95–102.

31 Duncan HF, El-Karim I, Dummer PMH, Whitworth J, Nagendrababu V. Factors that influence the outcome of pulpotomy in permanent teeth. *Int Endod J.* 2022;56:62–81.

32 Rothová M, Feng J, Sharpe PT, Peterková R, Tucker AS. Contribution of mesoderm to the developing dental papilla. *Int J Dev Biol.* 2011;55(1):59–64.

33 Aranha AM, Zhang Z, Neiva KG, Costa CA, Hebling J, Nor JE. Hypoxia enhances the angiogenic potential of human dental pulp cells. *J Endod.* 2010;36(10):1633–7.

34 Gomez-Sosa JF, Cardier JE, Caviedes-Bucheli J. The hypoxia-dependent angiogenic process in dental pulp. *J Oral Biosci.* 2022;64(4):381–91.

35 Orikasa S, Kawashima N, Tazawa K, Hashimoto K, Sunada-Nara K, Noda S, et al. Hypoxia-inducible factor 1alpha induces osteo/odontoblast differentiation of human dental pulp stem cells via Wnt/beta-catenin transcriptional cofactor BCL9. *Sci Rep.* 2022;12(1):682.

36 Dissanayaka WL, Han Y, Zhang L, Zou T, Zhang C. Bcl-2 overexpression and hypoxia synergistically enhance angiogenic properties of dental pulp stem cells. *Int J Mol Sci.* 2020;21(17):6159.

37 Fujii M, Kawashima N, Tazawa K, Hashimoto K, Nara K, Noda S, et al. Hypoxia-inducible factor 1alpha promotes interleukin 1beta and tumour necrosis factor alpha expression in lipopolysaccharide-stimulated human dental pulp cells. *Int Endod J.* 2020;53(5):636–46.

38 Ito K, Matsuoka K, Matsuzaka K, Morinaga K, Inoue T. Hypoxic condition promotes differentiation and mineralization of dental pulp cells in vivo. *Int Endod J.* 2015;48(2):115–23.

39 Li L, Zhu YQ, Jiang L, Peng W, Ritchie HH. Hypoxia promotes mineralization of human dental pulp cells. *J Endod.* 2011;37(6):799–802.

40 Gerli R, Secciani I, Sozio F, Rossi A, Weber E, Lorenzini G. Absence of lymphatic vessels in human dental pulp: a morphological study. *Eur J Oral Sci.* 2010;118(2):110–7.

41 Martin A, Gasse H, Staszyk C. Absence of lymphatic vessels in the dog dental pulp: an immunohistochemical study. *J Anat.* 2010;217(5):609–15.

42 Marchetti C, Piacentini C, Menghini P. Lymphatic vessels in inflamed human dental pulp. *Bull Group Int Rech Sci Stomatol Odontol.* 1990;33(3–4):155–9.

43 Matsumoto Y, Kato S, Miura M, Yanagisawa S, Shimizu M. Fine structure and distribution of lymphatic vessels in the human dental pulp: a study using an enzyme-histochemical method. *Cell Tissue Res.* 1997;288(1):79–85.

44 Matsumoto Y, Zhang B, Kato S. Lymphatic networks in the periodontal tissue and dental pulp as revealed by histochemical study. *Microsc Res Tech.* 2002;56(1):50–9.

45 Wisniewska K, Rybak Z, Szymonowicz M, Kuropka P, Kaleta-Kuratewicz K, Dobrzynski M. Detection of lymphatic vessels in dental pulp. *Biology (Basel).* 2022;11(5):635.

46 Bernick S. Lymphatic vessels of the human dental pulp. *J Dent Res.* 1977;56(1):70–7.

47 Oehmke MJ, Knolle E, Oehmke HJ. Lymph drainage in the human dental pulp. *Microsc Res Tech.* 2003;62(3):187–91.

48 Iijima T, Zhang JQ. Three-dimensional wall structure and the innervation of dental pulp blood vessels. *Microsc Res Tech.* 2002;56(1):32–41.

49 Moe K, Kettunen P, Kvinnsland IH, Luukko K. Development of the pioneer sympathetic innervation into the dental pulp of the mouse mandibular first molar. *Arch Oral Biol.* 2008;53(9):865–73.

50 Nair PN. Neural elements in dental pulp and dentin. *Oral Surg Oral Med Oral Pathol Oral Radiol Endod.* 1995;80(6):710–9.

51 Byers MR. Dental sensory receptors. *Int Rev Neurobiol.* 1984;25:39–94.

52 Koling A, Rask-Andersen H. Membrane junctions between odontoblasts and associated cells. A freeze-fracture study of the human odontoblastic cell layer with special reference to its nerve supply. *Acta Odontol Scand.* 1984;42(1):13–22.

53 Brannstrom M, Johnson G, Nordenvall KJ. Transmission and control of dentinal pain: resin impregnation for the desensitization of dentin. *J Am Dent Assoc.* 1979;99(4):612–8.

54 Couve E, Lovera M, Suzuki K, Schmachtenberg O. Schwann cell phenotype changes in aging human dental pulp. *J Dent Res.* 2018;97(3):347–55.

55 Ohkubo T, Shibata M, Yamada Y, Kaya H, Takahashi H. Role of substance P in neurogenic inflammation in the rat incisor pulp and the lower lip. *Arch Oral Biol.* 1993;38(2):151–8.

56 Killough SA, Lundy FT, Irwin CR. Substance P expression by human dental pulp fibroblasts: a potential role in neurogenic inflammation. *J Endod.* 2009;35(1):73–7.

57 Kim S. Neurovascular interactions in the dental pulp in health and inflammation. *J Endod.* 1990;16(2):48–53.

58 Okiji T, Jontell M, Belichenko P, Dahlgren U, Bergenholtz G, Dahlstrom A. Structural and functional association between substance P- and calcitonin gene-related peptide-immunoreactive nerves and accessory cells in the rat dental pulp. *J Dent Res.* 1997;76(12):1818–24.

59 Caviedes-Bucheli J, Munoz HR, Azuero-Holguin MM, Ulate E. Neuropeptides in dental pulp: the silent protagonists. *J Endod.* 2008;34(7):773–88.

60 Haas ET, Rowland K, Gautam M. Tooth injury increases expression of the cold sensitive TRP channel TRPA1 in trigeminal neurons. *Arch Oral Biol.* 2011;56(12):1604–9.

61 Jyvasjarvi E, Kniffki KD. Studies on the presence and functional properties of afferent C-fibers in the cat's dental pulp. *Proc Finn Dent Soc.* 1992;88(Suppl 1):533–42.

62 Sedgley CM, Messer HH. Are endodontically treated teeth more brittle? *J Endod.* 1992;18(7):332–5.

63 Tay FR, Gwinnett JA, Wei SH. Micromorphological spectrum from overdrying to overwetting acid-conditioned dentin in water-free acetone-based, single-bottle primer/adhesives. *Dent Mater.* 1996;12(4):236–44.

64 Sugimura R, Tsujimoto A, Hosoya Y, Fischer NG, Barkmeier WW, Takamizawa T, et al. Surface moisture influence on etch-and-rinse universal adhesive bonding. *Am J Dent.* 2019;32(1):33–8.

65 Pashley DH. Dentin-predentin complex and its permeability: physiologic overview. *J Dent Res.* 1985;64:613–20.

66 Cavalcanti BN, Otani C, Rode SM. High-speed cavity preparation techniques with different water flows. *J Prosthet Dent.* 2002;87(2):158–61.

67 Brodin P. Neurotoxic and analgesic effects of root canal cements and pulp-protecting dental materials. *Endod Dent Traumatol.* 1988;4(1):1–11.

68 Markowitz K, Moynihan M, Liu M, Kim S. Biologic properties of eugenol and zinc oxide-eugenol. A clinically oriented review. *Oral Surg Oral Med Oral Pathol.* 1992;73(6):729–37.

69 Sugiuchi A, Sano Y, Furusawa M, Abe S, Muramatsu T. Human dental pulp cells express cellular markers for inflammation and hard tissue formation in response to bacterial information. *J Endod.* 2018;44(6):992–6.

70 Tazawa K, Kawashima N, Kuramoto M, Noda S, Fujii M, Nara K, et al. Transient receptor potential ankyrin 1 is up-regulated in response to lipopolysaccharide via P38/mitogen-activated protein kinase in dental pulp cells and promotes mineralization. *Am J Pathol.* 2020;190(12):2417–26.

71 Chang YC, Yang SF, Huang FM, Liu CM, Tai KW, Hsieh YS. Proinflammatory cytokines induce cyclooxygenase-2 mRNA and protein expression in human pulp cell cultures. *J Endod.* 2003;29(3):201–4.

72 Ferreira DC, Brito DG, Cavalcanti BN. Cytokine production from human primary teeth pulp fibroblasts stimulated by different pulpotomy agents. *J Dent Child (Chic).* 2009;76(3):194–8.

73 Hahn CL, Best AM, Tew JG. Cytokine induction by *Streptococcus mutans* and pulpal pathogenesis. *Infect Immun.* 2000;68(12):6785–9.

74 Silva AC, Faria MR, Fontes A, Campos MS, Cavalcanti BN. Interleukin-1 beta and interleukin-8 in healthy and inflamed dental pulps. *J Appl Oral Sci.* 2009;17(5):527–32.

75 Tokuda M, Sakuta T, Fushuku A, Torii M, Nagaoka S. Regulation of interleukin-6 expression in human dental pulp cell cultures stimulated with Prevotella intermedia lipopolysaccharide. *J Endod.* 2001;27(4):273–7.

76 Yang LC, Tsai CH, Huang FM, Liu CM, Lai CC, Chang YC. Induction of interleukin-6 gene expression by pro-inflammatory cytokines and black-pigmented bacteroides in human pulp cell cultures. *Int Endod J.* 2003;36(5):352–7.

77 Yang X, Zhang S, Pang X, Fan M. Pro-inflammatory cytokines induce odontogenic differentiation of dental pulp-derived stem cells. *J Cell Biochem.* 2012;113(2):669–77.

78 Goldberg M, Farges JC, Lacerda-Pinheiro S, Six N, Jegat N, Decup F, et al. Inflammatory and immunological aspects of dental pulp repair. *Pharmacol Res.* 2008;58(2):137–47.

79 Lee S, Zhang QZ, Karabucak B, Le AD. DPSCs from inflamed pulp modulate macrophage function via the TNF-alpha/IDO axis. *J Dent Res.* 2016;95(11):1274–81.

80 Yang G, Ju Y, Liu S, Zhao S. Lipopolysaccharide upregulates the proliferation, migration, and odontoblastic differentiation of NG2(+) cells from human dental pulp in vitro. *Cell Biol Int.* 2019;43(11):1276–85.

81 Rechenberg DK, Galicia JC, Peters OA. Biological markers for pulpal inflammation: a systematic review. *PLoS One.* 2016;11(11):e0167289.

82 Arora S, Cooper PR, Friedlander LT, Rizwan S, Seo B, Rich AM, et al. Potential application of immunotherapy for modulation of pulp inflammation: opportunities for vital pulp treatment. *Int Endod J.* 2021;54(8):1263–74.

83 Chen S, Gluhak-Heinrich J, Wang YH, Wu YM, Chuang HH, Chen L, et al. Runx2, osx, and dspp in tooth development. *J Dent Res.* 2009;88(10):904–9.

84 Bei M, Kratochwil K, Maas RL. BMP4 rescues a non-cell-autonomous function of Msx1 in tooth development. *Development.* 2000;127(21):4711–8.

85 Bhargav A, Min KS, Wen Feng L, Fuh JYH, Rosa V. Taguchi's methods to optimize the properties and bioactivity of 3D printed polycaprolactone/mineral trioxide aggregate scaffold: theoretical predictions and experimental validation. *J Biomed Mater Res B Appl Biomater.* 2020;108(3):629–37.

86 D'Anto V, Cantile M, D'Armiento M, Schiavo G, Spagnuolo G, Terracciano L, et al. The HOX genes are expressed, in vivo, in human tooth germs: in vitro cAMP exposure of dental pulp cells results in parallel HOX network activation and neuronal differentiation. *J Cell Biochem.* 2006;97(4):836–48.

87 Duverger O, Zah A, Isaac J, Sun HW, Bartels AK, Lian JB, et al. Neural crest deletion of Dlx3 leads to major dentin defects through down-regulation of Dspp. *J Biol Chem.* 2012;287(15):12230–40.

88 Jiang L, Krongbaramee T, Lin X, Zhu M, Zhu Y, Hong L. microRNA-126 inhibits vascular cell adhesion molecule-1 and interleukin-1beta in human dental pulp cells. *J Clin Lab Anal.* 2022;36(5):e24371.

89 Kearney M, Duncan HF. Micro-RNA profiling in dental pulp cell cultures. *Methods Mol Biol.* 2023;2588:353–67.

90 Nara K, Kawashima N, Noda S, Fujii M, Hashimoto K, Tazawa K, et al. Anti-inflammatory roles of microRNA 21 in lipopolysaccharide-stimulated human dental pulp cells. *J Cell Physiol.* 2019;234(11):21331–41.

91 Yuan H, Zhao H, Wang J, Zhang H, Hong L, Li H, et al. MicroRNA let-7c-5p promotes osteogenic differentiation of dental pulp stem cells by inhibiting lipopolysaccharide-induced inflammation via HMGA2/PI3K/Akt signal blockade. *Clin Exp Pharmacol Physiol.* 2019;46(4):389–97.

92 Chakka LRJ, Vislisel J, Vidal CMP, Biz MT, Salem AK, Cavalcanti BN. Application of BMP-2/FGF-2 gene-activated scaffolds for dental pulp capping. *Clin Oral Investig.* 2020;24(12):4427–37.

2

Biological Basis for Vital Pulp Treatment

Fionnuala T. Lundy[1], *Lara T. Friedlander*[2], *and Paul R. Cooper*[2]

[1] *The Wellcome-Wolfson Institute for Experimental Medicine, School of Medicine, Dentistry and Biomedical Sciences, Queen's University Belfast, Belfast, Northern Ireland, UK*
[2] *Faculty of Dentistry, Sir John Walsh Research Institute, University of Otago, Dunedin, New Zealand*

Dental Pulp – Structure and Function

The dental pulp is a unique connective tissue containing cells and extracellular matrix (ECM), along with an extensive neuronal and vascular plexus, encased in a rigid dentine structure. The development of the dental pulp is outlined briefly below, along with the roles of the major cellular and structural components.

Development and Anatomy of the Dental Pulp

In embryological terms, the process of tooth development begins at around the fifth embryonic week (crown development) and continues after birth (root development). The initial stages of tooth development in the embryo commence as a result of a series of reciprocal interactions between the odontogenic epithelium and the neural crest-derived ectomesenchyme of the developing jaws (1, 2). These interactions play a fundamental role in tooth morphogenesis and regulate all aspects of tooth development including tooth morphogenesis, and the number, shape and spatial patterning of the teeth. Key signalling molecules act reiteratively during these processes to mediate crosstalk, including wingless-related integration site (Wnt), bone morphogenic protein (BMP), fibroblast growth factor (FGF), sonic hedgehog (Shh) and Ectodysplasin (Eda) (3).

Tooth development is a continuous process and therefore few completely distinct stages can be delineated. However, a key event for the initiation of tooth development is the formation of localized U-shaped thickenings, known as dental placodes (sixth embryonic week) within the primary epithelial bands, at the sites of the future dental arches of the embryonic mandible and maxilla. The first evidence of embryonic teeth is evident when the epithelial cells near the basement membrane multiply and invaginate into the underlying ectomesenchyme to give rise to the dental lamina in 10 areas of the upper arch and 10 areas of the lower arch. Each dental lamina is the origin of the tooth bud that will give rise to a tooth in the mandible and maxilla. Deciduous incisor and canine tooth buds are evident at the eighth embryonic week, and deciduous molar tooth buds are evident at the ninth week. In the bud stage, the ectodermal basement membrane progressively

Vital Pulp Treatment, First Edition. Edited by Henry F. Duncan and Ikhlas A. El-Karim.

invaginates into the underlying ectomesenchyme, in which the cells are closely packed around the epithelial bud. Transformation of the epithelial bud into a concave or cap-shaped structure initiates the establishment of the coronal architecture of the tooth. The cap, which consists of an epithelial outgrowth, is often called the enamel organ because it will later form the cells that produce enamel. The remainder of the tooth bud, known as the dental papilla, will give rise to the dentine and the pulp. An additional sac of cells, known as the dental follicle, surrounds the enamel organ and the dental papilla. The dental follicle contains the cells that give rise to the pulpal blood vessels and nerves. By the end of the cap stage, three different structures are apparent: the enamel organ, the dental papilla and the dental follicle. Within the enamel organ is the enamel knot, a transient structure that controls the morphogenesis of the dental cusps and determines the shape of the tooth at the bell stage. Two additional regions of the enamel organ are also apparent, the stratum intermedium and the stellate reticulum, both involved in facilitating enamel production.

A relatively large number of development changes occur during the transition from the cap stage to the bell stage and the cells of the enamel organ differentiate to perform specific functions. By this stage the enamel organ contains two layers of cuboidal cells named the inner and outer enamel epithelium. During the later bell stages, tooth morphogenesis is followed by a period of histodifferentiation, involving interactions between the cells of the inner enamel epithelium, which differentiate into pre-ameloblasts and those of the epithelial-mesenchyme, which differentiate into pre-odontoblasts. The pre-ameloblasts and pre-odontoblasts ultimately polarize and secrete enamel and dentine, respectively. The outer enamel epithelium differentiates to form the junctional epithelium between the tooth and the gingival tissue. The dental papilla cells differentiate into periodontal cells to form the cementum-periodontium-like tissues.

In the mature tooth, the dental pulp occupies the pulp chamber, pulp horns and radicular canals. Odontoblasts are subjacent to the dentine and are capable of detecting sensory stimuli (4). Sensory nerves also innervate the dental pulp, including projecting into the odontoblast layer and extending into the dentinal tubules. The majority of the pulp contains fibroblasts and the ECM, along with smaller numbers of stem cells and immune cells. The cells of the dental pulp are discussed below in greater detail, along with the ECM, pulpal innervation and vasculature.

Cells of the Dental Pulp

The dental pulp extends from a central chamber within the crown of the tooth into one or more root canals (depending on the type of tooth). The pulp is encased by dentine, and the relationship between the soft tissue of the dental pulp and the hard dentinal tissue has often been emphasized using the phrase the 'dentine-pulp complex'.

Odontoblasts

Located subjacent to the dentine, specialized cells known as odontoblasts line the pulp chamber and root canals. Odontoblasts are columnar, post-mitotic, polarized cells that are responsible for secreting a collagenous matrix, which mineralizes to form dentine. Dentine formation (dentinogenesis) occurs during tooth development, forming primary dentine at a rate of approximately 4 μm/day. Throughout their life span, quiescent odontoblasts synthesis secondary dentine, similar in structure and continuous with the primary dentine, at a much slower rate of approximately 0.4 μm/day. Secondary dentine is formed after the tooth has erupted and the root is fully formed. Tertiary dentine is produced in response to a carious lesion, injury or noxious reaction to dental materials. If the damage is mild, then the native odontoblast cells will synthesize tertiary dentine, in this case often referred to as reactionary dentine. However, more extensive damage will lead to the death of the odontoblasts in the local area of the lesion/injury, and in this case, the dentine is synthesized by odontoblast-like cells (5, 6). This type of tertiary dentine, formed by odontoblast-like cells, is often referred to as reparative dentine. The regulation and processes involved in dentinogenesis are discussed in greater detail below.

With their anatomical location in the outermost layer of the dental pulp, odontoblasts provide a natural barrier between mineralized dentine and the soft tissue of the dental pulp. Each odontoblast has a cellular process embedded in the mineralized dentinal tissue, giving dentine its tubular structure. The cell body of the odontoblast is located within the soft tissue of the pulp and is not encased in dentine (7). Evidence for the role of odontoblasts in forming the first line of defence in the dental pulp comes from their ability to detect a wide variety of pathogen-associated molecular pattern molecules (PAMPs), via the expression of pattern recognition receptors (PRRs) such as Toll-like receptors (TLRs) and nucleotide-oligomerization binding domain (NOD) receptors (8, 9). In addition to this defensive role, odontoblasts sense the external environment and can recognize thermal, mechanical and chemical stimuli via the expression of a variety of channels and receptors, including the transient receptor potential (TRP) channels (4, 10, 11) and piezo channels (12). Although sensory nerve fibres are known to innervate the odontoblast layer and dentinal tubules (13), the exact mechanism(s) of signal transduction from odontoblasts to sensory nerves remains to be fully elucidated. Some evidence indicates that ATP may play a role in this signal transduction (14); however, further studies are required to improve our understanding.

Fibroblasts

Dental pulp fibroblasts are the most abundant cells in the dental pulp and are responsible for synthesizing ECM proteins, such as collagen and fibronectin, as well as enzymes, including matrix metalloproteinases (MMPs), which are responsible for ECM turnover (15, 16). Pulp fibroblasts may also contribute to healing and inducing angiogenesis following injury by the expression of growth factors (GFs) such as vascular endothelial growth factor (VEGF) and FGF (17).

In addition to their well-recognized role in regulating the synthesis and turnover of the ECM, fibroblasts have defensive properties by virtue of their synthesis of complement system proteins (18). Fibroblasts also synthesize proinflammatory cytokines (19) and chemokines (20), and they express PRRs, suggesting their involvement in pathogen detection and the subsequent immune response (21). The synthesis of multiple GFs and cytokines by dental pulp fibroblasts also has a role in inducing the migration (22) and differentiation (23) of dental pulp stem cells (DPSCs) into odontoblast-like cells, which synthesize tertiary dentine in response to caries ingress or physical trauma.

The expression of some neuropeptides (24) and their receptors (25), provides a link between fibroblasts and the pulpal neurogenic inflammatory response (26). Indeed, neuropeptides have been shown to regulate the expression of angiogenic factors by pulp fibroblasts (27), providing further evidence for the wide range of functional proteins synthesized by pulp fibroblasts. The expression of the TRP channels by dental pulp fibroblasts (28) indicates they are able to sense the external milieu.

Stem Cells

Postnatal DPSCs were first identified in the dental pulp over 20 years ago and were shown to possess self-renewal capacity, multilineage differentiation capacity and clonogenic efficiency, with the ability to regenerate dentine-pulp-like complexes *in vivo* (29, 30). DPSCs are derived from the neural crest during development (31) and have the capacity to secrete neurotrophic factors (32) and differentiate into functional nerves (33, 34). Using genetic lineage tracing, Feng et al. described two locations for stem cells in the dental pulp; the perivascular region (pericytes) and peripheral nerve-associated glial cells (35). In the healthy dental pulp, stem cells are generally maintained in a quiescent state. As outlined above, odontoblasts will respond to injury or infection by synthesizing dentine to protect the underlying pulp tissue. However, if injury or infection is sufficient to cause the death of the odontoblasts in the local area, events may trigger the proliferation of resident stem cells to differentiate into odontoblast-like cells capable of tertiary, reactionary dentine secretion (35, 36). The cellular and molecular processes involved in this are described in greater detail below. Furthermore, DPSCs have also been reported to exhibit both immunomodulatory and antimicrobial functions. When cocultured with activated T cells, DPSCs were shown to decrease levels of proinflammatory cytokines, as well as increase levels of anti-inflammatory cytokines (37). Recently, the cytokines and GFs present in the secretome of DPSCs, including hepatocyte GF, angiopoietin-1, interleukin (IL)-6 and IL-8, were shown to have direct antibacterial activity against oral pathogens (38), indicating a novel role for stem cells in fighting infection.

Immune Cells

The dental pulp is served by a variety of resident and recruited immune cells. Following injury or ingress of caries, odontoblasts and sentinel immune cells within the pulp release cytokines and chemokines (39–41), some of which are involved in the recruitment and activation of additional immune cells from the bloodstream to the site of pulpal infection and inflammation (42). These immune cells aim to destroy and engulf the invading microorganisms, using a complex arsenal of antimicrobial peptides (AMPs) (43). A variety of immune cells, including monocytes, neutrophils, T cells and dendritic cells (DCs), are involved in the pulp's immune response and may become activated once bacterial antigens are captured following their diffusion through dentinal tubules to the pulp tissue (40, 44). The complex cellular and molecular processes involved in the pulp's immune response are described subsequently.

ECM

The cells of the dental pulp are located in a loose connective tissue, comprised mainly of collagen types I and III (45, 46), with much smaller amounts of type V collagen (47). Collagen fibrils are associated with non-collagenous proteins that play roles in either stabilizing the fibril network or participating as inhibitors or activators in the mineralization process. Fibronectin is the principal non-collagenous protein in the dental pulp, showing abundance within the odontoblast layer, around blood vessels and in the core of the dental pulp (46, 48). Proteoglycans, which are glycosylated proteins with covalently attached highly anionic glycosaminoglycans, are present in the dental pulp, as is the case in almost all connective tissue ECMs (46). Small leucine-rich proteoglycans are associated with collagen fibrils in dentine, whereas glycosaminoglycans contribute to collagen fibril structure. The family of non-collagenous proteins termed small integrin-binding ligand N-linked glycoproteins (SIBLINGS) play roles in regulating dentine formation and include; dentine sialoprotein (DSP), dentine phosphoprotein (DPP), dentine matrix protein-1 (DMP-1), bone sialoprotein (BSP), matrix extracellular phosphorglycoprotien (MEPE) and osteopontin (OPN) (49–51). Moreover, a complex array of GFs, cytokines, MMPs and neuropeptides are also detectable in the ECM and are implicated in pulpal homeostasis.

Nerves

The dental pulp is an extensively innervated tissue (52, 53). The majority of pulpal nerves are sensory trigeminal afferents that detect noxious stimuli in the dental pulp tissue and transmit signals to the central nervous system, which is perceived as pain. Sensory nerves innervate the entire dental pulp, including the odontoblast layer. Indeed, ultrastructural analysis suggests that sensory nerves also extend into the dentinal tubules in the inner portion of the dentine (13). Sensory nerve fibres are generally classified on the basis of their diameters and conduction velocities. 'A fibres' are myelinated nerves with large diameters and high conduction velocities, whereas 'C-fibres' are unmyelinated with smaller diameters and lower conduction velocities. The afferent sensory nerves that innervate the dental pulp include both A fibres and C-fibres, with approximately 87% of pulpal sensory nerves classed as unmyelinated C-fibres (54, 55), and the remaining 13% are classified as myelinated A fibres (93% Aδ and 7% Aβ). Interestingly, although nerves entering the tooth through the apical foramen tend to be myelinated, many of them lose their myelin sheath on entering the dental pulp, or as they course and branch through the radicular and coronal pulp tissues (56, 57).

Upon stimulation, sensory nerve fibres not only transmit pain to the central nervous system but also release neuropeptides, such as substance P (SP), neurokinin A and calcitonin gene-related peptide (CGRP) in the pulp tissue. Consequently, they contribute to the local neurogenic inflammatory response (26, 58). The remainder of the pulpal nerves are autonomic efferents that transmit signals from the central nervous system to the periphery. The autonomic (sympathetic and parasympathetic) nerves have been studied less comprehensively, but evidence suggests that the sympathetic nerves contribute to pulpal blood flow (59), and they may have sensory roles when the dental pulp is inflamed (60). There is also evidence that sympathetic nerves contribute to the recruitment and migration of inflammatory cells (61). Although there is no consensus regarding parasympathetic innervation of the dental pulp, it is worth noting that vasoactive intestinal polypeptide (VIP), considered to be a marker for parasympathetic nerves, has been demonstrated in the dental pulp (59, 62–64).

Vasculature

The dental pulp has a rich vascularity; however, in contrast to most other tissues, it lacks a collateral supply, meaning it is also vulnerable. A dense network of blood vessels perfuse the dental pulp to provide nutrition (65). Arterioles enter the apical foramen and ascend the central region of the pulp proper, branching to form a dense capillary network to bring oxygenated blood to the peripheral pulp tissue. A network of venules returns deoxygenated blood, via the apical foramen, to the circulation (66). During the pulpal inflammatory response to injury and infection, vasodilation of blood vessels and capillary proliferation will occur (67). Blood vessels in the dental pulp are in close association with nerves and pulpal blood flow is considered to be under neural local control (60). Recent evidence shows that the dental pulp lacks lymphatic vessels (68). Instead, the drainage of fluid within the pulp is likely to be governed by a tissue pressure gradient (driving pressure) and is transported in loose connective tissue gaps surrounding vessels and nerve fibres (68).

Ageing

Ageing reduces the dimensions and volume of the pulp chamber due to the accumulation of secondary and tertiary dentine. Deposition of dental cementum with increasing age narrows the apical foramen and decreases perfusion of the tissue and the extent of innervation. There is also some atrophy of the dental pulp tissue; a decline in the total number of pulp cells has been reported with ageing (69). Significant decreases in numbers of sub-odontoblast cells with ageing have been observed in rodent and human pulp (70, 71), and a progressive decrease in fibroblasts is considered to be part of the pulp ageing process in human teeth (71). The ageing of the pulp tissue is associated with reduced vascularity and is proposed to reduce blood flow and the draining capacity of the tissue, making it more vulnerable to circulatory failure (68).

Healing Capability of the Dental Pulp

As indicated above, and similar to other tissues around the body, the dentine-pulp complex has an innate ability to heal following disease or trauma. The response whereby new dental hard tissue is formed postnatally by the dental pulp tissue is termed tertiary dentinogenesis (Figure 2.1). This tertiary dentine provides a localized physical barrier beneath the site of injury and contributes to tissue integrity via repair and regenerative processes (72). Tertiary dentine can describe a range of hard tissue deposited including a regular tubular structure continuous with the developmentally derived primary and physiological secondary dentine, as well as a more dysplastic atubular matrix (73, 74). Importantly, the molecular and cellular processes responsible for the different tertiary dentine depositions vary significantly. Consequently, tertiary dentine is classified as being either reactionary or reparative (75), and this occurs in response to mild (e.g. slowly progressing carious lesions) or more severe (e.g. rapidly progressing carious lesions) external stimuli, respectively.

Reactionary dentine is stimulated in response to mild irritation and deposited by surviving primary odontoblasts (75). In contrast, in more severe injury where primary odontoblasts are lost, reparative dentine is deposited following the differentiation of a new generation of odontoblast-like cells. Interestingly, this local odontoblast death may occur in the absence of pulpal exposure but may be due to trauma or deep and rapidly progressing caries. A range of bioactive molecules are

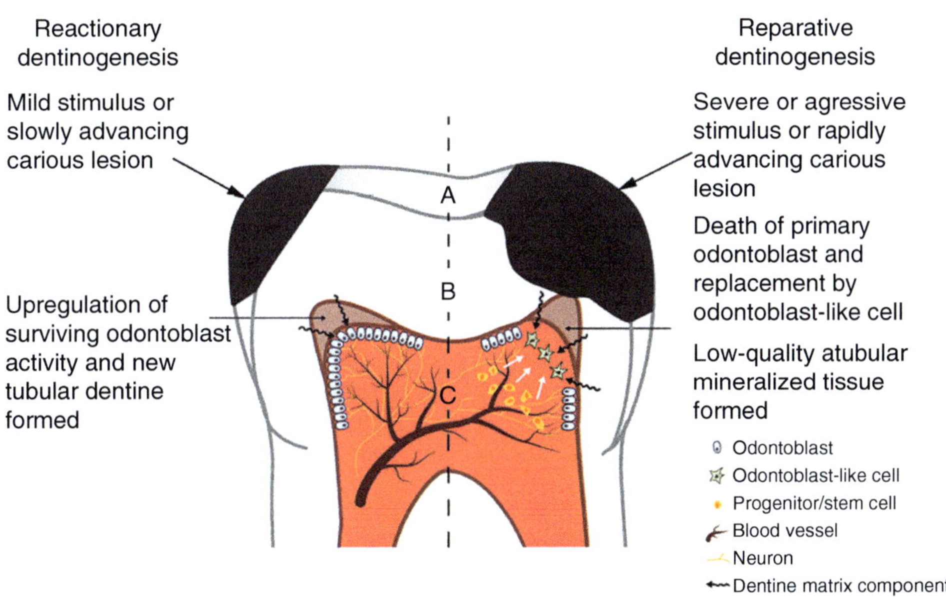

Figure 2.1 Schematic of the two types of tertiary dentine formation processes, reactionary and reparative dentinogenesis, formed in response to carious or traumatic lesions of differing intensities. Component tissues shown are A = Enamel; B = Dentine; C = Pulp.

important regulators and stimuli for both of these dentinogenic processes (76). Comparatively, reactionary dentinogenesis requires a less complex process as it involves only the re-stimulation of the existing primary odontoblasts to deposit dentine at a rate greater than that already observed during secondary dentinogenesis (77). However, reparative dentinogenesis involves the recruitment of progenitor dental pulp cells, which are subsequently signalled to differentiate into odontoblast-like cells (78). The stimulated reparative dentine differs from primary and secondary dentine in terms of the quality of the dentine deposited. It generally lacks a tubular structure, is an amorphous mineralized tissue bridge and may contain so-called 'tunnel' defects. The mineralized hard tissue deposited may be more similar to bone than it is to dentine (72, 74, 79, 80). Currently, there is significant debate as to the origin of the cells which deposit this mineralized bridge. Some researchers have proposed that this hard tissue occurs due to the activity of perivascular cells (81), fibroblasts (80) or fibrocytes (82) rather than cells that have been more traditionally termed odontoblast-like cells (83, 84). Interestingly, if pulpal fibroblasts were to produce the mineralized tissue in the reparative response, there would still need to be cytodifferentiation as these cells do not naturally produce hard tissues in their basal state. However, some evidence does exist that supports this cellular process being induced under appropriate conditions (85–88).

Whilst reactionary and reparative dentinogenesis is generally considered as occurring separately due to the disease or tissue stimulatory events present, some researchers have proposed that in relatively deep and active carious lesions, both processes may occur simultaneously (83). Indeed, in a dynamic and rapidly advancing carious lesion, active parts of the lesion may contain reactionary dentine formation, whereas, in more advanced areas of the lesion, reparative dentinogenesis may be present (89).

Molecular and Cellular Regulatory Processes in Tertiary Dentinogenesis

Bioactive Molecules

During primary and secondary dentinogenesis a plethora of bioactive molecules, termed dentine matrix components (DMCs), are deposited and archived within the dentine as the tooth develops and during dental tissue homeostasis. These DMCs include many GFs, cytokines, chemokines, MMPs as well as other bioactive molecule subclasses (83). DMCs are known to modulate a range of cellular processes important in tissue repair, including chemotaxis (84, 90, 91), angiogenesis (92), mineralization (91), stem cell recruitment (93) and neurogenesis (94). In particular, well-characterized GFs, which have been shown to be central to orchestrating and modulating dentine-pulp complex repair and regeneration, include members of the transforming GF (TGF) superfamily (95, 96) and insulin-like GFs (97, 98). Other GFs include angiogenesis-promoting molecules, such as VEGF, fibroblast GF-2 (FGF-2), platelet-derived GF (PDGF) and placenta GF (PlGF) (91, 99), as well as neurogenesis promoters including brain-derived neurotrophic factor (BDNF) and growth/differentiation factor 15 (GDF-15) (98).

As caries advance towards the pulp the dentine becomes progressively demineralized, and this results in the increased release of the archived DMCs (100). Interestingly, previous work has demonstrated that selected MMPs, including MMP-2, -8 -9 (101), are contained within the DMCs and are able to hydrolytically break the exposed dentine organic matrix (102) to generate potentially more potent bioactive molecules (103) that diffuse down the dentinal tubules and enter the pulp. These molecules have an important role in modulating the caries process and are known to be potent stimulators of tertiary dentine formation and other associated pulpal reparative processes, including angiogenesis and neurogenesis (97, 104). The holistic promotion of dentine-pulp complex repair is understood to be important due to the synergistic interaction of all component cells and tissue types (83).

The potential to therapeutically harness the bioactive DMCs has been a focus of considerable recent research activity (83). The use of several clinical reagents, treatments and chemicals, including ethylenediaminetetraacetic acid (EDTA) (90, 105), hydraulic calcium silicate cement (106), calcium hydroxide (105), dental adhesives (107) and ultrasonic agitation (108), to release DMCs have been explored. EDTA treatment of dentine promotes the migration and differentiation of DPSCs and remains the gold standard, with the TGF-β family members being used as key biomarkers demonstrating the release of the bioactives from the dentine (90). In contrast, 6% sodium hypochlorite (NaOCl) treatment of dentine has demonstrated a deleterious effect, particularly on the survival, viability and differentiation capability of DPSCs (109). This has led to clinical guidelines that balance disinfection with cellular vitality and recommend that irrigation with 1.5–3% NaOCl, followed by a final rinse of 17% EDTA, should be used for vital pulp treatment procedures (109, 110).

Importantly, the bioactive molecules can act synergistically at nanomolar concentrations to regulate many cellular processes. To stimulate the reactionary dentinogenic response, the DMCs directly act on the surviving primary odontoblasts to upregulate their dentine secretory and synthetic activity. However, as reparative dentinogenesis is more complex, bioactive molecules also regulate the progenitor cell recruitment process, proliferation and differentiation steps. Consequently, multifactorial signalling provides the flexibility required for the tissue and is required to invoke repair responses (84).

Cellular Responses

Cellular studies of tertiary dentinogenic responses have mainly focused on the role of odontoblasts (111) or the mesenchymal SC populations (112). Regeneration involves the replacement of tissue damaged by trauma or disease with that which resembles the native tissue, and pluri- or multi-potent stem cells under the regulation of growth and differentiation signals are required for this process. Several dental stem cell (SC) populations have been described including DPSCs, which comprise less than 5% of all pulp cells (30), as well as stem cells of the apical papilla (SCAP), stem cells from human exfoliated deciduous teeth (SHED), dental follicle stem cells (DFSCs) and periodontal ligament stem cells (PDLSCs) (113–117). Notably, several of these stem/progenitor cell populations have been proposed to contribute to dentine-pulp complex healing. In addition, animal models have also shown that there is the potential that SCs external to the tooth can be attracted to migrate into the pulp to enable tissue repair (35, 112). Indeed, recent data using bone-marrow fibrocytes have shown that they can migrate to the injured pulp to participate in early wound healing events including new blood vessel formation (82). It is evident that while there is a lack of consensus regarding the exact progenitor population involved in reparative dentinogenesis, marker expression analysis indicates that several cell types of mesenchymal origin may contribute to this process (118). Notably, at a molecular level, the relative influence of both dentine and pulp cell-derived factors on tertiary dentinogenesis is currently impossible to quantify; however, the healing process is likely influenced by their temporal bioavailability and the tissue environment (83).

Immune-Inflammatory Response in Dentine-Pulp Complex Repair – A Double-Edged Sword

While it is well known that the odontoblasts main function is regarded as being responsible for dentinogenesis, their immunocompetent role is also well described (119). During the early stages of caries and disease, the enamel and dentine become demineralized and soften due to the action of acids produced by the cariogenic bacteria (120). This process will further open up the porous tubular dentine, allowing bacterial products and components to traverse the hard tissue where they will initially be detected by receptors on the odontoblasts, leading to activation of the immune and inflammatory response beneath the lesion (121). If the carious environment is not appropriately arrested either by partial or complete caries excavation, the invading microbial biofilm will further evolve and will become mainly anaerobic in nature deeper within the pulp tissue (122–124). At the same time, the inflammatory response begins to amplify, and disease progression can lead to irreversible pulpitis, pulp necrosis and may ultimately result in apical periodontitis (125).

The molecular signalling response which occurs during the progressing infection is complex as it drives the host's defensive reaction within the pulpal tissue. In addition to the odontoblasts, pulpal cells including fibroblasts, stem cells, neurones and endothelial cells, express receptors which detect bacterial components. Members of the TLR family (TLRs 1-9) are shown to be present on many of the cell types within the pulp where they sense the presence of bacterial wall components, such as lipopolysaccharides (LPS) and lipoteichoic acids (LTA), and bacterial DNA (126–128). In particular, TLR2 and TL4 have important roles in early pulpitis and the innate immune response to bacterial infection. Specifically, TLR2 is involved in the recognition of peptidoglycans and LTA Gram-positive bacteria, while TLR4 mediates the effects of LPS on Gram-negative bacteria (39, 129). Once the bacterial ligand is bound, downstream intracellular signalling pathways are invoked, involving the nuclear factor kappa B (NF-kB) and mitogen activated protein (MAP) kinase (130) pathways. Consequently, AMPs which directly aim to kill the bacteria are released, as well as inflammatory regulating cytokines invoking immune cellular responses including cell recruitment, extravasation, activation, differentiation and antibody production by immune cells. Classic cytokines present during disease in the pulp include the IL-1α, -1β, -4, -6, -8, -10 and tumour necrosis factor (TNF-α) (131). It is only once the infection is removed or the microbial load reduced to a critical level, allowing a reparative host response, for example, following caries removal, that the inflammation becomes resolved and the levels of cytokines decrease towards levels present during tissue homeostasis. However, if this clinical outcome is not achieved, then chronic molecular inflammation will persist along with tissue swelling, pain and tissue necrosis. Under these conditions, the possibility of any tissue repair processes occurring is severely limited (132, 133).

The role of neurogenic inflammation within the pulp is also significant. As described above, the dental pulp is highly innervated with pulpal nerves located at sites of injury. Once activated during disease, these nerves contribute to inflammatory signalling by the release of neuropeptides (27, 59). Indeed, neuropeptides including SP, CGRP and VIP are upregulated in pulps containing deep carious lesions as well as in teeth with symptomatic pulpitis (58, 62, 134). It is understood that neuronal sprouting and activation of the complement system, which are associated with pulpal inflammation, along with the local release of neuropeptides, mediate an enhanced protective pain reflex as well as a neurogenic inflammatory response which aims to combat infection whilst facilitating tissue healing and repair (18). The locally released neuropeptides contribute to the regulation of pulpal blood flow and, along with angiogenic GFs, they can facilitate tissue healing (27, 60). Further, as previously indicated, neuropeptides exhibit antimicrobial activities against many endodontic pathogens, and these molecules may therefore be important in determining disease progression (135).

Immunological Response in the Dental Pulp

Comparable with other peripheral organs and tissues including the skin, gastrointestinal tract and lungs, the healthy dental pulp contains immunosensory leukocytes, such as macrophages, DCs, mast cells and T cells, which are able to detect disease-causing agents in the local environment and subsequently orchestrate the appropriate response (Figure 2.2) (40, 127, 136, 137). Indeed, studies

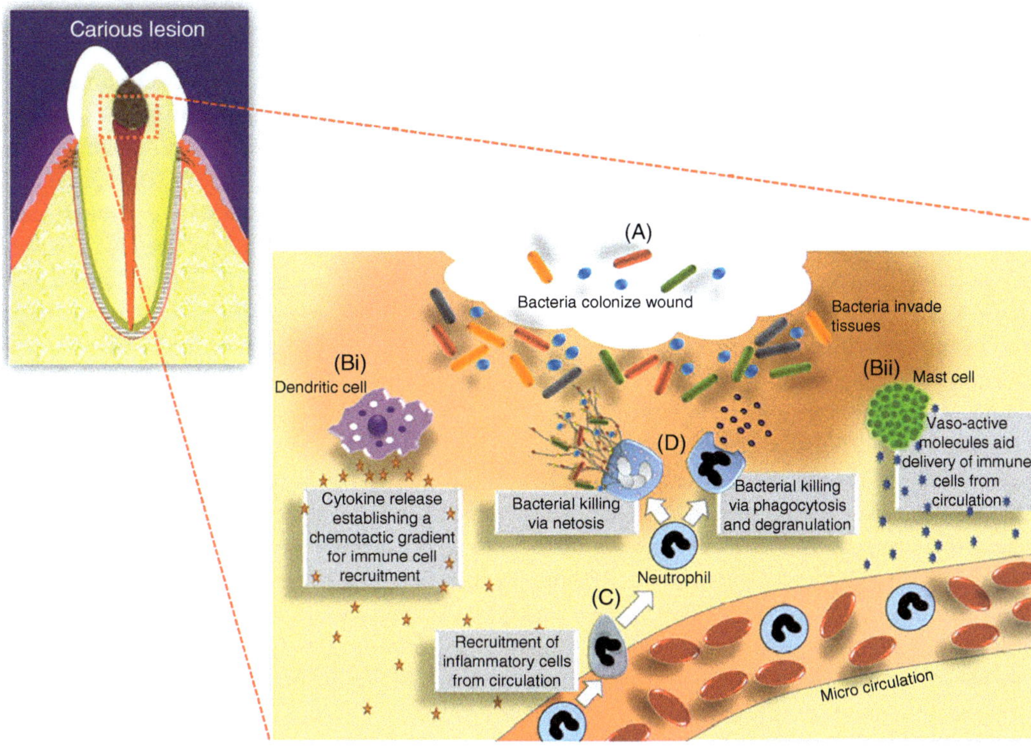

Figure 2.2 A schematic representation of the cellular and molecular immune processes involved in the dentine-pulp complex in response to carious infection. (A) Bacteria colonize and infect the dental wound and are subsequently detected by tissue-resident cells, including immune cells, such as (Bi) dendritic cells and (Bii) mast cells. Bioactive molecules and chemokines/cytokines are released, which generate signals and gradients to enable further immune cell recruitment and activation, such as (C) neutrophils, attracted from the bloodstream. Subsequently, neutrophils (D) utilize a range of bacterial killing mechanisms. The chronic cycle of the inflammatory response will continue while the infection remains. Macrophages can also remove bacteria and cellular debris, and enable the resolution of inflammation. Subsequently, wound healing processes can be invoked once conditions within the pulp become conducive. *Source:* Reproduced with permission Cooper et al. (136)/Elsevier.

have demonstrated that these immunosurveillance leukocytes can represent ~1% of the total cell population in human teeth (137). When pathogens are detected, leukocyte numbers significantly increase due to the signalling which occurs following the elevation of the molecular inflammatory process described in the previous section. This inflammation is aimed at being protective, with the ensuing immune response triggering the recruitment of additional leukocyte populations from the circulatory system. These leukocytes subsequently adhere to the endothelial cells lining the blood vessel walls and migrate out into the diseased site. The neutrophils are initially recruited to engulf and destroy the infecting bacteria; subsequently, there is a macrophage response which occurs following their development from monocytes, and this differentiation process is also regulated by the levels of the inflammatory molecules present. Notably, studies have reported on neutrophils and macrophages progressively increasing in diseased pulp tissue in response to irritants from the caries process (138, 139). Macrophages also phagocytose the infecting bacteria and this process then results in the recruitment and activation of T cells, resulting in an adaptive immune response which arises in association with the local DC activity. As described previously, DCs are initially in an immature state within the pulp, with odontoblast-derived chemokines being able to attract them to the site of the infectious lesion. Subsequently, DCs can then capture bacterial antigens from the local environment (39, 44, 140, 141), resulting in their maturation and subsequent migration to regional lymph nodes. Within this tissue, they then present the antigens to naive CD4+ T cells, resulting in their activation. Activated DCs express a plethora of cytokines that modulate both the innate and adaptive immune responses; consequently, DCs are considered key regulators of the defence reaction during infection. The activated naive CD4+ T cells, can differentiate into either effector CD4+ T helper cells, including Th1, Th2 or Th17 population subsets depending on the cytokine cocktail predominating within the tissue, or induced regulatory T (iTreg) cells. Notably, the different Th subsets also express different cytokines which can result in activation of different arms of the immune response, such as the regulation of humoral (immunoglobulin-mediated) immunity. Data has shown that T cell populations present in the pulp adapt and change as carious and pulpal disease progresses (128, 140, 142, 143).

Natural killer (NK) cells are also a well-characterized component of the innate immune response, and they have been identified in healthy rat molars and, recently, they have been shown to represent ~2.5% of the leukocytes present in human healthy pulp (137). Furthermore, natural killer T (NKT) cells, which are a subset of T cells, play a major role in the development of the Th1 versus Th2 immune axis and have also now been detected in healthy rat pulp. Notably, B cells are regarded as being present in relatively small numbers in healthy pulp tissue, although their numbers significantly increase during caries progression and in pulpitis (141, 144).

To avoid irreversible pulp damage, this complex immune response must be modulated to enable pathogen killing whilst minimizing local host tissue damage. Consequently, regulatory immune cells play a major role in this, and in particular, sub-populations of immature DCs, termed Tolerogenic (Tol)-DCs, are resistant to maturation (145, 146). These cells induce central and peripheral tolerance via several different mechanisms, such as T cell depletion or anergy, induced Treg (iTreg) cell differentiation from naive CD4+ T cells, and expression of a range of immunomodulatory mediators (147, 148). Notably, cytokines that are key to dampening the inflammatory response, include IL-10 and TGF-β, which suppress a range of immune cell functions. Interestingly, iTregs have been detected in diseased human pulps in relatively large numbers (149, 150). In addition, DCs expressing the immunomodulator, heme oxygenase-1 (HO-1), which protects cells against inflammatory and oxidative stress, have also been reported within pulps along with myeloid-derived suppressor cells (MDSCs), which exhibit a remarkable ability to regulate immune responses (151–154).

As discussed earlier, the pulpal inflammatory response is double-edged, and it is well known that chronic infection, with relatively high levels of inflammation, results in collateral host tissue damage due to the action of the immune cells targeted at killing the invading bacteria (128). Indeed, immune cells such as neutrophils and macrophages release tissue-degrading enzymes, such as MMPs, that are necessary for their recruitment and migration within tissues. For their antimicrobial killing activity, these cells release reactive oxygen species (ROS); however, these molecules can also cause significant collateral tissue damage. ROS are known to damage cell membranes, DNA and proteins, which can exacerbate cytokine release via activation of p38 MAP kinase and NF-kB intracellular signalling pathways. These events can perpetuate the inflammatory cycle (136). Interestingly, a novel bacterial killing and containment mechanism, termed neutrophil extracellular traps (NETs), has recently been reported. This mechanism involves the release of intracellular DNA adorned with AMPs; however, these structures have also been shown to be cytotoxic and proinflammatory. Consequently, their release into tooth tissue is also likely to contribute to the chronic inflammation observed in pulpal disease (136, 155).

Data indicates that not only is persistent and chronic inflammation damaging to the tissues, but it also directly impedes tissue repair processes. Consequently, pulp healing can only occur after the removal of the infection concomitant with a decrease in inflammation (40, 128). Studies *in vitro* and *in vivo* have indeed shown the biphasic nature of proinflammatory mediators (156) as relatively low levels of cytokines such as TNF-α and TGF-β, as well as ROS and bacterial LPS, can stimulate dental tissue repair mechanisms. However, when present at relatively high levels, they can exert deleterious effects, such as induction of cell death and tissue necrosis. Furthermore, stem cell differentiation processes important for tissue repair are directly inhibited by relatively high levels of proinflammatory molecules (40). Consequently, without clinical interventions, aimed at removing the source of inflammation and preserving pulpal vitality, the pulp will become infected, chronically inflamed and irreversibly damaged, necessitating either root canal treatment or extraction.

Notably, there are clinical translation opportunities in modulating the inflammation within pulp tissue. Calcium hydroxide [$Ca(OH)_2$] dental materials placed in direct contact with the pulp have long been recognized for their role in stimulating dental tissue repair by 'irritating' the pulp tissue and have achieved good long-term success (157–160). The high pH of the material is proposed to induce pulp cell death and a zone of superficial necrosis against vital pulp tissue, leading to a localized low-level inflammation which stimulates hard tissue repair and subsequently returns the tissue to a homeostatic state (159). While hard setting $Ca(OH)_2$ is relatively straightforward to use clinically and has remained the gold standard pulp capping material for many years, calcium silicate bioceramic materials are now considered best practice (161). Calcium hydroxide as a pulp capping material does not seal particularly well and undergoes dissolution over time, leaving a void beneath the restoration. Furthermore, the hard tissue barrier may be impaired in the presence of inflammation, and it is associated with 'tunnel defects', making the pulp prone to reinfection due to microleakage (74, 79). Randomized clinical trial studies comparing the calcium silicate pulp capping material, mineral trioxide aggregate (MTA) with hard setting $Ca(OH)_2$ indicates that MTA results in less pulpal inflammation, formation of a more predictable non-porous barrier and significantly less clinical failure than $Ca(OH)_2$ (79, 162).

Calcium silicate bioceramic materials, such as MTA and Biodentine, set with the release of calcium ions and show favourable clinical healing and success (163–165). The repair mechanism associated with MTA has also been attributed to its ability to stimulate a temporary localized tissue cytokine burst, which involves the release of IL-1α, IL-1β, IL-2, IL-6 and IL-8, from hard tissue-forming cells. The molecular and cellular stimulatory action of this type of material may explain how it promotes dental tissue repair (166, 167). Other studies are now using this knowledge of the immune and inflammatory response to exploit the interaction between inflammation and regeneration by developing novel materials which modulate these processes. Biodentine, a tricalcium silicate-based material, has been shown to exert anti-inflammatory molecular effects *in vitro*, which promote tissue healing. Although Biodentine has previously been shown to reduce inflammatory-induced TRPA1 expression and functional responses (168), particularly those mediated by TNF-α (169), the range of mechanisms responsible for this material's modulatory effects have, however, yet to be fully identified (170). More recently, premixed bioceramic putty materials have been introduced, which provide a homogenous consistency and are comparable to MTA in terms of clinical use, good biocompatibility, bridge formation and minimal inflammation; however, fully understand molecular responses and long-term clinical studies are needed (171, 172).

The application of naturally derived therapeutic inflammatory modulators is also being explored for use adjunctively or by incorporation into dental materials to promote tissue healing and facilitate restoration longevity. Dental resin placement is known to generate significant tissue-damaging

ROS; consequently, studies have reported on the incorporation of powerful antioxidants, such as *N*-acetylcysteine (NAC), into these materials to protect pulp cells. Notably, beneficially NAC may also exert antibacterial activity targeted against multispecies endodontic biofilms (173, 174). Consequently, these modified restorative materials may better combat infection whilst modulating inflammation to create a conducive environment to enable dental tissue repair. Other studies are also reporting on the anti-inflammatory effects of naturally derived compounds within the diseased pulp. For example, pachymic acid, a bioactive derived from mushroom, *Formitopsis niagra*, exerts an anti-inflammatory effect whilst promoting odontogenic differentiation (175). Studies have also started to consider the use of immuno-modulatory therapies, such as the application of anti-cytokine molecules, for the treatment pulp of inflammation. Indeed, similarities with other chronic inflammatory diseases, such as psoriasis, inflammatory bowel diseases and rheumatoid arthritis, which are also characterized by an excessive molecular and cellular immune response along with microbial-association and hard-soft tissue destructive pathologies, have been highlighted. The development and therapeutic success of anti-cytokine treatment in these diseases indicates the potential for use of this class of therapeutic molecule in pulpal disease. However, further work is required to determine whether this therapeutic approach will be efficacious as an adjunctive treatment in pulpal disease (176).

Combined, the studies described above indicate that there remains plenty of work still to be undertaken to fully characterize the molecular and cellular components involved in healthy and diseased pulp tissue. However, clearly there are opportunities for future development of new vital pulp treatments and smart restorative materials which can work with the complex host cell and tissue responses to promote dental tissue healing and repair.

Diagnostics for Pulpal Disease

As outlined above, the immunological and cellular responses of the pulp to injury aim to be defensive and promote tissue healing and repair. As such, the extent of pulpal inflammation varies depending on the severity of tissue injury, the level of microbial contamination and the individual host response. Bacterial by-products and/or bacterial toxins will generally evoke a mild or moderate inflammatory response. However, severe pulpal inflammation will be evident upon invasion of the dental pulp tissue by microorganisms associated with the development of a deep carious lesion (132). Although the inflammatory response is a protective mechanism, it also has destructive elements, such as pain, and the nature of the pulpal pain experienced will vary depending on the microflora and the type and extent of inflammation (128, 177). In biological terms, the intensity of pain (mild, moderate, severe) experienced is determined by the number and types of nerve fibres stimulated, as well as by the frequency of firing of the nerves. Of the two major types of sensory nerve present, the myelinated A-delta nerve fibres are fast-conducting (conduction velocity of 12–30 m/s) and, located in the peripheral pulp, give rise to sharp, transient pain in response to stimuli. Conversely, the unmyelinated C-fibres are slow-conducting (conduction velocity of 0.5–2 m/s) and are located in the central pulp where they give rise to a spontaneous, dull, throbbing pain (178, 179).

Pain symptoms reported by the patient often challenge the clinician's diagnosis because they rely on subjective tests, which do not accurately or objectively determine the degree of inflammation, or the ability of the inflamed dental pulp to heal (180, 181). The clinical diagnosis of the status of the dental pulp in teeth compromised by caries, or by trauma is generally determined by sensibility and vitality testing of the pulp, using electric pulp testing, cold testing, heat testing, as well as percussion sensitivity and intraoral radiography (161, 182). It is well-recognized that there are inadequacies in these clinical methods currently used to diagnose the status of the dental pulp (180). Although these approaches continue to be used routinely in clinical practice, there is no consensus on their utility in assessing the inflammatory status of the dental pulp (182), and indeed, it has been reported by systematic review that evidence for their use in diagnosing the health status of the dental pulp is inadequate (180). Furthermore, in histological studies of the dental pulp, a relationship between the pain reported, the severity of inflammation and the signs and symptoms of pulpitis has not been unequivocally demonstrated (181, 183, 184). Moreover, classification of pulpitis as reversible or irreversible (185) on the basis of current clinical diagnostic methods is problematic. Systematic reviews and vital pulp treatment studies have shown that the clinical outcomes are very good following carious pulp exposure in cases of reversible pulpitis (163, 186) and that maintaining the vitality of at least part of the pulp is also possible in teeth displaying signs and symptoms of irreversible pulpitis (172, 187). Robust diagnostic methods, potentially involving biomarkers that more accurately reflect the inflammatory status of the dental pulp, are required to guide case selection for minimal intervention and more predictable treatment outcomes. To date, several primary studies have investigated different biomolecules in pulpitis that could be used as diagnostic biomarkers (188–190). In addition, three systematic reviews have reported on biomarker expression during pulpal inflammation (191–193). Inflammatory mediators are amongst the leading candidates for use as future biomarkers since levels of inflammatory mediators are reportedly low in healthy pulp tissue and rise significantly following a robust inflammatory response to trauma and/or infection. Ultimately, biomarkers could become a diagnostic tool for pulp vitality that would aid prognosis and guide less invasive treatments. Teeth with pulpitis that have a biological profile closer to that of a clinically normal pulp could be identified more predictably for conservative management such as vital pulp treatment, thereby avoiding invasive treatments, additional costs, and importantly, prolonging the restorative lifecycle of teeth.

Future Vital Pulp Treatments

In addition to considering the use of anti-inflammatory and tissue-protective approaches described above to preserve pulp vitality, a variety of other areas are being explored, which may result in the development of new therapeutics. Data on the application of a combination of antibiotic-based pastes and inducing a blood clot to act as a scaffold (194, 195) has indicated that this approach enables repair but not tissue regeneration (196, 197). Further, the European Society of Endodontology (ESE) position statement and clinical guideline for revitalization procedures supports the use of calcium hydroxide as an intracanal medicament rather than antibiotics (110). Consequently, attention has now shifted to treatments which enable the biological response by using methods which locally release bioactive DMCs (Figure 2.3), including GFs and signalling molecules, including irrigants, medicaments and materials (90, 106, 198). In addition, the application of concentrated blood products, such as platelet-rich plasma (PRP) and platelet-rich fibrin (PRF), has been explored (199). These materials can provide a rich supply of endogenous GFs (200), and when delivered therapeutically, they form natural fibrin gels which act as scaffolds to stimulate hard and soft-tissue healing (201). While they represent an attractive autologous and locally sourced supply of GFs, key disadvantages to their use are that they require a 'chairside' centrifuge, specialist reagents and expertise, as well as phlebotomy skills, which increases costs and invasiveness of the treatment (199). Furthermore, to improve the physical properties of PRP, it may need to be combined with other materials such as hydrogels in order to regulate its

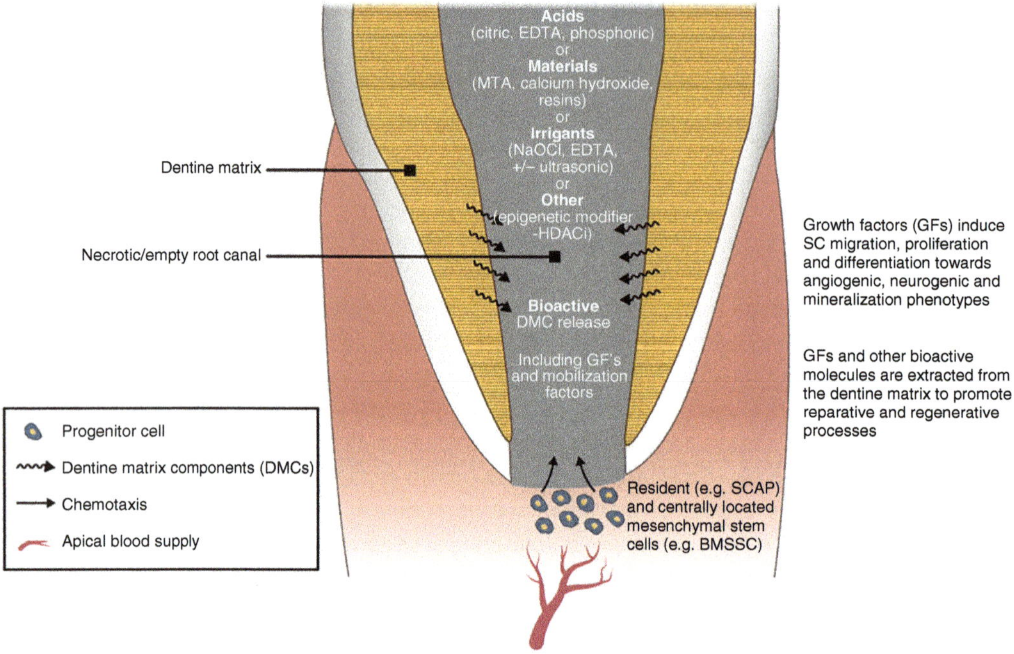

Figure 2.3 Schematic representation of the interaction between dentine matrix components (DMCs) and a range of etchants, irrigants, dental materials and epigenetic modifying agents. The release of DMCs stimulates cellular processes central to dentine-pulp complex tissue regeneration. *Source:* Reproduced with permission Duncan et al. (198)/Springer Nature.

degradation and bioactivity (201). In comparison, PRF provides a biodegradable fibrin scaffold structure (202) but requires the addition of anticoagulants to regulate GF release (203). A recent systematic review has indicated that there is potentially no difference between PRP, PRF and blood clotting alone approaches when comparing the outcome measures of increased dentinal wall thickening and root closure in treated teeth (204).

As indicated above, stem cells within the pulp can provide an opportunity to heal and regenerate the tissue. However, suitable scaffolds which either support their delivery or recruitment, i.e. cell-homing and enable cell proliferation and differentiation, are required (205). The use of a range of natural and synthetically derived materials which exhibit specific mechanical and structural properties is currently being explored. These scaffolds also need to provide appropriate environmental cues for tissue regeneration and facilitate the supply of sufficient nutrients to the cells; hence, vascular-promoting properties are considered key (205, 206). Scaffolds also need to enable cell adhesion and cell-cell interactions to enable complex tissue formation. Their biodegradation and ability to not provoke significant immune or cytotoxic responses are also important properties (207).

Natural scaffolds include PRP and PRF, as described above, however, scaffolds which incorporate collagen exhibit good tensile strength, cell adhesion and cell migratory properties (208). Indeed, the inclusion of key GFs in collagen scaffolds can promote cell recruitment and population as well as enable neovascularization (209). Chitin, a primary and natural component of the exoskeletons of crustaceans such as crabs or shrimps can also be used to develop chitosan scaffolds via deacetylation chemical processes. The product generated is non-toxic, absorbable, antibacterial and has bioinductive properties for both dental hard and soft tissues (210) and combined in a hydrogel it may hold potential for dental pulp regeneration (211). Silk fibroin-based scaffolds have unique mechanical and biocompatible properties and are biodegraded relatively slowly, enabling their replacement by newly formed host tissue (212, 213). Alginate hydrogels can be derived from seaweed and can be further modified by the inclusion of arginine-glycineaspartic acid (RGD) motifs to enable cell adhesion, proliferation and differentiation for enhanced bioinductivity when placed clinically (214).

There are also a variety of chemically synthesized polymer scaffolds developed for use in pulp regeneration (215). Significantly, these have been engineered to degrade more slowly *in vivo* when compared with natural scaffolds. Polylactic acid (PLA) is a biocompatible and biodegradable polymer which has been shown to support the adherence and proliferation of DPSCs (216). Poly-L-lactic acid (PLLA) scaffolds exhibit an increased pore size which facilitates cell proliferation and differentiation of DPSCs (217, 218). Polyglycolic acid (PGA) scaffolds are biocompatible, and their degradation is tunable *in vivo* when combined with polylactic-*co*-glycolic acid (PLGA) (219).

Synthetic ECM scaffolds utilize hydrogel systems to enable them to be delivered into narrow and difficult-to-access locations such as inside a pulp chamber or root canal. These hydrogels can be formed using thermal, ionic interaction, physical cross-linking, photo-polymerization and chemical cross-linking processing (220). Notably, this enables these hydrogels to act as cell and/or GF delivery systems. Indeed, PuraMatrix™, can spontaneously polymerize under normal physiological conditions and has been used for DPSC proliferation and odontoblast-like cell differentiation with suitable GFs (221). Due to its mechanical properties, firmer hydrogels, such as ones derived from gelatin-methacryloyl (GelMA), can stimulate cell proliferation and differentiation of both endothelial cells and odontoblast-like cells *in vitro* (222).

The use of bioprinted scaffolds are at the forefront regenerative medicine and dental tissue engineering research (223) and may provide potential for the regeneration of the dentine-pulp complex. This technology offers the ability to customize a scaffold to an individual and to incorporate cells and bioactive molecules to enhance its properties. Further, the advances in 4D printing techniques indicate that these scaffolds may change functionality under cues from a range of different environments, for example, in response to temperature or pH (224). Within the clinical environment, this may offer potential in future for the controlled release of drugs or angiogenic GFs, which until now has been problematic (225).

Clearly, studies into new vital pulp treatments represent a highly active research area with the need for collaborations between clinicians and basic biological, chemical and physical scientists to underpin future developments necessary for patient benefit. Indeed, it is also evident that in order for the field to progress, we need a thorough understanding of the molecular and cellular biology of the dentine-pulp complex in terms of its development, homeostasis, immune response and its innate ability to heal.

References

1 Cobourne MT, Sharpe PT. Tooth and jaw: molecular mechanisms of patterning in the first branchial arch. *Arch Oral Biol.* 2003;48(1):1–14.

2 Tucker A, Sharpe P. The cutting-edge of mammalian development; how the embryo makes teeth. *Nat Rev Genet.* 2004;5(7):499–508.

3 Balic A, Thesleff I. Tissue interactions regulating tooth development and renewal. *Curr Top Dev Biol.* 2015;115:157–86.

4 El Karim IA, Linden GJ, Curtis TM, About I, McGahon MK, Irwin CR, et al. Human odontoblasts express functional thermo-sensitive TRP channels: implications for dentin sensitivity. *Pain.* 2011;152(10):2211–23.

5 Bjørndal L. The caries process and its effect on the pulp: the science is changing and so is our understanding. *Pediatr Dent.* 2008;30(3):192–6.

6 Bjørndal L, Darvann T. A light microscopic study of odontoblastic and non-odontoblastic cells involved in tertiary dentinogenesis in well-defined cavitated carious lesions. *Caries Res.* 1999;33(1):50–60.

7 Frank RM. Ultrastructure of human dentine 40 years ago—progress and perspectives. *Arch Oral Biol.* 1999;44(12):979–84.

8 Farges JC, Keller JF, Carrouel F, Durand SH, Romeas A, Bleicher F, et al. Odontoblasts in the dental pulp immune response. *J Exp Zool B Mol Dev Evol.* 2009;312b(5):425–36.

9 Yumoto H, Hirao K, Hosokawa Y, Kuramoto H, Takegawa D, Nakanishi T, et al. The roles of odontoblasts in dental pulp innate immunity. *Jpn Dent Sci Rev.* 2018;54(3):105–17.

10 Tazawa K, Ikeda H, Kawashima N, Okiji T. Transient receptor potential melastatin (TRPM) 8 is expressed in freshly isolated native human odontoblasts. *Arch Oral Biol.* 2017;75:55–61.

11 Wen W, Que K, Zang C, Wen J, Sun G, Zhao Z, et al. Expression and distribution of three transient receptor potential vanilloid(TRPV) channel proteins in human odontoblast-like cells. *J Mol Histol.* 2017;48(5–6):367–77.

12 Sato M, Ogura K, Kimura M, Nishi K, Ando M, Tazaki M, et al. Activation of mechanosensitive transient receptor potential/piezo channels in odontoblasts generates action potentials in cocultured isolectin B(4)-negative medium-sized trigeminal ganglion neurons. *J Endod.* 2018;44(6):984–91. e2.

13 Carda C, Peydró A. Ultrastructural patterns of human dentinal tubules, odontoblasts processes and nerve fibres. *Tissue Cell.* 2006;38(2):141–50.

14 Egbuniwe O, Grover S, Duggal AK, Mavroudis A, Yazdi M, Renton T, et al. TRPA1 and TRPV4 activation in human odontoblasts stimulates ATP release. *J Dent Res.* 2014;93(9):911–7.

15 Álvarez-Vásquez JL, Castañeda-Alvarado CP. Dental pulp fibroblast: a star cell. *J Endod.* 2022;48(8):1005–19.

16 Martinez EF, Araújo VC. In vitro immunoexpression of extracellular matrix proteins in dental pulpal and gingival human fibroblasts. *Int Endod J.* 2004;37(11):749–55.

17 Tran-Hung L, Mathieu S, About I. Role of human pulp fibroblasts in angiogenesis. *J Dent Res.* 2006;85(9):819–23.

18 Chmilewsky F, About I, Chung SH. Pulp fibroblasts control nerve regeneration through complement activation. *J Dent Res.* 2016;95(8):913–22.

19 Matsushima K, Ohbayashi E, Takeuchi H, Hosoya S, Abiko Y, Yamazaki M. Stimulation of interleukin-6 production in human dental pulp cells by peptidoglycans from Lactobacillus casei. *J Endod.* 1998;24(4):252–5.

20 Sipert CR, Morandini AC, Dionísio TJ, Machado MA, Oliveira SH, Campanelli AP, et al. In vitro regulation of CCL3 and CXCL12 by bacterial by-products is dependent on site of origin of human oral fibroblasts. *J Endod.* 2014;40(1):95–100.

21 Hirao K, Yumoto H, Takahashi K, Mukai K, Nakanishi T, Matsuo T. Roles of TLR2, TLR4, NOD2, and NOD1 in pulp fibroblasts. *J Dent Res.* 2009;88(8):762–7.

22 Howard C, Murray PE, Namerow KN. Dental pulp stem cell migration. *J Endod.* 2010;36(12):1963–6.

23 Sakai VT, Zhang Z, Dong Z, Neiva KG, MacHado MAAM, Shi S, et al. SHED differentiate into functional odontoblasts and endothelium. *J Dent Res.* 2010;89(8):791–6.

24 Killough SA, Lundy FT, Irwin CR. Substance P expression by human dental pulp fibroblasts: a potential role in neurogenic inflammation. *J Endod.* 2009;35(1):73–7.

25 Killough SA, Lundy FT, Irwin CR. Dental pulp fibroblasts express neuropeptide Y Y1 receptor but not neuropeptide Y. *Int Endod J.* 2010;43(10):835–42.

26 Lundy FT, Linden GJ. Neuropeptides and neurogenic mechanisms in oral and periodontal inflammation. *Crit Rev Oral Biol Med.* 2004;15(2):82–98.

27 El Karim IA, Linden GJ, Irwin CR, Lundy FT. Neuropeptides regulate expression of angiogenic growth factors in human dental pulp fibroblasts. *J Endod.* 2009;35(6):829–33.

28 El Karim IA, Linden GJ, Curtis TM, About I, McGahon MK, Irwin CR, et al. Human dental pulp fibroblasts express the "cold-sensing" transient receptor potential channels TRPA1 and TRPM8. *J Endod.* 2011;37(4):473–8.

29 Gronthos S, Brahim J, Li W, Fisher LW, Cherman N, Boyde A, et al. Stem cell properties of human dental pulp stem cells. *J Dent Res.* 2002;81(8):531–5.

30 Gronthos S, Mankani M, Brahim J, Robey PG, Shi S. Postnatal human dental pulp stem cells (DPSCs) in vitro and in vivo. *Proc Natl Acad Sci U S A.* 2000;97(25):13625–30.

31 Achilleos A, Trainor PA. Neural crest stem cells: discovery, properties and potential for therapy. *Cell Res.* 2012;22(2):288–304.

32 Sugimura-Wakayama Y, Katagiri W, Osugi M, Kawai T, Ogata K, Sakaguchi K, et al. Peripheral nerve regeneration by secretomes of stem cells from human exfoliated deciduous teeth. *Stem Cells Dev.* 2015;24(22):2687–99.

33 Arthur A, Rychkov G, Shi S, Koblar SA, Gronthos S. Adult human dental pulp stem cells differentiate toward functionally active neurons under appropriate environmental cues. *Stem Cells.* 2008;26(7):1787–95.

34 Clarke R, Monaghan K, About I, Griffin CS, Sergeant GP, El Karim I, et al. TRPA1 activation in a human sensory neuronal model: relevance to cough hypersensitivity? *Eur Respir J.* 2017;50(3):1700995.

35 Feng J, Mantesso A, De Bari C, Nishiyama A, Sharpe PT. Dual origin of mesenchymal stem cells contributing to organ growth and repair. *Proc Natl Acad Sci U S A.* 2011;108(16):6503–8.

36 Kaukua N, Shahidi MK, Konstantinidou C, Dyachuk V, Kaucka M, Furlan A, et al. Glial origin of mesenchymal stem cells in a tooth model system. *Nature.* 2014;513(7519):551–4.

37 Demircan PC, Sariboyaci AE, Unal ZS, Gacar G, Subasi C, Karaoz E. Immunoregulatory effects of human dental pulp-derived stem cells on T cells: comparison of transwell co-culture and mixed lymphocyte reaction systems. *Cytotherapy.* 2011;13(10):1205–20.

38 Ravenscroft H, El Karim I, Krasnodembskaya AD, Gilmore B, About I, Lundy FT. Novel antibacterial properties of the human dental pulp multipotent mesenchymal stromal cell secretomp. *Am J Pathol.* 2022;192(6):956–69.

39 Keller JF, Carrouel F, Colomb E, Durand SH, Baudouin C, Msika P, et al. Toll-like receptor 2 activation by lipoteichoic acid induces differential production of pro-inflammatory cytokines in human odontoblasts, dental pulp fibroblasts and immature dendritic cells. *Immunobiology.* 2010;215(1):53–9.

40 Farges JC, Alliot-Licht B, Renard E, Ducret M, Gaudin A, Smith AJ, et al. Dental pulp defence and repair mechanisms in dental caries. *Mediators Inflamm.* 2015;2015:230251.

41 Farges JC, Carrouel F, Keller JF, Baudouin C, Msika P, Bleicher F, et al. Cytokine production by human odontoblast-like cells upon Toll-like receptor-2 engagement. *Immunobiology.* 2011;216(4):513–7.

42 Kolaczkowska E, Kubes P. Neutrophil recruitment and function in health and inflammation. *Nat Rev Immunol.* 2013;13(3):159–75.

43 Lundy FT, Irwin CR, McLean DF, Linden GJ, El Karim IA. Natural antimicrobials in the dental pulp. *J Endod.* 2020;46(9s):S2–9.

44 Farges JC, Romeas A, Melin M, Pin JJ, Lebecque S, Lucchini M, et al. TGF-beta1 induces accumulation of dendritic cells in the odontoblast layer. *J Dent Res.* 2003;82(8):652–6.

45 Lechner JH, Kalnitsky G. The presence of large amounts of type III collagen in bovine dental pulp and its significance with regard to the mechanism of dentinogenesis. *Arch Oral Biol.* 1981;26(4):265–73.

46 Linde A. The extracellular matrix of the dental pulp and dentin. *J Dent Res.* 1985;64:523–9.

47 Tsuzaki M, Yamauchi M, Mechanic GL. Bovine dental pulp collagens: characterization of types III and V collagen. *Arch Oral Biol.* 1990;35(3):195–200.

48 Karjalainen S, Söderling E, Pelliniemi L, Foidart JM. Immunohistochemical localization of types I and III collagen and fibronectin in the dentine of carious human teeth. *Arch Oral Biol.* 1986;31(12):801–6.

49 Fisher LW, Torchia DA, Fohr B, Young MF, Fedarko NS. Flexible structures of SIBLING proteins, bone sialoprotein, and osteopontin. *Biochem Biophys Res Commun.* 2001;280(2):460–5.

50 He G, Dahl T, Veis A, George A. Nucleation of apatite crystals in vitro by self-assembled dentin matrix protein 1. *Nat Mater.* 2003;2(8):552–8.

51 Qin C, Baba O, Butler WT. Post-translational modifications of sibling proteins and their roles in osteogenesis and dentinogenesis. *Crit Rev Oral Biol Med.* 2004;15(3):126–36.

52 Cadden SW, Lisney SJ, Matthews B. Thresholds to electrical stimulation of nerves in cat canine tooth-pulp with A beta-, A delta- and C-fibre conduction velocities. *Brain Res.* 1983;261(1):31–41.

53 Reader A, Foreman DW. An ultrastructural qualitative investigation of human intradental innervation. *J Endod.* 1981;7(4):161–8.

54 Nair PN, Luder HU, Schroeder HE. Number and size-spectra of myelinated nerve fibers of human premolars. *Anat Embryol (Berl).* 1992;186(6):563–71.

55 Nair PN, Schroeder HE. Number and size spectra of non-myelinated axons of human premolars. *Anat Embryol (Berl).* 1995;192(1):35–41.

56 Bae YC, Yoshida A. Ultrastructural basis for craniofacial sensory processing in the brainstem. *Int Rev Neurobiol.* 2011;97:99–141.

57 Henry MA, Luo S, Levinson SR. Unmyelinated nerve fibers in the human dental pulp express markers for myelinated fibers and show sodium channel accumulations. *BMC Neurosci.* 2012;13:29.

58 Awawdeh L, Lundy FT, Shaw C, Lamey PJ, Linden GJ, Kennedy JG. Quantitative analysis of substance P, neurokinin A and calcitonin gene-related peptide in pulp tissue from painful and healthy human teeth. *Int Endod J.* 2002;35(1):30–6.

59 El Karim IA, Lamey PJ, Linden GJ, Awawdeh LA, Lundy FT. Caries-induced changes in the expression of pulpal neuropeptide Y. *Eur J Oral Sci.* 2006;114(2):133–7.

60 Olgart L. Neural control of pulpal blood flow. *Crit Rev Oral Biol Med.* 1996;7(2):159–71.

61 Haug SR, Heyeraas KJ. Modulation of dental inflammation by the sympathetic nervous system. *J Dent Res.* 2006;85(6):488–95.

62 Caviedes-Bucheli J, Muñoz HR, Azuero-Holguín MM, Ulate E. Neuropeptides in dental pulp: the silent protagonists. *J Endod.* 2008;34(7):773–88.

63 Luthman J, Luthman D, Hökfelt T. Occurrence and distribution of different neurochemical markers in the human dental pulp. *Arch Oral Biol.* 1992;37(3):193–208.

64 Rodd HD, Boissonade FM. Comparative immunohistochemical analysis of the peptidergic innervation of human primary and permanent tooth pulp. *Arch Oral Biol.* 2002;47(5):375–85.

65 Zhang JQ, Nagata K, Iijima T. Scanning electron microscopy and immunohistochemical observations of the vascular nerve plexuses in the dental pulp of rat incisor. *Anat Rec.* 1998;251(2):214–20.

66 Kishi Y, Shimozato N, Takahashi K. Vascular architecture of cat pulp using corrosive resin cast under scanning electron, microscopy. *J Endod.* 1989;15(10):478–83.

67 Trowbridge HO. Pathogenesis of pulpitis resulting from dental caries. *J Endod.* 1981;7(2):52–60.
68 Berggreen E, Wiig H, Virtej A. Fluid transport from the dental pulp revisited. *Eur J Oral Sci.* 2020;128(5):365–8.
69 Bernick S, Nedelman C. Effect of aging on the human pulp. *J Endod.* 1975;1(3):88–94.
70 Murray PE, Matthews JB, Sloan AJ, Smith AJ. Analysis of incisor pulp cell populations in Wistar rats of different ages. *Arch Oral Biol.* 2002;47(10):709–15.
71 Murray PE, Stanley HR, Matthews JB, Sloan AJ, Smith AJ. Age-related odontometric changes of human teeth. *Oral Surg Oral Med Oral Pathol Oral Radiol Endod.* 2002;93(4):474–82.
72 Duncan HF, Cooper PR, Smith AJ. Dissecting dentine–pulp injury and wound healing responses: consequences for regenerative endodontics. *Int Endod J.* 2019;52(3):261–6.
73 Kuttler Y. Classification of dentine into primary, secondary, and tertiary. *Oral Surg Oral Med Oral Pathol.* 1959;12(8):996–9.
74 Cox CF, Subay RK, Ostro E, Suzuki S, Suzuki SH. Tunnel defects in dentin bridges: their formation following direct pulp capping. *Oper Dent.* 1996;21(1):4–11.
75 Smith AJ, Cassidy N, Perry H, Begue-Kirn C, Ruch JV, Lesot H. Reactionary dentinogenesis. *Int J Dev Biol.* 1995;39(1):273–80.
76 Smith AJ, Murray PE, Sloan AJ, Matthews JB, Zhao S. Trans-dentinal stimulation of tertiary dentinogenesis. *Adv Dent Res.* 2001;15:51–4.
77 Bjørndal L, Simon S, Tomson PL, Duncan HF. Management of deep caries and the exposed pulp. *Int Endod J.* 2019;52(7):949–73.
78 Tziafas D. Characterization of odontoblast-like cell phenotype and reparative dentin formation in vivo: a comprehensive literature review. *J Endod.* 2019;45(3):241–9.
79 Nair PNR, Duncan HF, Pitt Ford TR, Luder HU. Histological, ultrastructural and quantitative investigations on the response of healthy human pulps to experimental capping with mineral trioxide aggregate: a randomized controlled trial. *Int Endod J.* 2008;41(2):128–50.
80 Ricucci D, Loghin S, Lin LM, Spångberg LSW, Tay FR. Is hard tissue formation in the dental pulp after the death of the primary odontoblasts a regenerative or a reparative process? *J Dent.* 2014;42(9):1156–70.
81 Tecles O, Laurent P, Zygouritsas S, Burger A-S, Camps J, Dejou J, et al. Activation of human dental pulp progenitor/stem cells in response to odontoblast injury. *Arch Oral Biol.* 2005;50(2):103–8.
82 Yoshiba N, Edanami N, Tohma A, Takeuchi R, Ohkura N, Hosoya A, et al. Detection of bone marrow-derived fibrocytes in human dental pulp repair. *Int Endod J.* 2018;51(11):1187–95.
83 Smith AJ, Duncan HF, Diogenes A, Simon S, Cooper PR. Exploiting the bioactive properties of the dentin-pulp complex in regenerative endodontics. *J Endod.* 2016;42(1):47–56.
84 Smith AJ, Scheven BA, Takahashi Y, Ferracane JL, Shelton RM, Cooper PR. Dentine as a bioactive extracellular matrix. *Arch Oral Biol.* 2012;57(2):109–21.
85 Ronchetti I, Boraldi F, Annovi G, Cianciulli P, Quaglino D. Fibroblast involvement in soft connective tissue calcification. *Front Genet.* 2013;4:22.
86 Yamamoto K, Kishida T, Nakai K, Sato Y, Kotani S-i, Nishizawa Y, et al. Direct phenotypic conversion of human fibroblasts into functional osteoblasts triggered by a blockade of the transforming growth factor-β signal. *Sci Rep.* 2018;8(1):8463.
87 Yamamoto K, Kishida T, Sato Y, Nishioka K, Ejima A, Fujiwara H, et al. Direct conversion of human fibroblasts into functional osteoblasts by defined factors. *Proc Natl Acad Sci U S A.* 2015;112(19):6152–7.
88 Mizoshiri N, Kishida T, Yamamoto K, Shirai T, Terauchi R, Tsuchida S, et al. Transduction of Oct6 or Oct9 gene concomitant with Myc family gene induced osteoblast-like phenotypic conversion in normal human fibroblasts. *Biochem Biophys Res Commun.* 2015;467(4):1110–6.

89 Bjørndal L. Presence or absence of tertiary dentinogenesis in relation to caries progression. *Adv Dent Res.* 2001;15(1):80–3.

90 Galler KM, Widbiller M, Buchalla W, Eidt A, Hiller KA, Hoffer PC, et al. EDTA conditioning of dentine promotes adhesion, migration and differentiation of dental pulp stem cells. *Int Endod J.* 2016;49(6):581–90.

91 Tomson PL, Lumley PJ, Alexander MY, Smith AJ, Cooper PR. Hepatocyte growth factor is sequestered in dentine matrix and promotes regeneration-associated events in dental pulp cells. *Cytokine.* 2013;61(2):622–9.

92 Zhang R, Cooper PR, Smith G, Nör JE, Smith AJ. Angiogenic activity of dentin matrix components. *J Endod.* 2011;37(1):26–30.

93 Fayazi S, Takimoto K, Diogenes A. Comparative evaluation of chemotactic factor effect on migration and differentiation of stem cells of the apical papilla. *J Endod.* 2017;43(8):1288–93.

94 Marquardt LM, Ee X, Iyer N, Hunter D, Mackinnon SE, Wood MD, et al. Finely tuned temporal and spatial delivery of GDNF promotes enhanced nerve regeneration in a long nerve defect model. *Tissue Eng Part A.* 2015;21(23–24):2852–64.

95 Cassidy N, Fahey M, Prime SS, Smith AJ. Comparative analysis of transforming growth factor-beta isoforms 1–3 in human and rabbit dentine matrices. *Arch Oral Biol.* 1997;42(3):219–23.

96 Galler KM, Buchalla W, Hiller KA, Federlin M, Eidt A, Schiefersteiner M, et al. Influence of root canal disinfectants on growth factor release from dentin. *J Endod.* 2015;41(3):363–8.

97 Finkelman RD, Mohan S, Jennings JC, Taylor AK, Jepsen S, Baylink DJ. Quantitation of growth factors IGF-I, SGF/IGF-II, and TGF-beta in human dentin. *J Bone Miner Res.* 1990;5(7):717–23.

98 Duncan HF, Smith AJ, Fleming GJ, Reid C, Smith G, Cooper PR. Release of bio-active dentine extracellular matrix components by histone deacetylase inhibitors (HDACi). *Int Endod J.* 2017;50(1):24–38.

99 Roberts-Clark DJ, Smith AJ. Angiogenic growth factors in human dentine matrix. *Arch Oral Biol.* 2000;45(11):1013–6.

100 Dung SZ, Gregory RL, Li Y, Stookey GK. Effect of lactic acid and proteolytic enzymes on the release of organic matrix components from human root dentin. *Caries Res.* 1995;29(6):483–9.

101 Chaussain C, Boukpessi T, Khaddam M, Tjaderhane L, George A, Menashi S. Dentin matrix degradation by host matrix metalloproteinases: inhibition and clinical perspectives toward regeneration. *Front Physiol.* 2013;4:308.

102 Mazzoni A, Tjäderhane L, Checchi V, Di Lenarda R, Salo T, Tay FR, et al. Role of dentin MMPs in caries progression and bond stability. *J Dent Res.* 2015;94(2):241–51.

103 Okamoto M, Takahashi Y, Komichi S, Cooper PR, Hayashi M. Dentinogenic effects of extracted dentin matrix components digested with matrix metalloproteinases. *Sci Rep.* 2018;8(1):10690.

104 Bègue-Kirn C, Smith AJ, Loriot M, Kupferle C, Ruch JV, Lesot H. Comparative analysis of TGF beta s, BMPs, IGF1, msxs, fibronectin, osteonectin and bone sialoprotein gene expression during normal and in vitro-induced odontoblast differentiation. *Int J Dev Biol.* 1994;38(3):405–20.

105 Graham L, Cooper PR, Cassidy N, Nor JE, Sloan AJ, Smith AJ. The effect of calcium hydroxide on solubilisation of bio-active dentine matrix components. *Biomaterials.* 2006;27(14):2865–73.

106 Tomson PL, Grover LM, Lumley PJ, Sloan AJ, Smith AJ, Cooper PR. Dissolution of bio-active dentine matrix components by mineral trioxide aggregate. *J Dent.* 2007;35(8):636–42.

107 Ferracane JL, Cooper PR, Smith AJ. Dentin matrix component solubilization by solutions of pH relevant to self-etching dental adhesives. *J Adhes Dent.* 2013;15(5):407–12.

108 Widbiller M, Eidt A, Hiller KA, Buchalla W, Schmalz G, Galler KM. Ultrasonic activation of irrigants increases growth factor release from human dentine. *Clin Oral Investig.* 2017;21(3):879–88.

109 Martin DE, De Almeida JFA, Henry MA, Khaing ZZ, Schmidt CE, Teixeira FB, et al. Concentration-dependent effect of sodium hypochlorite on stem cells of apical papilla survival and differentiation. *J Endod.* 2014;40(1):51–5.

110 European Society of Endodontology. European Society of Endodontology position statement: revitalization procedures. *Int Endod J.* 2016;49(8):717–23.

111 Simon S, Smith AJ, Lumley PJ, Berdal A, Smith G, Finney S, et al. Molecular characterization of young and mature odontoblasts. *Bone.* 2009;45(4):693–703.

112 Frozoni M, Zaia AA, Line SR, Mina M. Analysis of the contribution of nonresident progenitor cells and hematopoietic cells to reparative dentinogenesis using parabiosis model in mice. *J Endod.* 2012;38(9):1214–9.

113 Miura M, Gronthos S, Zhao M, Lu B, Fisher LW, Robey PG, et al. SHED: stem cells from human exfoliated deciduous teeth. *Proc Natl Acad Sci U S A.* 2003;100(10):5807–12.

114 Seo BM, Miura M, Gronthos S, Bartold PM, Batouli S, Brahim J, et al. Investigation of multipotent postnatal stem cells from human periodontal ligament. *Lancet.* 2004;364(9429):149–55.

115 Sonoyama W, Liu Y, Yamaza T, Tuan RS, Wang S, Shi S, et al. Characterization of the apical papilla and its residing stem cells from human immature permanent teeth: a pilot study. *J Endod.* 2008;34(2):166–71.

116 Huang GTJ, Gronthos S, Shi S. Mesenchymal stem cells derived from dental tissues vs. those from other sources: their biology and role in regenerative medicine. *J Dent Res.* 2009;88(9):792–806.

117 Morsczeck C, Völlner F, Saugspier M, Brandl C, Reichert TE, Driemel O, et al. Comparison of human dental follicle cells (DFCs) and stem cells from human exfoliated deciduous teeth (SHED) after neural differentiation in vitro. *Clin Oral Investig.* 2009;14:1–8.

118 Simon S, Smith AJ. Regenerative endodontics. *Br Dent J.* 2014;216(6):E13.

119 Couve E, Osorio R, Schmachtenberg O. The amazing odontoblast: activity, autophagy, and aging. *J Dent Res.* 2013;92(9):765–72.

120 Takahashi N, Nyvad B. The role of bacteria in the caries process: ecological perspectives. *J Dent Res.* 2011;90(3):294–303.

121 Veerayutthwilai O, Byers MR, Pham TT, Darveau RP, Dale BA. Differential regulation of immune responses by odontoblasts. *Oral Microbiol Immunol.* 2007;22(1):5–13.

122 Warfvinge J, Bergenholtz G. Healing capacity of human and monkey dental pulps following experimentally-induced pulpitis. *Endod Dent Traumatol.* 1986;2(6):256–62.

123 Nadkarni MA, Caldon CE, Chhour KL, Fisher IP, Martin FE, Jacques NA, et al. Carious dentine provides a habitat for a complex array of novel Prevotella-like bacteria. *J Clin Microbiol.* 2004;42(11):5238–44.

124 Chhour KL, Nadkarni MA, Byun R, Martin FE, Jacques NA, Hunter N. Molecular analysis of microbial diversity in advanced caries. *J Clin Microbiol.* 2005;43(2):843–9.

125 Ricucci D, Siqueira JF Jr, Loghin S, Lin LM. Pulp and apical tissue response to deep caries in immature teeth: a histologic and histobacteriologic study. *J Dent.* 2017;56:19–32.

126 Kawai T, Akira S. The role of pattern-recognition receptors in innate immunity: update on Toll-like receptors. *Nat Immunol.* 2010;11(5):373–84.

127 Farges JC, Alliot-Licht B, Baudouin C, Msika P, Bleicher F, Carrouel F. Odontoblast control of dental pulp inflammation triggered by cariogenic bacteria. *Front Physiol.* 2013;4:326.

128 Galler KM, Weber M, Korkmaz Y, Widbiller M, Feuerer M. Inflammatory response mechanisms of the dentine–pulp complex and the periapical tissues. *Int J Mol Sci.* 2021;22(3):1480.

129 Mutoh N, Tani-Ishii N, Tsukinoki K, Chieda K, Watanabe K. Expression of Toll-like receptor 2 and 4 in dental pulp. *J Endod.* 2007;33(10):1183–6.

130 Martinho FC, Leite FR, Chiesa WM, Nascimento GG, Feres M, Gomes BP. Signaling pathways activation by primary endodontic infectious contents and production of inflammatory mediators. *J Endod.* 2014;40(4):484–9.

131 McLachlan JL, Sloan AJ, Smith AJ, Landini G, Cooper PR. S100 and cytokine expression in caries. *Infect Immun.* 2004;72(7):4102–8.

132 Ricucci D, Siqueira JF, Li Y, Tay FR. Vital pulp therapy: histopathology and histobacteriology-based guidelines to treat teeth with deep caries and pulp exposure. *J Dent.* 2019;86:41–52.

133 Bjørndal L, Demant S, Dabelsteen S. Depth and activity of carious lesions as indicators for the regenerative potential of dental pulp after intervention. *J Endod.* 2014;40(4, Suppl):S76–81.

134 El Karim IA, Lamey PJ, Ardill J, Linden GJ, Lundy FT. Vasoactive intestinal polypeptide (VIP) and VPAC1 receptor in adult human dental pulp in relation to caries. *Arch Oral Biol.* 2006;51(10):849–55.

135 El Karim IA, Linden GJ, Orr DF, Lundy FT. Antimicrobial activity of neuropeptides against a range of micro-organisms from skin, oral, respiratory and gastrointestinal tract sites. *J Neuroimmunol.* 2008;200(1–2):11–6.

136 Cooper PR, Chicca IJ, Holder MJ, Milward MR. Inflammation and regeneration in the dentin-pulp complex: net gain or net loss? *J Endod.* 2017;43(9s):S87–s94.

137 Gaudin A, Renard E, Hill M, Bouchet-Delbos L, Bienvenu-Louvet G, Farges JC, et al. Phenotypic analysis of immunocompetent cells in healthy human dental pulp. *J Endod.* 2015;41(5):621–7.

138 Cooper PR, Holder MJ, Smith AJ. Inflammation and regeneration in the dentin-pulp complex: a double-edged sword. *J Endod.* 2014;40(4):S46–51.

139 Hahn CL, Liewehr FR. Innate immune responses of the dental pulp to caries. *J Endod.* 2007;33(6):643–51.

140 Okiji T, Jontell M, Belichenko P, Bergenholtz G, Dahlström A. Perivascular dendritic cells of the human dental pulp. *Acta Physiol Scand.* 1997;159(2):163–9.

141 Onoé K, Yanagawa Y, Minami K, Iijima N, Iwabuchi K. Th1 or Th2 balance regulated by interaction between dendritic cells and NKT cells. *Immunol Res.* 2007;38(1–3):319–32.

142 Abbas AK. The control of T cell activation vs. tolerance. *Autoimmun Rev.* 2003;2(3):115–8.

143 Bedoya SK, Lam B, Lau K, Larkin J 3rd. Th17 cells in immunity and autoimmunity. *Clin Dev Immunol.* 2013;2013:986789.

144 Kawashima N, Wongyaofa I, Suzuki N, Kawanishi HN, Suda H. NK and NKT cells in the rat dental pulp tissues. *Oral Surg Oral Med Oral Pathol Oral Radiol Endod.* 2006;102(4):558–63.

145 Tanoue T, Umesaki Y, Honda K. Immune responses to gut microbiota-commensals and pathogens. *Gut Microbes.* 2010;1(4):224–33.

146 Banchereau J, Steinman RM. Dendritic cells and the control of immunity. *Nature.* 1998;392(6673):245–52.

147 Morelli AE, Thomson AW. Tolerogenic dendritic cells and the quest for transplant tolerance. *Nat Rev Immunol.* 2007;7(8):610–21.

148 Li H, Shi B. Tolerogenic dendritic cells and their applications in transplantation. *Cell Mol Immunol.* 2015;12(1):24–30.

149 Zhu J, Yamane H, Paul WE. Differentiation of effector CD4 T cell populations (*). *Annu Rev Immunol.* 2010;28:445–89.

150 Bruno KF, Silva JA, Silva TA, Batista AC, Alencar AHG, Estrela C. Characterization of inflammatory cell infiltrate in human dental pulpitis. *Int Endod J.* 2010;43(11):1013–21.

151 Chauveau C, Rémy S, Royer PJ, Hill M, Tanguy-Royer S, Hubert FX, et al. Heme oxygenase-1 expression inhibits dendritic cell maturation and proinflammatory function but conserves IL-10 expression. *Blood.* 2005;106(5):1694–702.

152 Gabrilovich DI, Nagaraj S. Myeloid-derived suppressor cells as regulators of the immune system. *Nat Rev Immunol.* 2009;9(3):162–74.

153 Dugast AS, Haudebourg T, Coulon F, Heslan M, Haspot F, Poirier N, et al. Myeloid-derived suppressor cells accumulate in kidney allograft tolerance and specifically suppress effector T cell expansion. *J Immunol.* 2008;180(12):7898–906.

154 Drujont L, Carretero-Iglesia L, Bouchet-Delbos L, Beriou G, Merieau E, Hill M, et al. Evaluation of the therapeutic potential of bone marrow-derived myeloid suppressor cell (MDSC) adoptive transfer in mouse models of autoimmunity and allograft rejection. *PLoS One.* 2014;9(6):e100013.

155 Holder MJ, Wright HJ, Couve E, Milward MR, Cooper PR. Neutrophil extracellular traps exert potential cytotoxic and proinflammatory effects in the dental pulp. *J Endod.* 2019;45(5): 513–20.e3.

156 Inoue T, Shimono M. Repair dentinogenesis following transplantation into normal and germ-free animals. *Proc Finn Dent Soc.* 1992;88(Suppl 1):183–94.

157 Nyborg H. Healing processes in the pulp on capping; a morphologic study; experiments on surgical lesions of the pulp in dog and man. *Acta Odontol Scand.* 1955;13(Suppl 16):1–130.

158 Cvek M. A clinical report on partial pulpotomy and capping with calcium hydroxide in permanent incisors with complicated crown fracture. *J Endod.* 1978;4(8):232–7.

159 Schröder U. Effects of calcium hydroxide-containing pulp-capping agents on pulp cell migration, proliferation, and differentiation. *J Dent Res.* 1985;64:541–8.

160 Dammaschke T, Leidinger J, Schäfer E. Long-term evaluation of direct pulp capping-treatment outcomes over an average period of 6.1 years. *Clin Oral Investig.* 2010;14(5):559–67.

161 European Society of Endodontology. European Society of Endodontology position statement: management of deep caries and the exposed pulp. *Int Endod J.* 2019;52(7):923–34.

162 Hilton TJ, Ferracane JL, Mancl L. Comparison of CaOH with MTA for direct pulp capping: a PBRN randomized clinical trial. *J Dent Res.* 2013;92(Suppl 7):S16.

163 Bogen G, Kim JS, Bakland LK. Direct pulp capping with mineral trioxide aggregate: an observational study. *J Am Dent Assoc.* 2008;139(3):305–15.

164 Natale LC, Rodrigues MC, Xavier TA, Simões A, de Souza DN, Braga RR. Ion release and mechanical properties of calcium silicate and calcium hydroxide materials used for pulp capping. *Int Endod J.* 2015;48(1):89–94.

165 Awawdeh L, Al-Qudah A, Hamouri H, Chakra RJ. Outcomes of vital pulp therapy using mineral trioxide aggregate or biodentine: a prospective randomized clinical trial. *J Endod.* 2018;44(11):1603–9.

166 Koh ET, McDonald F, Pitt Ford TR, Torabinejad M. Cellular response to mineral trioxide aggregate. *J Endod.* 1998;24(8):543–7.

167 Mitchell PJ, Pitt Ford TR, Torabinejad M, McDonald F. Osteoblast biocompatibility of mineral trioxide aggregate. *Biomaterials.* 1999;20(2):167–73.

168 El Karim IA, McCrudden MT, McGahon MK, Curtis TM, Jeanneau C, Giraud T, et al. Biodentine reduces tumor necrosis factor alpha-induced TRPA1 expression in odontoblastlike cells. *J Endod.* 2016;42(4):589–95.

169 El Karim I, McCrudden MT, Linden GJ, Abdullah H, Curtis TM, McGahon M, et al. TNF-α-induced p38MAPK activation regulates TRPA1 and TRPV4 activity in odontoblast-like cells. *Am J Pathol.* 2015;185(11):2994–3002.

170 Giraud T, Jeanneau C, Rombouts C, Bakhtiar H, Laurent P, About I. Pulp capping materials modulate the balance between inflammation and regeneration. *Dent Mater.* 2019;35(1):24–35.

171 Song W, Li S, Tang Q, Chen L, Yuan Z. In vitro biocompatibility and bioactivity of calcium silicate-based bioceramics in endodontics. *Int J Mol Med.* 2021;48(1):128.

172 Taha NA, Al-khatib H. 4-Year follow-up of full pulpotomy in symptomatic mature permanent teeth with carious pulp exposure using a stainproof calcium silicate–based material. *J Endod.* 2022;48(1):87–95.

173 Yamada M, Kojima N, Paranjpe A, Att W, Aita H, Jewett A, et al. N-acetyl cysteine (NAC)-assisted detoxification of PMMA resin. *J Dent Res.* 2008;87(4):372–7.

174 Choi YS, Kim C, Moon JH, Lee JY. Removal and killing of multispecies endodontic biofilms by N-acetylcysteine. *Braz J Microbiol.* 2018;49(1):184–8.

175 Lee YH, Lee NH, Bhattarai G, Kim GE, Lee IK, Yun BS, et al. Anti-inflammatory effect of pachymic acid promotes odontoblastic differentiation via HO-1 in dental pulp cells. *Oral Dis.* 2013;19(2):193–9.

176 Arora S, Cooper PR, Friedlander LT, Rizwan S, Seo B, Rich AM, et al. Potential application of immunotherapy for modulation of pulp inflammation: opportunities for vital pulp treatment. *Int Endod J.* 2021;54(8):1263–74.

177 Zheng J, Wu Z, Niu K, Xie Y, Hu X, Fu J, et al. Microbiome of deep dentinal caries from reversible pulpitis to irreversible pulpitis. *J Endod.* 2019;45(3):302–9. e1.

178 Närhi M, Bjørndal L, Pigg M, Fristad I, Haug SR. Acute dental pain I: pulpal and dentinal pain. *Nor Tannlegeforen Tid.* 2016;126:10–8.

179 Lundy FT, El Karim I, Scheven BA. Current and future views on pulpal pain and neurogenesis. In: Duncan HF, Cooper PR (eds.) Clinical Approaches in Endodontic Regeneration: Current and Emerging Therapeutic Perspectives, Springer International Publishing, Cham, 2019, 19–36.

180 Mejàre IA, Axelsson S, Davidson T, Frisk F, Hakeberg M, Kvist T, et al. Diagnosis of the condition of the dental pulp: a systematic review. *Int Endod J.* 2012;45(7):597–613.

181 Ricucci D, Loghin S, Siqueira JF. Correlation between clinical and histologic pulp diagnoses. *J Endod.* 2014;40(12):1932–9.

182 Levin LG. Pulp and periradicular testing. *J Endod.* 2013;39(3 Suppl):S13–9.

183 Seltzer S, Bender IB, Ziontz M. The dynamics of pulp inflammation: correlations between diagnostic data and actual histologic findings in the pulp. *Oral Surg Oral Med Oral Pathol.* 1963;16:846–71.

184 Dummer PM, Hicks R, Huws D. Clinical signs and symptoms in pulp disease. *Int Endod J.* 1980;13(1):27–35.

185 American Association of Endodontists. Endodontic Diagnosis 2013 [22 Mar 2023]. Available from: https://www.aae.org/specialty/wpcontent/. . ./sites/. . ./endodonticdiagnosisfall2013.pdf

186 Cushley S, Duncan HF, Lappin MJ, Chua P, Elamin AD, Clarke M, et al. Efficacy of direct pulp capping for management of cariously exposed pulps in permanent teeth: a systematic review and meta-analysis. *Int Endod J.* 2021;54(4):556–71.

187 Cushley S, Duncan HF, Lappin MJ, Tomson PL, Lundy FT, Cooper P, et al. Pulpotomy for mature carious teeth with symptoms of irreversible pulpitis: a systematic review. *J Dent.* 2019;88:103158.

188 Brizuela C, Meza G, Mercadé M, Inostroza C, Chaparro A, Bravo I, et al. Inflammatory biomarkers in dentinal fluid as an approach to molecular diagnostics in pulpitis. *Int Endod J.* 2020;53(9):1181–91.

189 Zehnder M, Wegehaupt FJ, Attin T. A first study on the usefulness of matrix metalloproteinase 9 from dentinal fluid to indicate pulp inflammation. *J Endod.* 2011;37(1):17–20.

190 Al-Natour B, Rankin R, McKenna R, McMillan H, Zhang SD, About I, et al. Identification and validation of novel biomarkers and therapeutics for pulpitis using connectivity mapping. *Int Endod J.* 2021;54(9):1571–80.

191 Zanini M, Meyer E, Simon S. Pulp inflammation diagnosis from clinical to inflammatory mediators: a systematic review. *J Endod.* 2017;43(7):1033–51.

192 Rechenberg DK, Galicia JC, Peters OA. Biological markers for pulpal inflammation: a systematic review. *PLoS One.* 2016;11(11):e0167289.

193 Hirsch V, Wolgin M, Mitronin AV, Kielbassa AM. Inflammatory cytokines in normal and irreversibly inflamed pulps: a systematic review. *Arch Oral Biol.* 2017;82:38–46.

194 Banchs F, Trope M. Revascularization of immature permanent teeth with apical periodontitis: new treatment protocol? *J Endod.* 2004;30(4):196–200.

195 Kim SG, Malek M, Sigurdsson A, Lin LM, Kahler B. Regenerative endodontics: a comprehensive review. *Int Endod J.* 2018;51(12):1367–88.

196 Alobaid AS, Cortes LM, Lo J, Nguyen TT, Albert J, Abu-Melha AS, et al. Radiographic and clinical outcomes of the treatment of immature permanent teeth by revascularization or apexification: a pilot retrospective cohort study. *J Endod.* 2014;40(8):1063–70.

197 Eramo S, Natali A, Pinna R, Milia E. Dental pulp regeneration via cell homing. *Int Endod J.* 2018;51(4):405–19.

198 Duncan HF, Kobayashi Y, Shimizu E. Growth factors and cell homing in dental tissue regeneration. *Curr Oral Health Rep.* 2018;5(4):276–85.

199 Murray PE. Platelet-rich plasma and platelet-rich fibrin can induce apical closure more frequently than blood-clot revascularisation for the regeneration of immature permanent teeth: a meta-analysis of clinical efficacy. *Front Bioeng Biotechnol.* 2018;6:139.

200 Albanese A, Licata ME, Polizzi B, Campisi G. Platelet-rich plasma (PRP) in dental and oral surgery: from the wound healing to bone regeneration. *Immun Ageing.* 2013;10(1):23.

201 Rodriguez IA, Growney Kalaf EA, Bowlin GL, Sell SA. Platelet-rich plasma in bone regeneration: engineering the delivery for improved clinical efficacy. *BioMed Res Int.* 2014;2014:392398.

202 Hotwani K, Sharma K. Platelet rich fibrin – a novel acumen into regenerative endodontic therapy. *Restor Dent Endod.* 2014;39(1):1–6.

203 Simonpieri A, Del Corso M, Vervelle A, Jimbo R, Inchingolo F, Sammartino G, et al. Current knowledge and perspectives for the use of platelet-rich plasma (PRP) and platelet-rich fibrin (PRF) in oral and maxillofacial surgery part 2: bone graft, implant and reconstructive surgery. *Curr Pharm Biotechnol.* 2012;13(7):1231–56.

204 Lolato A, Bucchi C, Taschieri S, Kabbaney AE, Fabbro MD. Platelet concentrates for revitalization of immature necrotic teeth: a systematic review of the clinical studies. *Platelets.* 2016;27(5):383–92.

205 Bottino MC, Pankajakshan D, Nör JE. Advanced scaffolds for dental pulp and periodontal regeneration. *Dent Clin North Am.* 2017;61(4):689–711.

206 O'Brien FJ. Biomaterials & scaffolds for tissue engineering. *Mater Today.* 2011;14(3):88–95.

207 Moussa DG, Aparicio C. Present and future of tissue engineering scaffolds for dentin-pulp complex regeneration. *J Tissue Eng Regen Med.* 2019;13(1):58–75.

208 Rozario T, DeSimone DW. The extracellular matrix in development and morphogenesis: a dynamic view. *Dev Biol.* 2010;341(1):126–40.

209 Yang JW, Zhang YF, Wan CY, Sun ZY, Nie S, Jian SJ, et al. Autophagy in SDF-1α-mediated DPSC migration and pulp regeneration. *Biomaterials.* 2015;44:11–23. https://doi.org/10.1016/j.biomaterials.2014.12.006.

210 Matsunaga T, Yanagiguchi K, Yamada S, Ohara N, Ikeda T, Hayashi Y. Chitosan monomer promotes tissue regeneration on dental pulp wounds. *J Biomed Mater Res A.* 2006;76(4):711–20.

211 Moreira MS, Sarra G, Carvalho GL, Gonçalves F, Caballero-Flores HV, Pedroni ACF, et al. Physical and biological properties of a chitosan hydrogel scaffold associated to photobiomodulation therapy for dental pulp regeneration: an in vitro and in vivo study. *BioMed Res Int.* 2021;2021:6684667.

212 Kuboyama N, Kiba H, Arai K, Uchida R, Tanimoto Y, Bhawal UK, et al. Silk fibroin-based scaffolds for bone regeneration. *J Biomed Mater Res B Appl Biomater.* 2013;101(2):295–302.

213 Meinel L, Hofmann S, Karageorgiou V, Kirker-Head C, McCool J, Gronowicz G, et al. The inflammatory responses to silk films in vitro and in vivo. *Biomaterials.* 2005;26(2):147–55.

214 Sharma S, Srivastava D, Grover S, Sharma V. Biomaterials in tooth tissue engineering: a review. *J Clin Diagn Res.* 2014;8(1):309–15.

215 Gathani KM, Raghavendra SS. Scaffolds in regenerative endodontics: a review. *Dent Res J (Isfahan).* 2016;13(5):379–86.

216 Chandrahasa S, Murray PE, Namerow KN. Proliferation of mature ex vivo human dental pulp using tissue engineering scaffolds. *J Endod.* 2011;37(9):1236–9.

217 Karageorgiou V, Kaplan D. Porosity of 3D biomaterial scaffolds and osteogenesis. *Biomaterials.* 2005;26(27):5474–91.

218 Conde CM, Demarco FF, Casagrande L, Alcazar JC, Nör JE, Tarquinio SB. Influence of poly-L-lactic acid scaffold's pore size on the proliferation and differentiation of dental pulp stem cells. *Braz Dent J.* 2015;26(2):93–8.

219 Singhal AR, Agrawal CM, Athanasiou KA. Salient degradation features of a 50:50 PLA/PGA scaffold for tissue engineering. *Tissue Eng.* 1996;2(3):197–207.

220 Zhao F, Yao D, Guo R, Deng L, Dong A, Zhang J. Composites of polymer hydrogels and nanoparticulate systems for biomedical and pharmaceutical applications. *Nanomaterials (Basel).* 2015;5(4):2054–130.

221 Cavalcanti BN, Zeitlin BD, Nör JE. A hydrogel scaffold that maintains viability and supports differentiation of dental pulp stem cells. *Dent Mater.* 2013;29(1):97–102.

222 Athirasala A, Lins F, Tahayeri A, Hinds M, Smith AJ, Sedgley C, et al. A novel strategy to engineer pre-vascularized full-length dental pulp-like tissue constructs. *Sci Rep.* 2017;7(1):3323.

223 Chung JJ, Im H, Kim SH, Park JW, Jung Y. Toward biomimetic scaffolds for tissue engineering: 3D printing techniques in regenerative medicine. *Front Bioeng Biotechnol.* 2020;8:586406.

224 Gao B, Yang Q, Zhao X, Jin G, Ma Y, Xu F. 4D bioprinting for biomedical applications. *Trends Biotechnol.* 2016;34(9):746–56.

225 Piva E, Silva AF, Nör JE. Functionalized scaffolds to control dental pulp stem cell fate. *J Endod.* 2014;40(4 Suppl):S33–40.

3

Pulpal Diagnosis

Johnah C. Galicia[1] *and Asma A. Khan*[2]

[1] *College of Dentistry, Manila Central University, EDSA-Monumento, Caloocan City, Philippines*
[2] *Department of Endodontics, School of Dentistry, UT Health San Antonio, San Antonio, TX, USA*

Introduction

Over the last few years, there has been a significant shift towards maintaining the dental pulp (1–4). From a research perspective, this push can be viewed as a triumph resulting from years of data gathering to understand the biology of the dental pulp.

To practice a conservative approach in the treatment of pulpitis, an accurate diagnostic method that is quick, non-invasive and quantifiable should be available for chairside use. This test should be able to stage pulpal inflammation accurately, ideally identifying the threshold between pulp tissue that can be saved and tissue that cannot. However, clinicians have had to rely on tests that have been shown over decades to correlate poorly with the histopathology of the pulp (5–9).

The current diagnostic techniques using thermal and electric pulp testers have good sensitivity and specificity in eliciting a positive response on teeth with vital tissues (10, 11). The lingering predicament with these tests is their inability to stage the severity of pulpal disease. In teeth with vital pulp tissue, eliciting a reliable and unambiguous response using these tests is often achieved without too much complexity. The problem lies in determining the extent of inflammation, which these tests cannot decipher. Another concern with the currently used clinical sensibility tests like thermal and electric pulp testing (EPT) is the purpose that these tests were designed for. Rather than measuring blood flow, which is the hallmark of tissue vitality, these tests stimulate nerves. An assumption is made that a positive response to these tests means that vital pulp tissue remains; however, it has been suggested that nerve tissue can remain even after necrosis of the pulp tissue and associated blood vessels (12). In this scenario, a positive response to EPT or cold is a misleading measure of pulp vitality. A more common misleading scenario is of teeth which have recently been traumatized and do not respond to cold or EPT, even though the pulp is vital and a blood supply remains.

Advocates of vital pulp treatment (VPT) and minimally invasive endodontics strongly support a change in diagnostic terminology to better reflect the extent of pulpitis (2). With currently available terminologies, the fate of the dental pulp is categorically dictated by the clinician's educated interpretation of the patient's subjective description of the sensation elicited by the tests. Traditionally, the dental pulp can either be kept intact or removed entirely based on the diagnostic

Vital Pulp Treatment, First Edition. Edited by Henry F. Duncan and Ikhlas A. El-Karim.

terminology emanating from the results of the tests (13). Future efforts should be shifted towards developing non-invasive, biologically-based pulpal diagnostic techniques that accurately measure the extent of pulpal inflammation and towards introducing diagnostic terminologies that favour conservative treatment of the dental pulp.

Diagnoses of Pulpal Status and Their Associated Diagnostic Terminologies

Medical diagnosis is the process of determining which disease or condition explains a person's symptoms and signs, but for pulpitis, this is not exactly the same. Although it is an inflammatory disease, generally caused by bacterial infection, the diagnosis of pulpitis has remained a conundrum for reasons including the anatomical location of the dental pulp and limitations of current diagnostic tools (14, 15). Over the years, different classifications and diagnostic systems have been advocated for pulpitis, reflecting the challenges and lack of consensus amongst experts (12). Although histology is the gold standard in diagnosis, attempts to classify pulp disease based on histology and symptoms failed due to the lack of correlation (7, 9) and because the pulp must be removed in order to examine it histologically. A more pragmatic approach based on signs and symptoms was introduced, and a different classification was proposed (12). The American Association of Endodontists (AAE) called for a consensus on classification and terminology used for pulp disease that resulted in the current widely used classification (13). This classification describes pulpitis as reversible, indicating that the inflammation should resolve following appropriate management, or irreversible, indicating that the inflamed pulp is considered incapable of healing and for which root canal treatment is indicated. These terms, however, do not take into consideration the current evidence showing that in carious teeth, pulpal inflammation and necrosis may be locally limited to the pulpal tissue adjacent to the carious lesion, while the rest of the pulp remains relatively normal (6). Furthermore, an improved understanding of pulp biology provides evidence of the regenerative capabilities of the pulp. We now know that pulpal inflammation is part of the healing response of the pulp to infectious or noxious stimuli. With the advent of hydraulic calcium silicate cement materials, VPT can be used to predictably save at least part of the pulp in teeth which were preoperatively diagnosed with "irreversible pulpitis" (16, 17).

For these reasons, calls have been made to revise the existing pulpitis terminology and a proposed classification in which the level of pulpitis was graded and described as mild, moderate and severe was introduced (2). This new classification proposed for the first time VPT as an option for treating different stages of pulpits and that root canal treatment can be reserved for cases with advanced pulpal inflammation in which pulpal haemorrhage cannot be controlled during the operative procedure. The classification, however, needs to be validated, and results from recent studies showed that preoperative symptoms could be used to predict the outcome that teeth with moderate pulpits can be successfully treated with partial pulpotomy compared with teeth with severe pulpitis (18) (Table 3.1).

The Diagnostic Process

Obtaining an accurate diagnosis is essential for the provision of appropriate treatment. The pulpal diagnostic process requires the gathering of information via detailed history taking, followed by thorough clinical examination and application of special investigations. The objective of pulpal

Table 3.1 Current classifications systems of pulpitis.

Wolters et al. 2017	Hashem et al. 2015	AAE 2013
Initial pulpitis Heightened but not lengthened response to the cold test, not sensitive to percussion and no spontaneous pain	*Mild reversible pulpitis* Patients' descriptions of sensitivity to hot, cold and sweet lasting ≤15–20 seconds and settling spontaneously	*Reversible pulpitis* Discomfort is experienced when a stimulus such as cold or sweet is applied and goes away within a couple of seconds following the removal of the stimulus
Mild pulpitis Heightened and lengthened reaction to cold, warm and sweet stimuli that can last ≤20 seconds but then subsides, possibly percussion sensitive	*Severe reversible pulpitis* Increased pain for more than several minutes and needing oral analgesics	*Symptomatic irreversible pulpitis* Characteristics may include sharp pain upon thermal stimulus, lingering pain (often ≥30 seconds stimulus removal), spontaneity (unprovoked pain) and referred pain. Sometimes, the pain may be accentuated by postural changes such as lying down or bending over, and over-the-counter analgesics are typically ineffective
Moderate pulpitis Clear symptoms, strong, heightened and prolonged reaction to cold, which can last for minutes, possibly percussion sensitive and spontaneous dull pain that can be more or less suppressed with pain medication	*Irreversible pulpitis* Persistent dull throbbing pain, sharp spontaneous pain and tenderness to percussion or pain exacerbated by lying down	
Severe pulpitis Severe spontaneous pain and clear pain reaction to warmth and cold stimuli, often, sharp to dull throbbing pain; patients have trouble sleeping because of the pain (gets worse when lying down). Tooth is very sensitive to touch and percussion		*Asymptomatic irreversible pulpitis* No clinical symptoms and usually respond normally to thermal testing but may have had trauma or deep caries that would likely result in exposure following removal

diagnosis is to determine the condition of the dental pulp, i.e. not just in an absolute sense (vital versus non-vital), but also the degree of pulp inflammation if present.

Pain History

Obtaining a detailed pain history is an important component of patient assessment and the overall diagnostic process. The mnemonic OPQRST is commonly used in the medical field and can easily be adapted to dental pain as well. In this mnemonic, O stands for onset of event, P stands for palliation/provocation, Q is quality, R is region/radiation, S is severity and T is time when the pain started. Patients who have inflamed pulps may present with a chief complaint of spontaneous pain or one that is only elicited by cold or hot stimuli. Although subjective, the nature, duration and onset of pain are important factors that can help determine whether pulpitis is reversible or irreversible. Severe pain (19), history of previous pain (20) and presence of spontaneous pain (6, 20) have been considered to be poor prognostic factors and often associated with severe inflammation suggestive of irreversible pulpitis. On the other hand, non-spontaneous pain in response to thermal changes often indicate reversible pulp inflammation.

Pain can be reported as a symptom in the patient history but can also be elicited as a sign during clinical examination. For example, tenderness to percussion and pain on thermal stimuli can be of diagnostic value. In cases where the patients have severe spontaneous pain, the resulting afferent barrage results in central sensitization (increased responsiveness of neurons of the central nervous system) and referred pain, making diagnosis challenging. This was elegantly demonstrated in a clinical study in which patients presenting for endodontic treatment were asked to localize the symptomatic tooth (21). Patients who did not have percussion sensibility (i.e. those who only had pulpal pain) were less likely to accurately localize the right tooth as compared to those who had percussion sensitivity (30% versus 89.1%). Notably, in patients who did not have percussion sensitivity, the pain intensity was inversely correlated with the patients' ability to accurately localize the right tooth (21).

Relying on only pain symptoms for diagnosis can be misleading. It should be emphasized that pain is subjective, and pulpitis can be painless in approximately 40% of cases (22), while it was also shown that 40% of cases with salvageable pulps were associated with pain (19). In addition, most patients who presented with a toothache usually have odontogenic pain (and not pain referred to the teeth from a non-odontogenic source). However, astute clinicians understand that non-odontogenic pain can also be perceived by the patient as a toothache. These sources of non-odontogenic pain include the muscles of mastication, temporomandibular joint, maxillary sinus and cardiac tissues (23–25).

Pulp Sensitivity/Sensibility Testing

The patient's response to pulp sensibility tests plays a critical role in determining the diagnosis and subsequent treatment. However, the lack of standardized methods for performing these tests results in unpredictable results and misinterpretation. Commonly performed sensibility tests are done with thermal (cold and heat) or electrical stimuli. Cold testing is often done using refrigerant spray (1,1,1,2-tetrafluoroethane), and there are many variations in how the test is performed (for example, the size of the cotton pellet, how long the pellet is applied for, the location where the cotton pellet is placed, etc.). This noxious cold stimulus is not physiological and elicits a painful response, which is subjectively reported by the patient. The interpretation of the patients' response by the clinician is neither quantitative nor is objective. There continues to be a lack of a uniform consensus on what constitutes an exacerbated and/or lingering response as compared with a so-called 'normal' response. Heat is used less commonly to determine pulpal status, being only used when the chief complaint is that hot foods elicit pain or as a test of last resort. This test is commonly done after isolation with a dental dam and by rinsing the tooth with hot water or using a rubber wheel to generate heat. Unfortunately, there is a lack of consensus regarding the ideal temperature or duration of the stimulus. Electrical pulp testing (EPT) is another common diagnostic test that is recommended for routine use in combination with thermal tests (26). This non-physiological stimulus is essentially used to determine the responsiveness of the nerves innervating the pulp. It cannot be used to detect the presence or extent of inflammation.

Diagnostic Accuracy of Sensibility Tests

The ability of sensitivity tests to accurately determine the vitality of the dental pulp and, to some degree, the pulpal condition has been summarized in a recent systematic review (14). The accuracy of these tests was determined by measuring their sensitivity, specificity and diagnostic odd ratio (DOR) using histology or direct inspection of the pulp as a reference standard. Among the thermal tests, cold had the highest accuracy, 0.85–0.95 (27). The accuracy of the EPT was reported to be in the range of 0.75–0.90 (10, 27), and for the heat test, the accuracy was 0.86 (28). The result of the review concurs with that of Mainkar and Kim 2018 (11), in which, adjusted accuracy of 0.84, 0.82 and 0.72, was reported for cold, EPT and heat test respectively. Using a combination of tests has, however, been shown to improve diagnostic accuracy, with a high DOR reported for combined use of cold and EPT (14), suggesting that both should be used in combination in clinical practice, particularly if there is doubt on the performance of individual tests.

Other Diagnostic Tests

In addition to thermal and electric tests, assessing pulp vitality with pulse oximetry has also been suggested. Pulse oximetry has a reported accuracy of 97% (11, 14) in assessing pulp vitality and is considered a reliable tool; however, to date, there is no pulse oximeter device licensed for dental use to suggest its routine use in practice. The studies using pulse oximetry have modified a medical device which cannot be employed in dental clinics. Another test, the laser doppler flowmeter, offers the advantage of measuring blood flow in the dental pulp as a definitive marker of vitality with an equally high reported accuracy of 97% (11); however, laser doppler is technique sensitive and does not work well if the tooth is heavily restored. While these diagnostics were developed decades ago, they are not used in clinical practice. One reason could potentially be that there has been no significant progress in developing new diagnostic terms that offer a more accurate description of pulpal status and the expected results of the sensibility testing.

Radiographic Examination

Although radiographs have limited diagnostic value in pulpitis, they provide vital information that assists in the overall diagnostic and treatment planning process. Radiographic assessment of caries depth as well as clinical indicators of its activity (e.g. symptoms, progression rate and colour), should be used to assist clinical decision-making for VPT. Intraoral periapical radiographs are valuable tool for the assessment of periapical tissues, pulpal and radicular calcification, root resorption and bone levels. Cone-beam computed tomography has been reported to be helpful in order to identifying pulpitis with more advanced symptomatic pulpitis more likely to show apical rarefaction (29); however, the value of this has been questioned as even vital teeth with radiographically visible radiolucencies can heal after VPT (30).

The methods described above can be used to determine with some accuracy if the pulp is vital or necrotic (14) but have limited ability in their capacity to accurately describe the degree of pulpal inflammation and healing potential of the pulp. Therefore, a need exists for the development of new pulp tests based on pulpal disease markers to inform decision-making for VPT (31). In the absence of clinically available molecular tests of inflammation, the colour and intensity of pulp bleeding on exposure may provide a crude measure or surrogate marker of inflammation (32) and capacity to recover after treatment (3, 33), although at present evidence to support arrest of pulpal bleeding affecting treatment outcome in limited (18).

Preoperative Diagnosis versus Direct Observation

The recent position statement by the AAE recommends a methodical approach to assessing the pulpal condition directly through visual examination after exposure rather than relying on a preoperative diagnosis to determine the fate of the dental pulp (3). This recommendation is well aligned with recent calls to review the current endodontic diagnostic nomenclature and terminology and with a renewed impetus towards maintaining pulp vitality (1, 2, 34, 35). That said, visualization of the pulp may only give limited information that could be of prognostic benefit.

The goal of direct observation is to remove the inflamed or necrotic part of the dental pulp under aseptic conditions. This is followed by an immediate placement of a well-sealing permanent restoration. With this in mind and in lieu of a treatment plan that is a result of a preoperative diagnosis, the dental pulp is managed conservatively. The subjectivity of the preoperative pulpal diagnostic testing results divides pulpitis into 'reversible' and 'irreversible' and, consequently, its treatment into the removal of the aetiology alone or pulpectomy. However, there is mounting evidence that even with a preoperative diagnosis of irreversible pulpitis, direct visualization of the pulp and performing pulpotomy under optimal conditions can result in favourable outcomes (36).

Clinical to Molecular Diagnostic Tests: Possibilities and Challenges

The dental pulp is an immunocompetent tissue with cytokines, cell surface receptors and other protein markers, which are differentially expressed in inflamed pulps compared with normal pulps (37–43). Gene and protein expression studies support the dynamic immunocompetence of the dental pulp (44–46). A microarray study showed an association between over- or under-expressed genes and pulpal status when the patient was being treated for pulpitis at chairside (44).

Besides being immunocompetent, the dental pulp is not in an isolated environment but rather a reactive tissue that communicates with its surrounding environment. The neural and vascular supply of the endodontium and periodontium are functionally and anatomically connected (47, 48). Therefore, a local neurogenic spread of the inflammatory response can occur from the pulp to the surrounding periodontal tissues (49). Furthermore, there is an overlap in the identified bacterial species in the progression from gingivitis to periodontitis as well as pulpitis to apical periodontitis (20). These findings provide a snapshot of the potential use of inflammatory markers to differentiate normal from inflamed pulp and to quantify the level of inflammation with appropriate controls and techniques.

Among the substrates that are being explored for diagnostic purposes are the gingival crevicular fluid (GCF) and the dentinal fluid (DF). GCF can be extracted non-invasively, while access through the dentine will be required to collect DF. Further to being invasive, the collection of DF is challenging due to the small volume of analyte available. The biological differences in the GCF and DF between healthy and inflamed, symptomatic dental pulp have been assessed extensively in a systematic review by Rechenberg and co-authors (50). The GCF presented increased levels of various biomarkers during tooth pain (49, 51, 52). A marked decrease in the levels of these biomarkers was noted after endodontic treatment compared with pre-treatment levels.

The exploratory use of biomarkers such as matrix metalloproteases, substance P, Interleukin-8, neurokinin-A and others as tools to diagnose not only the vitality of the dental pulp but also to stage the severity of the inflammation has been carried out but is limited in scope (53–57). There has been a distinct lack of commercial drive to explore the possibility of using protein-rich oral fluids as biologically-based diagnostic tools. This is not surprising because of the challenges posed by clinical research, primarily in acquiring participants, the cost and time required to undertake these studies as well as participant drop-outs (58). These challenges are magnified in endodontic clinical studies, especially in biomarker research using oral fluids because of contamination from periodontal fluids and blood, challenges in identifying and collecting pulp tissue from appropriate control teeth, and the limited volume of vital tissue that can be collected from inflamed dental pulps. A recent systematic review highlighted further issues with biomarkers for pulpal diagnosis that further delay progress in the field (59). The review aimed to calculate sensitivity, specificity and DOR of previously investigated pulpitis biomarkers and to determine if biomarker levels discriminate between clinical diagnoses of pulpitis based on presence or absence of spontaneous pain. As shown in Table 3.2, IL-8 and IL-6 can discriminate with high accuracy between healthy pulps and that with irreversible pulpitis. None, however, of the biomolecule's studies can differentiate between reversible and irreversible pulpitis, where the distinction is needed most.

The decision to treat the dental pulp depends heavily on the results of sensibility testing, which, as discussed before, may correlate poorly with the actual histopathology of the dental pulp under examination. In addition, these clinical testing methods are non-standardized and not objective. As a

Table 3.2 Summary findings and evidence certainty for all outcomes using GRADE (59).

Outcomes	Impact	№ of participants (studies)	Certainty of the evidence (GRADE)
Diagnostic accuracy: healthy versus pulpitis with spontaneous pain	The inflammatory cytokines IL-6 and IL-8 have high sensitivity, specificity and DOR to discriminate between healthy and pulpits with spontaneous pain suggestive of IRP, while the diagnostic accuracy of TNFα and IL-1β is low	IL-6: 4 studies; 69 healthy; 108 IRP IL-8: 4 studies; 77 healthy; 91 IRP 5 studies; 100 healthy; 134 IRP IL-1β: 3 studies; 44 healthy; 50 IRP	IL-6 ⊕⊕◯◯ (b,c,d) Low IL-8 ⊕⊕◯◯ (b,c,d) Low TNF α⊕◯◯◯ (c,d) Very low IL-1β⊕⊕◯◯ (b,c,d) Low
Diagnostic accuracy: pulpitis with spontaneous versus non-spontaneous pain	None of the biomarkers showed high sensitivity, specificity or DOR to discriminate between pulpitis and spontaneous versus non-spontaneous pain. IL-6 showed moderate DOR with very wide Confidence Interval (CI) and no significant difference in standardized mean between spontaneous versus non-spontaneous pain	IL-6: 2 studies; 77 RP 72 IRP IL-8: 2 studies; 77 RP 72 IRP IL-1β: 2 studies; 37 RP 33 IRP TNFα: 2 studies; 77 RP 72 IRP	⊕◯◯◯(c,d) Very low ⊕◯◯◯(c,d) Very low ⊕◯◯◯(c,d) Very low ⊕◯◯◯(c,d) Very low
Evaluate if the level of biomarkers correlates with and can predict VPT outcomes	Limited data suggests high levels of active-matrix metalloproteinase 9 (MMP-9) correlate with poorer outcomes of full coronal pulpotomy	MMP-9: 1 study; 40 IRP, 10 healthy	⊕◯◯◯(c,d) Very low

(Continued)

Table 3.2 (Continued)

Outcomes	Impact	№ of participants (studies)	Certainty of the evidence (GRADE)

GRADE Working Group grades of evidence:

High certainty: We are very confident that the true effect lies close to that of the estimate of the effect.

Moderate certainty: We are moderately confident in the effect estimate. The true effect is likely to be close to the estimate of the effect, but there is a possibility that it is substantially different.

Low certainty: Our confidence in the effect estimate is limited. The true effect may be substantially different from the estimate of the effect.

Very low certainty: We have very little confidence in the effect estimate. The true effect is likely to be substantially different from the estimate of the effect

Downgraded due to high risk of bias on randomization and selection of reported results.

Observational studies upgraded due to effect size.

Downgraded due to lack of precision (small sample size)

Observational studies graded as low

With permission from Karrar et al. (59)/John Wiley & Sons.

consequence, endodontic diagnosis in many clinical situations can be challenging, and the resulting treatment becomes a defensive reaction to simply extirpate the dental pulp. This dilemma is exacerbated when clinical diagnosis becomes difficult in real-case scenarios where the patient cannot identify the offending tooth in the arch, and the potential offending tooth has a full coverage restoration (which makes pulp sensibility testing difficult) or a history of recent trauma, among others.

Measuring biomarker expression rather than relying on subjective responses to sensibility testing may lead to a biologically based diagnostic tool that can stage pulpal inflammation, which typically progresses from the coronal to the apical pulp (Figure 3.1). However, In the

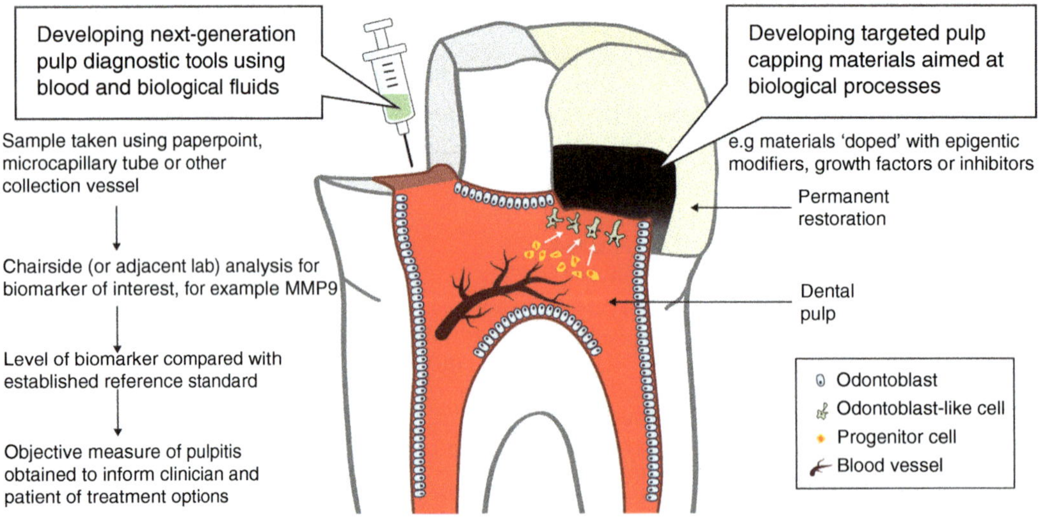

Figure 3.1 Illustration of potential next-generation pulp diagnostic tests and customized therapeutics. Reproduced with permission from Duncan (31).

absence of a clinical biomarker test to stage pulpitis into initial, mild, moderate and severe inflammation (2, 33), direct observation of the dental pulp using magnification is recommended (3). The European Society of Endodontology's position statement on the management of deep caries and exposed pulp (33) recommends a detailed pain history and meticulous clinical examination supplemented with a high-quality periapical radiograph and pulp sensibility testing using low-temperature cold testing in combination with EPT are necessary to assess the status of the pulp. The routine use of Cone Beam Computed Tomography (CBCT) is not justified for assessing pulpitis. Vital pulps should be considered reversibly inflamed when the tooth is symptomless or has sharp pain of short duration (<30 seconds), while irreversible pulpitis (partial or complete) is characterized by episodes of spontaneous, radiating pain that lingers after removal of the stimulus.

Conclusion

Although fundamental for the provision of appropriate treatment, arriving at an accurate diagnosis of pulp disease is still challenging and problematic in everyday clinical practice. Relying on subjective patients' symptoms and diagnostic tools that are not fit for purpose are the major issues that need to be addressed in future research in methods for pulpal diagnosis. Advances in pulp biology and molecular diagnostics should be utilized for the development of novel chairside tests that can accurately determine the degree of pulp inflammation and the healing potential of the tissue that need to be maintained.

References

1 Philip N, Suneja B. Minimally invasive endodontics: a new era for pulpotomy in mature permanent teeth. *Br Dent J.* 2022;233(12):1035–41.

2 Wolters WJ, Duncan HF, Tomson PL, Karim IE, McKenna G, Dorri M, et al. Minimally invasive endodontics: a new diagnostic system for assessing pulpitis and subsequent treatment needs. *Int Endod J.* 2017;50(9):825–9.

3 AAE position statement on vital pulp therapy. *J Endod.* 2021;47(9):1340–4.

4 Taha NA, About I, Sedgley CM, Messer HH. Conservative management of mature permanent teeth with carious pulp exposure. *J Endod.* 2020;46(9S):S33–41.

5 Hasler JE, Mitchell DF. Painless pulpitis. *J Am Dent Assoc* This controlled study evaluated the relationship between objective clinical findings and histopathologic findings in asymptomatic human teeth with suspected painless pulpitis. 1970;81(3):671–7.

6 Ricucci D, Loghin S, Siqueira JF Jr. Correlation between clinical and histologic pulp diagnoses. *J Endod.* 2014;40(12):1932–9.

7 Seltzer S, Bender IB, Ziontz M. The dynamics of pulp inflammation: correlations between diagnostic data and actual histologic findings in the pulp. *Oral Surg Oral Med Oral Pathol* "This study was designed to determine the diagnostic usefulness of common endodontic tests through retrospective evaluation of studies in which histologic examinations were performed." 1963;16(7):846–71.

8 Hyman JJ, Cohen ME. The predictive value of endodontic diagnostic tests. *Oral Surg Oral Med Oral Pathol.* 1984;58(3):343–6.

9 Johnson RH, Dachi SF, Haley JV. Pulpal hyperemia—a correlation of clinical and histologic data from 706 teeth. *J Am Dent Assoc.* 1970;81(1):108–17.

10 Jespersen JJ, Hellstein J, Williamson A, Johnson WT, Qian F. Evaluation of dental pulp sensibility tests in a clinical setting. *J Endod.* 2014;40(3):351–4.

11 Mainkar A, Kim SG. Diagnostic accuracy of 5 dental pulp tests: a systematic review and meta-analysis. *J Endod.* 2018;44(5):694–702.

12 Abbott PV, Yu C. A clinical classification of the status of the pulp and the root canal system. *Aust Dent J.* 2007;52(1 Suppl):S17–31.

13 Glickman GN. AAE consensus conference on diagnostic terminology: background and perspectives. *J Endod.* 2009;35(12):1619–20.

14 Donnermeyer D, Dammaschke T, Lipski M, Schafer E. Effectiveness of diagnosing pulpitis: a systematic review. *Int Endod J.* 2022;56:296–325.

15 Mejare IA, Axelsson S, Davidson T, Frisk F, Hakeberg M, Kvist T, et al. Diagnosis of the condition of the dental pulp: a systematic review. *Int Endod J.* 2012;45(7):597–613.

16 Asgary S, Eghbal MJ, Fazlyab M, Baghban AA, Ghoddusi J. Five-year results of vital pulp therapy in permanent molars with irreversible pulpitis: a non-inferiority multicenter randomized clinical trial. *Clin Oral Investig.* 2015;19(2):335–41.

17 Shallal-Ayzin M, Trinh T, Yeung W, Tawil PZ, Haggerty CL, Wu D, et al. A prospective analysis of the correlation between postoperative pain and vital pulp therapy. *Front Dent Med.* 2021;2:647417.

18 Careddu R, Duncan HF. A prospective clinical study investigating the effectiveness of partial pulpotomy after relating preoperative symptoms to a new and established classification of pulpitis. *Int Endod J.* 2021;54(12):2156–72.

19 Dummer PM, Hicks R, Huws D. Clinical signs and symptoms in pulp disease. *Int Endod J.* 1980;13(1):27–35.

20 Cisneros-Cabello R, Segura-Egea JJ. Relationship of patient complaints and signs to histopathologic diagnosis of pulpal condition. *Aust Endod J.* 2005;31(1):24–7.

21 McCarthy PJ, McClanahan S, Hodges J, Bowles WR. Frequency of localization of the painful tooth by patients presenting for an endodontic emergency. *J Endod.* 2010;36(5):801–5.

22 Michaelson PL, Holland GR. Is pulpitis painful? *Int Endod J.* 2002;35(10):829–32.

23 Danesh-Sani SH, Danesh-Sani SA, Zia R, Faghihi S. Incidence of craniofacial pain of cardiac origin: results from a prospective multicentre study. *Aust Dent J.* 2012;57(3):355–8.

24 Kreiner M, Okeson JP. Toothache of cardiac origin. *J Orofac Pain.* 1999;13(3):201–7.

25 Wright EF. Referred craniofacial pain patterns in patients with temporomandibular disorder. *J Am Dent Assoc.* 2000;131(9):1307–15.

26 European Society of Endodontology (ESE). Quality guidelines for endodontic treatment: consensus report of the European Society of Endodontology. *Int Endod J.* 2006;39(12):921–30.

27 Kamburoğlu K, Paksoy CA. The usefulness of standard endodontic diagnostic tests in establishing pulpal status. *Pain Clin.* 2005;17(2):157–65.

28 Farid H, Khan FR, Pasha L, Shinwari MS. Are pulp sensibility tests still sensible? *J Ayub Med Coll Abbottabad.* 2015;27(4):874–7.

29 Abella F, Patel S, Duran-Sindreu F, Mercade M, Bueno R, Roig M. Evaluating the periapical status of teeth with irreversible pulpitis by using cone-beam computed tomography scanning and periapical radiographs. *J Endod.* 2012;38(12):1588–91.

30 Taha NA, Khazali MA. Partial pulpotomy in mature permanent teeth with clinical signs indicative of irreversible pulpitis: a randomized clinical trial. *J Endod.* 2017;43(9):1417–21.

31 Duncan HF. Present status and future directions—vital pulp treatment and pulp preservation strategies. *Int Endod J.* 2022;55(Suppl 3):497–511.

32 Matsuo T, Nakanishi T, Shimizu H, Ebisu S. A clinical study of direct pulp capping applied to carious-exposed pulps. *J Endod.* 1996;22(10):551–6.

33 European Society of Endodontology developed b, Duncan HF, Galler KM, Tomson PL, Simon S, El-Karim I, et al. European Society of Endodontology position statement: management of deep caries and the exposed pulp. *Int Endod J.* 2019;52(7):923–34.

34 Galicia JC, Peters OA. Proposal for a new diagnostic terminology to describe the status of the dental pulp. *Int Endod J.* 2021;54(8):1415–6.

35 Rechenberg DK, Zehnder M. Call for a review of diagnostic nomenclature and terminology used in Endodontics. *Int Endod J.* 2020;53(10):1315–7.

36 Lin LM, Ricucci D, Saoud TM, Sigurdsson A, Kahler B. Vital pulp therapy of mature permanent teeth with irreversible pulpitis from the perspective of pulp biology. *Aust Endod J.* 2020; 46(1):154–66.

37 Caviedes-Bucheli J, Camargo-Beltran C, Gomez-la-Rotta AM, Moreno SC, Abello GC, Gonzalez-Escobar JM. Expression of calcitonin gene-related peptide (CGRP) in irreversible acute pulpitis. *J Endod.* 2004;30(4):201–4.

38 Caviedes-Bucheli J, Gutierrez-Guerra JE, Salazar F, Pichardo D, Moreno GC, Munoz HR. Substance P receptor expression in healthy and inflamed human pulp tissue. *Int Endod J.* 2007;40(2):106–11.

39 Caviedes-Bucheli J, Lombana N, Azuero-Holguin MM, Munoz HR. Quantification of neuropeptides (calcitonin gene-related peptide, substance P, neurokinin A, neuropeptide Y and vasoactive intestinal polypeptide) expressed in healthy and inflamed human dental pulp. *Int Endod J.* 2006;39(5):394–400.

40 Huang GT, Lee HW, Lee HS, Lee GH, Huh SY, Choi GW, et al. Localization of substance P-induced upregulated interleukin-8 expression in human dental pulp explants. *Int Endod J.* 2008;41(2):100–7.

41 Huang GT, Potente AP, Kim JW, Chugal N, Zhang X. Increased interleukin-8 expression in inflamed human dental pulps. *Oral Surg Oral Med Oral Pathol Oral Radiol Endod.* 1999;88(2):214–20.

42 Jiang HW, Zhang W, Ren BP, Zeng JF, Ling JQ. Expression of toll like receptor 4 in normal human odontoblasts and dental pulp tissue. *J Endod.* 2006;32(8):747–51.

43 Wu Q, Li S, Li R, Chen X, Guo L, Zheng Y. The detection of pro-inflammatory cytokines in exudates from dental pulp tissues. *Cytokine.* 2022;153:155846.

44 Galicia JC, Henson BR, Parker JS, Khan AA. Gene expression profile of pulpitis. *Genes Immun.* 2016;17(4):239–43.

45 Paakkonen V, Tjaderhane L. High-throughput gene and protein expression analysis in pulp biologic research: review. *J Endod.* 2010;36(2):179–89.

46 Tete S, Mastrangelo F, Scioletti AP, Tranasi M, Raicu F, Paolantonio M, et al. Microarray expression profiling of human dental pulp from single subject. *Clin Invest Med.* 2008;31(2):E55–61.

47 Capra NF, Anderson KV, Pride JB, Jones TE. Simultaneous demonstration of neuronal somata that innervate the tooth pulp and adjacent periodontal tissues, using two retrogradely transported anatomic markers. *Exp Neurol.* 1984;86(1):165–70.

48 Vertucci FJ, Williams RG. Furcation canals in the human mandibular first molar. *Oral Surg Oral Med Oral Pathol.* 1974;38(2):308–14.

49 Avellan NL, Sorsa T, Tervahartiala T, Forster C, Kemppainen P. Experimental tooth pain elevates substance P and matrix metalloproteinase-8 levels in human gingival crevice fluid. *Acta Odontol Scand.* 2008;66(1):18–22.

50 Rechenberg DK, Galicia JC, Peters OA. Biological markers for pulpal inflammation: a systematic review. *PLoS One.* 2016;11(11):e0167289.

51 Karapanou V, Kempuraj D, Theoharides TC. Interleukin-8 is increased in gingival crevicular fluid from patients with acute pulpitis. *J Endod.* 2008;34(2):148–51.

52 Shin SJ, Lee W, Lee JI, Baek SH, Kum KY, Shon WJ, et al. Matrix metalloproteinase-8 and substance P levels in gingival crevicular fluid during endodontic treatment of painful, nonvital teeth. *Oral Surg Oral Med Oral Pathol Oral Radiol Endod.* 2011;112(4):548–54.

53 Akbal Dincer G, Erdemir A, Kisa U. Comparison of neurokinin A, substance P, interleukin 8, and matrix metalloproteinase-8 changes in pulp tissue and gingival crevicular fluid samples of healthy and symptomatic irreversible pulpitis teeth. *J Endod.* 2020;46(10):1428–37.

54 Golbasi F, Erdemir A, Kisa U. Comparison of ADAMTS levels in pulp tissue samples of healthy and symptomatic irreversible pulpitis teeth. *J Endod.* 2022;48(4):496–501.

55 Zhang F, Liu E, Radaic A, Yu X, Yang S, Yu C, et al. Diagnostic potential and future directions of matrix metalloproteinases as biomarkers in gingival crevicular fluid of oral and systemic diseases. *Int J Biol Macromol.* 2021;188:180–96.

56 Awawdeh L, Lundy FT, Shaw C, Lamey PJ, Linden GJ, Kennedy JG. Quantitative analysis of substance P, neurokinin A and calcitonin gene-related peptide in pulp tissue from painful and healthy human teeth. *Int Endod J.* 2002;35(1):30–6.

57 Mente J, Petrovic J, Gehrig H, Rampf S, Michel A, Schurz A, et al. A prospective clinical pilot study on the level of matrix metalloproteinase-9 in dental pulpal blood as a marker for the state of inflammation in the pulp tissue. *J Endod.* 2016;42(2):190–7.

58 Ellis E, Riegel B, Hamon M, Carlson B, Jimenez S, Parkington S. The challenges of conducting clinical research: one research team's experiences. *Clin Nurse Spec.* 2001;15(6):286–92. quiz 93-4.

59 Karrar RN, Cushley S, Duncan HF, Lundy FT, Abushouk SA, Clarke M, et al. Molecular biomarkers for objective assessment of symptomatic pulpitis: a systematic review and meta-analysis. *Int Endod J.* 2023;56:1160–77. https://doi.org/10.1111/iej.13950.

4

Vital Pulp Treatment Modalities

The Management of Deep Caries Using Selective and Non-Selective Removal of Carious Tissue, Stepwise Excavation and Indirect Pulp Capping

Helena Fransson[1] *and Lars Bjørndal*[2]

[1] *Department of Endodontics, Faculty of Odontology, Malmö University, Malmö, Sweden*
[2] *Cariology and Endodontics, Section of Clinical Oral Microbiology, Department of Odontology, Faculty of Health and Medical Sciences, University of Copenhagen, Copenhagen, Denmark*

Introduction

When you first become a dentist and perhaps later pursue a career within a specialty, you are or should be in your comfort zone. You are supposed to make qualified judgements and decisions and carry out the treatments that are expected and evidence-based. You are an expert in the field. However, acquired expertise is not permanent as the considered best choice of treatment for a given health state may change over time, perhaps due to the impact of new research or a change in the demographics of the population. Within endodontics, the tradition has been to address two main domains: the exposed vital pulp or the infected, necrotic root canal system associated with apical periodontitis. In short, the prevention or treatment of apical periodontitis has been the focus of endodontics. The question arises as to how far back in the disease development we would like to go to prevent apical periodontitis. Does it include excavation of carious tissue in order to prevent pulp exposure?

Often, pulp inflammation has been described without the associated cause (1). In this chapter, we will focus on caries being the cause of inflammation, as it is one of the main indications for endodontic treatment (2, 3). An insight into the dynamics of the pulp inflammation due to progressing stages of caries is presented. Instead of simply presenting a case with a deep carious lesion being the cause of further treatment, it seems relevant to describe the carious lesion in more detail. Is it possible to introduce a threshold for deciding on the need for an invasive pulp treatment, or would the prognosis of the tooth be improved if pulp exposure was avoided?

It is perhaps the norm that dentists limiting their practice to endodontics only receive referrals on root canal treatments that often have already been initiated; perhaps an emergency treatment has been performed or attempts to negotiate the root canals have been made. It is tempting to suggest that these dentists rarely perform primary carious-tissue removal close to the pulp, even though such a dentist should have extensive theoretical knowledge about the pulp and its healing capacity. However, there is a trend within the endodontic field that dentists and endodontists should also have knowledge on the treatment when pulp exposure should be avoided. This is important not only for pre- and postgraduate students but also for the trained endodontist in educating and training general dentists.

The development and updating of clinical guidelines are examples of ways to help dentists to keep up with any changes regarding established treatments and to inform about potential new

Vital Pulp Treatment, First Edition. Edited by Henry F. Duncan and Ikhlas A. El-Karim.

treatment concepts. In this chapter, recently updated publications on evidence and guidelines on the treatment of deep carious lesions will be included. From the perspective of a general dental practitioner, this should form part of being an engaged and motivated dentist. It is, however, a difficult task to implement new knowledge and change the behaviours or traditions related to treatment. At the beginning of this chapter, we will present the treatment modalities as well as the indications based on a pragmatic subdivision of an extensive carious lesion into three classes.

Vital Pulp Treatment Modalities Aiming Not to Expose the Pulp

Based on understanding the biological concepts behind treatment recommendations, the goal is to provide the reader with tools to adopt a minimally invasive approach, such as the vital pulp treatments in teeth with well-defined deep carious lesions, as outlined in Table 4.1.

Indications – A Pragmatic Subdivision of Extensive Carious Lesions

For the management of extensive carious lesions, the clinical dilemma is obvious, as the presence of infected dentine is not an objective clinical measure. Concomitantly, it is not possible to monitor the degree of pulpal inflammation at the chairside based on the patient's symptoms or other clinical findings (5). So what is meant by a 'deep carious lesion'. The traditional wording of 'complete' and 'partial' removal of carious tissue is not precise and has unclear elements, and you may speculate on what is actually meant when the words are used. Is it the partial removal of microorganisms or demineralized dentine?

Table 4.1 Definitions of the vital pulp treatment modalities presented in this chapter were modified after a position paper from the European Society of Endodontology (4).

Treatment	Definition
Non-selective caries removal	Complete removal of soft and firm carious dentine from the periphery and central aspects of the cavity until hard dentine is reached
Selective caries removal	A collective name for several treatments: selective caries removal in one-stage and stepwise excavation
Selective caries removal in one-stage	Application of a biomaterial onto a dentine barrier in an indirect one-stage selective carious-tissue removal technique. Removal of soft or firm dentine. Immediate placement of a permanent restoration
Stepwise excavation	Application of a biomaterial in an indirect two-stage selective carious-tissue removal technique. Temporary restoration placement between visits and re-entry after 6–12 mo. The first stage involves selective carious removal to soft dentine to the extent that it facilitates proper placement of a temporary restoration, and the second stage involves removal to firm dentine – the final placement of a permanent restoration
Indirect pulp capping	Application of a biomaterial onto a thin dentine barrier in a one-stage carious-tissue removal technique generally to hard dentine. Leaves neither soft nor firm carious dentine behind. Considered more aggressive than selective carious-tissue removal in one-stage and stepwise excavation. However, if the excavation is successful, pulp exposure is avoided. The problem is that the frequency of unintended exposures will be more frequent than for selective caries removal in one-stage or stepwise excavation

Source: Adapted from the European Society of Endodontology.

The International Caries Consensus Collaboration have carried out a comprehensive qualitative analysis of the nomenclature for excavation and treatment options, attempting to simplify the topic and making it more suitable for dental practice (6, 7). This practice-based terminology on carious-tissue removal is based on the features of the carious tissue and presented in Figure 4.1 (8).

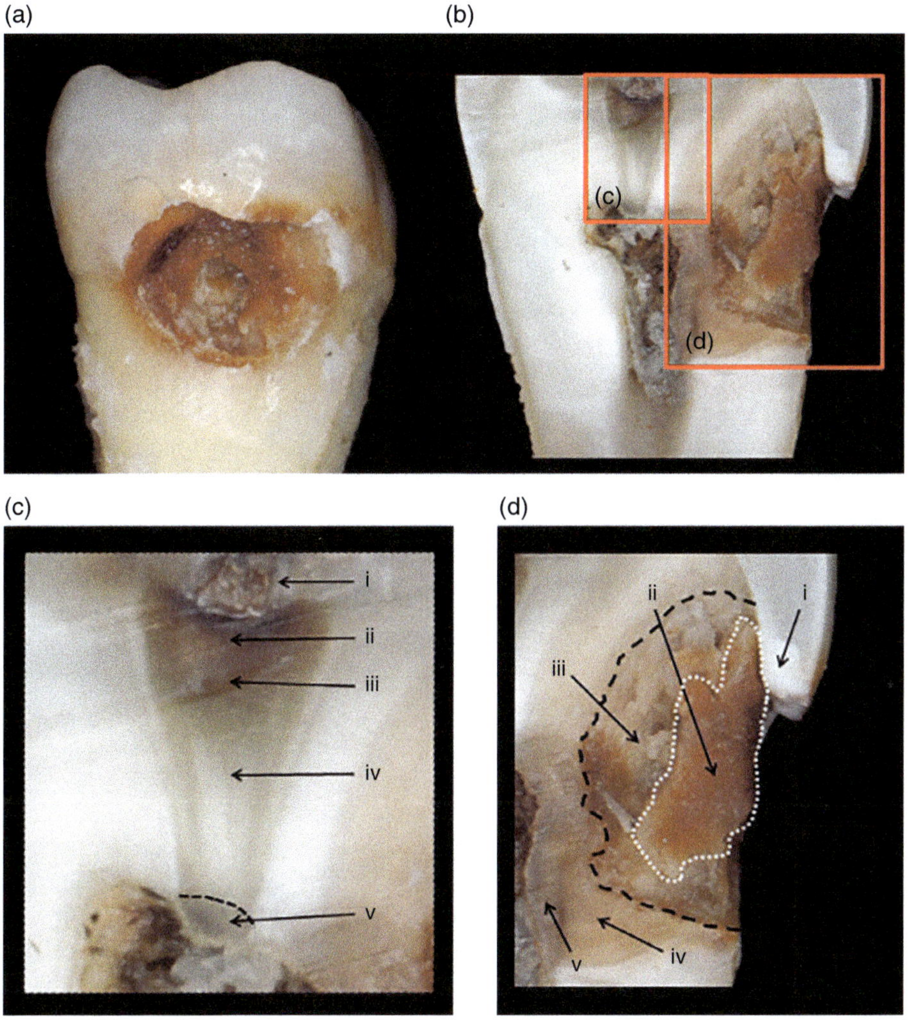

Figure 4.1 Macroscopic view of an extracted tooth with a proximal extensive carious lesion (a) and a longitudinal mesial/distal axial crosscut (b). Higher magnification shows the pre-cavitated enamel-dentine lesion (c) originating from the occlusal surface with the following zones: i = demineralized enamel, ii = black/dark brown discolouration of demineralized dentine, iii = light brown discolouration of demineralized dentine (the darker zones reflects areas of arrested caries), iv = hypermineralized dentine equivalent to zone of sclerosis, v = tertiary dentine. The proximal carious lesion (d) with the following zones: i = retrograde enamel demineralization, which typically is seen in the proximity to the open dentine lesion, ii = soft, dark brown dentine, iii = destructed dentine, iv = pulp close demineralized dentine, v = tertiary dentine. Selective removal to soft or firm dentine would be in the area iv. Selective removal to soft dentine should not be interpreted as a stop excavating within the destructed dentine, as seen in iii, as this area is too soft. The definition of soft is that it can be excavated with minimum resistance to a hand excavator, and firm would be resistant to hand instrumentation. *Source:* John Wiley & Sons, Inc.

The common subdivision of caries diagnoses in thirds, denoting *caries superficialis*, *media* and *profunda* is a widely accepted terminology (9). However, for extensive carious lesions, the diagnosis *caries profunda* can further be subdivided into three classes, which could be related to evidence-based treatments (10).

Caries Profunda 1

Radiographic features: This stage is defined as a lesion penetrating 2/3–3/4 of the dentine, with a radiopaque zone separating the advancing front of the lesion and the pulp.

Histologic features: Microorganisms are located in the carious dentine. Evidence of chronic pulp inflammation, but not associated with invasion of microorganisms into the pulp cavity (Figure 4.2).

Recommended treatment: Selective carious removal in one step to either soft or firm dentine (Figure 4.3e–h). This particular lesion class is most often treated with a selective caries removal strategy (11–13).

Caries Profunda 2

Radiographic features: This stage, described as *deep* caries, is defined as a lesion penetrating 3/4 or more of the dentine, but still with a radiopaque zone separating the advancing front of the lesion and the pulp.

Histologic features: Microorganisms are located in the carious dentine. Evidence of chronic pulp inflammation with a low probability of the presence of invading microorganisms in the pulp cavity (Figure 4.2).

Recommended treatment: Stepwise excavation (Figure 4.3a–d). Evidence for selective carious removal in one step to either soft or firm dentine is available but mainly based on children and adolescent patients. See also Table 4.1 (13).

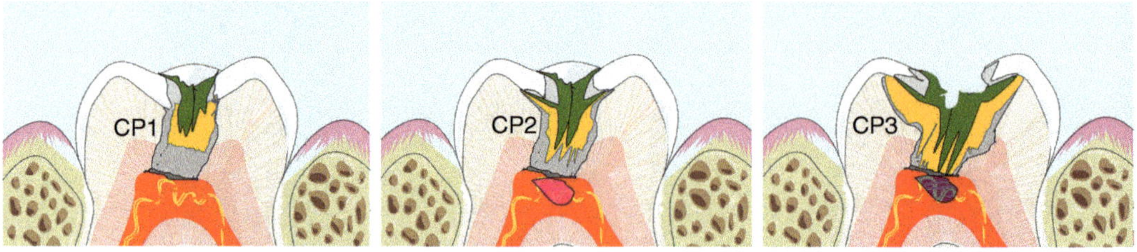

Figure 4.2 Schematic drawing of a cavitated coronal carious lesion. In Caries Profunda (CP) 1, the microorganisms are located in the carious dentine. There is evidence of pulp inflammation, but microorganisms are not invaded into the pulp cavity. Without any intervention, the process will develop, and in CP2, the bulk of microorganisms are still located in the carious dentine, and there is pulp inflammation, as indicated by the pink zone. At this stage, there is a low probability of invading microorganisms in the pulp cavity. However, from this point, a spread along the enamel-dentine junction is noted. In CP3, the carious lesion has progressed further, and microorganisms are in the carious lesion extending into the tertiary dentine and are also present within the pulp cavity (purple zone). The pulpal status includes severe inflammation, and the pulp in the proximity of the carious lesion is partially or fully necrotic. At CP3, a pulp invasive treatment is needed. Green indicates cariogenic microbiota and yellow dentine demineralization. Light grey reflects demineralized enamel, and dark grey is the hypermineralized zone in the dentine. A basic sketch is available from smart.servier.com. *Source:* With permission from Karger.

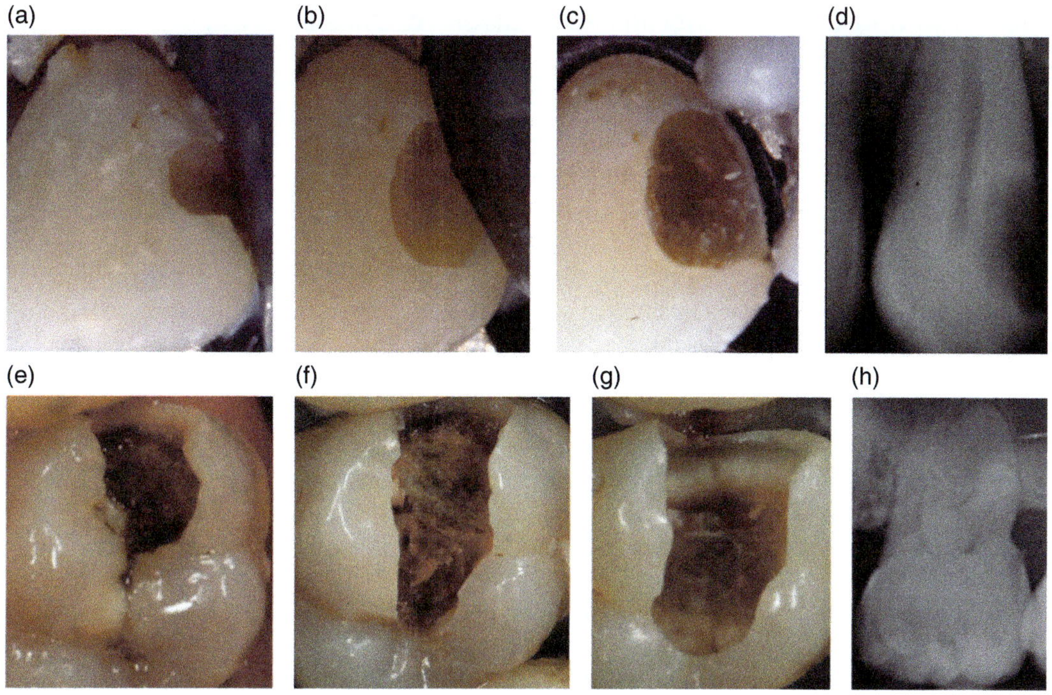

Figure 4.3 Two teeth, one treated with stepwise excavation and the other with selective caries removal in one stage. Approximal carious lesion in a maxillary canine planned for stepwise excavation (a). After the first stage selective carious removal to soft dentine to an extent that facilitates proper placement of a temporary restoration (b). Following a treatment interval and removal of temporary restoration the retained dentine is darker reflecting lesion arrestment. The periphery of the cavity should be excavated to hard dentine in order to facilitate the proper placement of a temporary restoration (c). The carious lesion before treatment is categorized as a radiographically well-defined deep carious lesion penetrating to the pulpal quarter but with a radiopaque zone separating the carious lesion to the pulp (d). Maxillary molar with an 'open' lesion environment planned for selective caries removal in one stage (e). Parts of the overlaying enamel have been removed. Note the outermost disintegrated carious dentine with a dark brown, dry and soft appearance (f). Completion of selective removal using burs and hand excavator to firm dentine. The periphery of the cavity should be excavated to hard dentine in order to facilitate the proper placement of a temporary restoration (g). The carious lesion before treatment is categorized as a radiographically well-defined carious lesion penetrating to the middle third of the dentine (h). *Source:* Lim et al. (11)/Reproduced from Springer Nature.

Caries Profunda 3

Radiographic features: This stage, described as *extremely deep* caries, is defined as a lesion penetrating the entire thickness of the dentine without a radiopaque zone separating the advancing front of the lesion and the pulp.

Histologic features: Microorganisms are located in the carious dentine, tertiary dentine and within the pulp cavity. The pulpal status includes severe inflammation associated with partial or full necrosis in the pulp cavity (Figure 4.2).

Recommended treatment: Pulpectomy or root canal treatment. Pulpotomy including partial pulpotomy may also be considered, but comparative studies with longer follow-up are lacking (14–16).

Understanding Caries Pathology – A Reason to 'Dare' Leaving Carious Dentine Behind

The Non-cavitated Enamel-Dentine Lesion

Dental tissues represent a unique entity that, over a lifetime, sustains its physiological properties despite a multitude of various external stimuli and/or injuries affecting the tooth surface. The enamel layer is not considered a tissue but a secretory product from past ameloblast cells that have laid down a matrix that is systematically packed with rod and inter-rod enamel. Ultrastructurally, these enamel crystals are oriented in different directions. The enamel layer is not a solid barrier but allows for a transportation route along the direction of the enamel crystals, making it possible to transfer external stimuli from the periphery of the enamel into the dentine in an exceptionally organized manner. On this basis, the early topographic signs of carious enamel demineralization (the 'white spot lesion') is considered a time-dependent development (17, 18). The reason for the 3D configuration with the cone-shaped approximal enamel lesion is due to a time difference between the central versus the peripheral parts of the enamel. That is, the central and deepest lesion penetration reflects the oldest part of the lesion, where the cariogenic biofilm has been located for the longest time. This is seen subjacent to the approximal contact area, whereas the peripheral part can be interpreted as the youngest lesion front, hence the site of the youngest biofilm accumulation (19).

As the lesion progresses towards the enamel–dentine junction, there is a notable early response from the dentine–pulp complex. In fact, even before the demineralization has reached the enamel–dentine junction, it has been suggested that cells in the odontoblast-predentine region, including the subodontoblastic cells, respond to noxious stimuli (20, 21). This demonstrates that the enamel should not be seen as an absolute physical barrier.

As the non-cavitated enamel lesion develops closer to the dentine, the next reaction is initiated with the mineral content increasing within the dentinal tubules. Many of the thousands of dentinal tubules with their finger-like projections will respond to an early cariogenic stimulus, but when the odontoblast cell responds, it may resemble an accelerated ageing process. This process is restricted to a local area subjacent to the enamel lesion. Notably, at this non-cavitated stage of lesion penetration, no pH drop has created dentine mineral loss yet, making it plausible that the early dentine mineral increase seen within the dentinal tubules could be related to a cellular reaction and not purely a chemo-physical reprecipitation of dissolved mineral.

When the demineralized enamel reaches the enamel–dentine junction, the first *clinical* visible signs of dentine mineral loss appear as a yellow-brownish discolouration of the dentinal matrix. Evidence indicates that as long as there is an intact rod-/inter-rod structure separating the surface biofilm aligning the enamel from the dentine, the number of microorganisms reaching the dentine does not have as significant influence on the severity of caries progression. Although studies show early invaders of microorganisms into subjacent dentine even in non-cavitated enamel (22, 23), such patterns do not represent the typical microbial spread into carious dentine, being more likely associated with a gradual breakdown of the enamel layer (24, 25). From this, it is understood that the odontoblast cells respond to a very shallow carious lesion by trying to defend the pulp from penetrating bacterial products.

As the growth of the enamel lesion extends laterally, the peripheral and less advanced aspects eventually reach the enamel–dentine junction, repeating the sequence of events, developing a hypermineralized/translucent zone and demineralizing dentine (19).

Overall, the progression of the enamel–dentine lesion takes place from the enamel surface and is guided along the enamel rods.

As the extent of dentine demineralization increases, it is suggested that bioactive dentine matrix components fossilized in the primary dentine matrix during development are released and participate in the tertiary dentinogenesis process (26).

Notably, even before many microorganisms have invaded the dentine, a rather complex series of pulp-dentinal responses have occurred without any severe pulp inflammation.

The Approximal and Occlusal Cavitated Carious Lesion

The microbiological ecosystem within the carious lesions penetrates deeper and deeper as the demineralized enamel breaks down. A cavity is eventually formed, mainly due to the forces from mastication. The characteristics of the cavitated enamel lesion where the dentine is clinically exposed comprise several ecologically important elements:

- The dentine is invaded by a significant number of microorganisms.
- The possibility of cleaning and removing the cariogenic biofilm is compromised, leading to an undisturbed progression, a so-called 'closed' ecosystem (27).
- The focus of a microbial spread is no longer from the enamel surface along the microstructures of the enamel layer but spreads into the dentinal tubules as well as the gap created at the enamel–dentine junction due to shrinkage of the demineralized dentine, also described as retrograde demineralization (Figure 4.2).
- In untreated extensive occlusal lesions, the undermined enamel breaks down; the growth condition for the biofilm may then change considerably, creating a so-called 'open' lesion environment showing temporary signs of caries arrest (Figure 4.4).

Additional consequences of the above changes are that when microorganisms invade the dentine, it is always with a zone of non-infected demineralized dentine ahead, both at the lateral front as well as in the advancing central front. Unfortunately, it has long been a clinical dilemma to define the border where the infected dentine ends and the demineralized but non-infected dentine begins. More than 50 years ago, Fusayama and co-workers (28, 29) carried out a series of studies trying to characterize the infected versus the affected zones of carious dentine, providing more evidence to the concept of leaving affected dentine behind. The innermost affected dentine, although having altered consistency, did not need to be removed, as it had the potential to remineralize (30). In addition, the concept of separating the excavation procedure into two stages in teeth with deep carious lesions raised the understanding about the possibility of leaving infected dentine in the most pulpal part of the cavity and sealing the cavity with a restoration. Bacterial samples from the carious dentine indicated a clear reduction in the infection status just by a superficial removal of infected dentine (31). In other words, changing the cariogenic environment without completely removing all infected carious dentine and restoring the tooth with a well-placed 'tight' seal has proven to be an accepted treatment concept for initiating arrestment of the carious lesion. During this process, the carious dentine darkens markedly through the Maillard reaction (32).

The extent of bacterial invasion into the pulp cavity has been illustrated by the classical study by Reeves and Stanley (33), showing that when the microorganisms enter the innermost tertiary dentine, there were histological signs of severe pulp inflammation, considered irreversible. However, in a clinical context, it has been unclear when exactly this could occur during excavation. In other words, this classical study did not study a correlation between the radiographic depth of

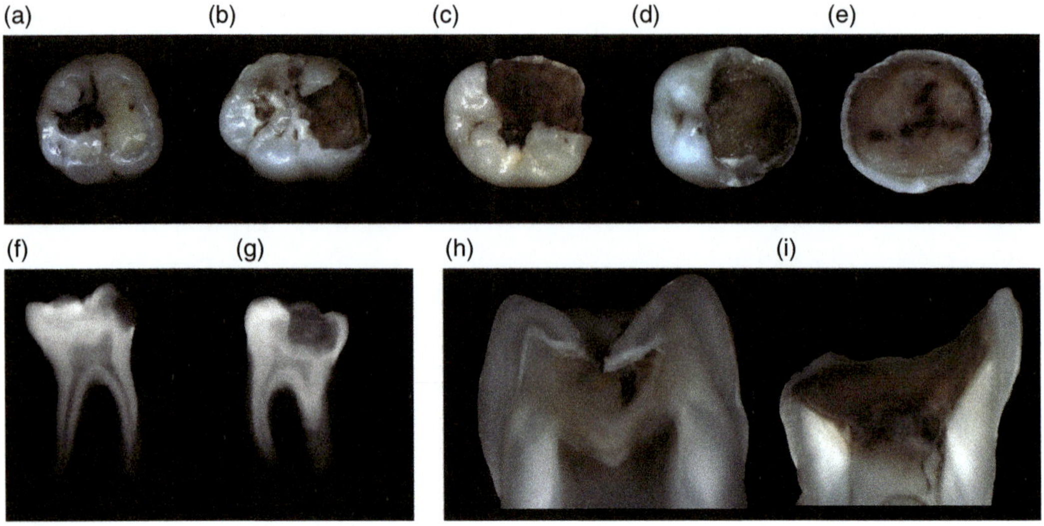

Figure 4.4 The degree of openness is defined as the involvement in the carious lesion of between 1 and 5 tooth surfaces (a–e). Well-defined radiographic penetration depth: (f) a deep carious lesion has reached the pulpal quarter of the dentine with a zone of radiopaque dentine between the lesion and the pulp. (g) An extremely deep carious lesion penetrates the entire thickness of the dentine. States related to carious activity: (h) a closed lesion environment with retrograde demineralization seen as a white line of demineralization undermining the enamel. The underlying demineralized dentine is light/yellow, and clear signs of biofilm accumulation are noted. (i) An open lesion environment with darkening of the demineralized dentine, only plaque accumulation in the central part of the specimen, where the carious lesion has exposed the pulp chamber. *Source:* With permission from the International Endodontic Journal published by John Wiley & Sons Ltd.

the carious lesion and the degree of bacterial penetration. Recently, a combined analysis of the microbial profile in two well-defined extensive stages of carious lesion formations provided some insights concerning the threshold when microorganisms can be present in the pulp cavity and, thus, the need for a more invasive approach than any selective removal (34).

Cavitated Deep and Extremely Deep Carious Lesions

As the carious lesion progresses, the infected advancing front also progresses, but typically with an innermost zone of demineralized dentine without microorganisms. Based on a sample of freshly extracted teeth, the bacterial penetration is confined to primary dentine in well-defined deep lesions without reaching the pulp, as shown in Figure 4.5.

In summary, a deep carious lesion in the pulpal quarter with a radiopaque zone separating the lesion from the pulp tends to have no bacteria. It is without signs of necrosis or severe inflammatory infiltrate. In contrast, severe inflammatory infiltrates and partial necrosis are typically seen in teeth with deep carious lesions with no radiopaque zone separating the lesion from the pulp. Moreover, the pulp inflammation is often located in the coronal part of the pulp, indicating that even in severely infected pulp cavities, the radicular pulp can appear without histological signs of inflammation.

Untreated carious lesions change their ecosystem over time, and it is recognized that the growth condition for the cariogenic biofilm may change dramatically. As described above, a temporary clinical arrest of lesion activity can take place due to a sudden breakdown of undermined enamel and the creation of a much more open environment (Figure 4.4a–e); the open exposed dentine becomes darker and also harder (35). The darkening of exposed carious dentine is also a very

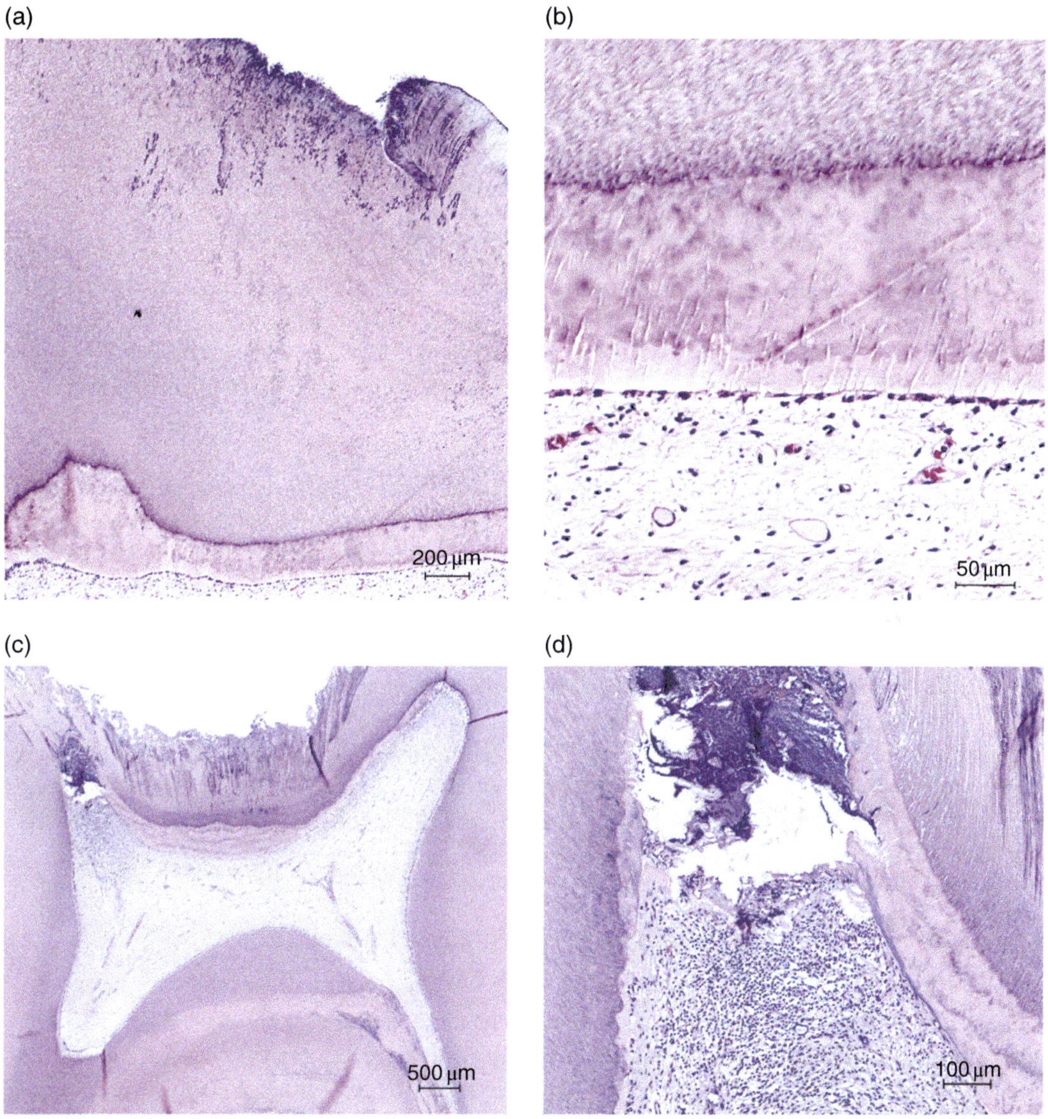

Figure 4.5 (a) Histological features of a well-defined deep lesion. (b) Detail shows that the bacteria have not reached the pulp. The tertiary dentine is partly atubular, and the pulp has no inflammatory infiltrate. (c) The bacteria have reached tertiary dentine in the extremely deep carious lesion. (d) Detail showing the region as partly necrotic and with a subjacent inflammatory infiltrate. Haematoxylin and Eosin stain. *Source:* With permission from the International Endodontic Journal published by John Wiley & Sons Ltd.

familiar sign in root carious lesions (36, 37). Histologically, the inflammatory infiltrates may still be present but accompanied by the formation of tertiary reactionary dentine formation.

Consequences of Changing the Cariogenic Ecosystem – Knowhow for Less Invasive Treatments

In principle, the sequence of events following the breakdown of enamel in an occlusal carious lesion is utilized when treating deep carious lesions with a less invasive removal technique. By removing the superficial parts of the cavitated lesion, the dentist is creating an environment with a substantial change in the microbial ecosystem. Over time, this change will affect the colour, consistency and moisture of the carious dentine.

Enhanced tertiary dentine deposition is expected as well, but it is difficult to confirm and monitor by radiographs. However, it is relevant to be aware of tertiary dentine formation, as it is a natural consequence of the pulpal defence.

Formation of Intra-Pulpal Cartilage-Like and Hyperplastic Tissue in the Pulp

The formation of ectopic mineralized cartilage-like tissue can be observed in the pulp as a late response to inflammation in advanced carious lesions (38). The cartilage-like tissue occurs in different places: (i) close towards necrotic pulp tissue; (ii) attached to the walls of the pulp chamber but with a clearly discernible difference between primary dentine and newly formed tissue; and (iii) embedded within the inflamed pulpal tissue (Figure 4.6).

This tissue resembles so-called heterotopic mineralization, also seen in other severely injured parts of the body where necrosis and inflammation are apparent (39). It seems linked to complex interactions between immune cells and pulpal stroma cells rather than to a direct upregulation of the odontoblast expected during normal reactionary dentinogenesis (38). Decades ago, Baume (40) discussed the phenotypic presence of atubular dentine and denoted it as fibrodentine. It can be speculated that the cartilage-like tissue seen within the pulp may eventually mineralize further to become fibrodentine.

Concomitantly, with the appearance of a cartilage-like tissue pulp polyps can be present in open lesion environments (in extremely deep lesions) (Figure 4.7) (34). The formation of a pulp polyp demonstrates yet another way the pulp can attempt to demarcate an external stimulus, even following a long history of a previously progressing carious lesion. The polyps may comprise vascular and inflamed tissue. The polyp can vary from very small to large extensions outside the pulp chamber and histologically can be with or without a stratified squamous epithelium barrier (34).

Intra-Pulpal Mineralized Tissue – A Sign of Pulp Pathology and Avoidance of Non-exposing Treatments?

Endodontists recognize intra-pulpal mineralization as a sign of pulp pathology (41); however, it has not been accepted as an integrated part of the diagnostic process of assessing the state of the pulp. The implementation of this could provide added information within an unresolved task of estimating the severity of pulp inflammation. For example, when assessing teeth with an unclear diagnosis, the presence of intra-pulpal mineralization could possibly indicate irreversible or at least more severe pulpal damage and a reason for not opting for a non-exposure carious-tissue removal procedure.

Outcomes

As previously stated, there is no diagnostic method, sign or symptom, which can accurately identify all teeth in which the caries process has inflicted irreversible rather than reversible damage; therefore, some of these treatments will fail (5). A safety-first approach is to treat every case with pulpectomy and root canal treatment (Figure 4.8). Root canal treatment of teeth with a vital pulp can, under ideal conditions, be performed with a good prognosis, but epidemiological studies of root canal treatments predominately performed by general dental practitioners showed that

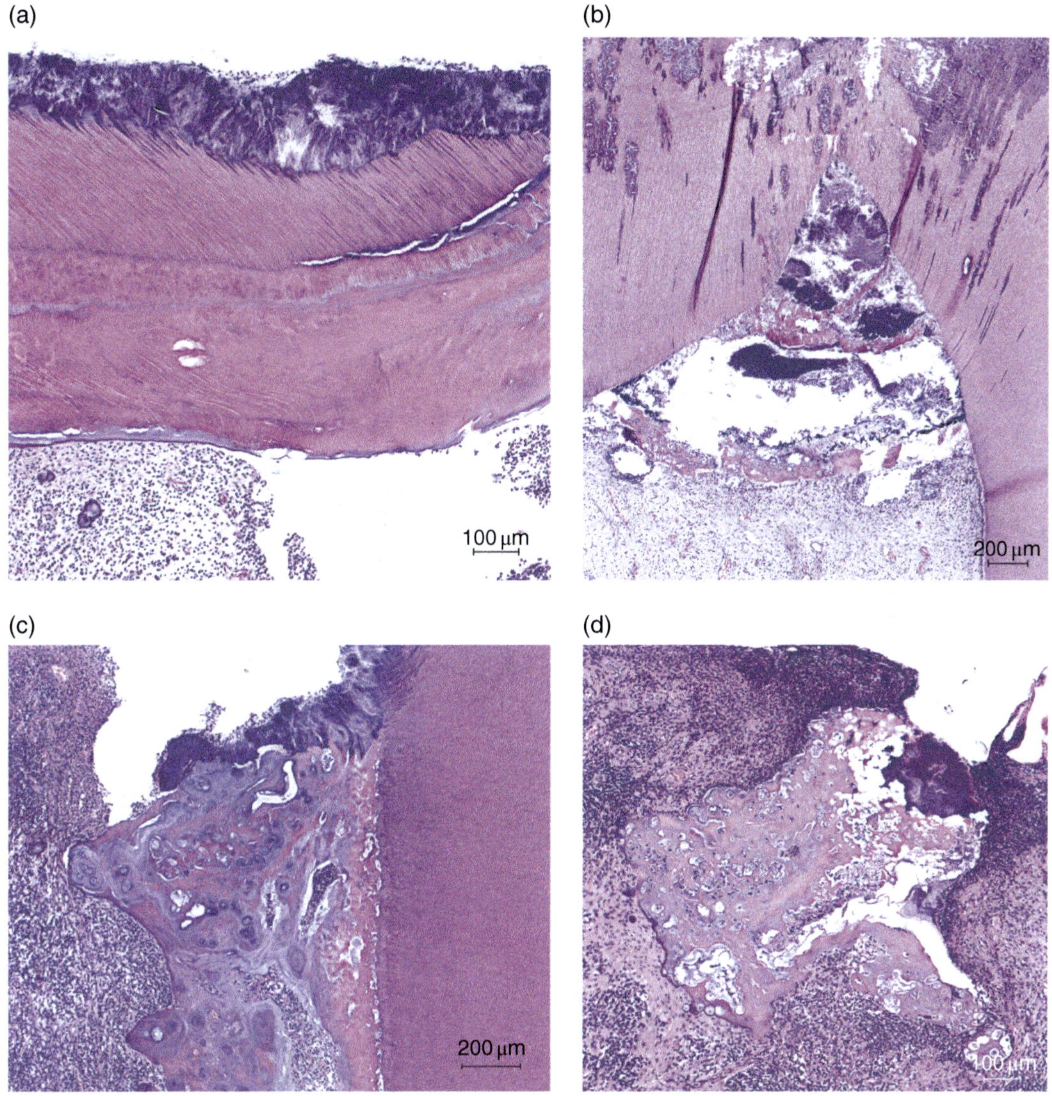

Figure 4.6 Hard tissue and/or ectopic connective tissue: (a) tertiary dentine with tubular and atubular areas formed in layers, of which the first zone underneath primary dentine is mainly tubular in appearance. The surface of carious dentine is covered with biofilm. There are three clear patterns of ectopic connective tissue formation: (b) towards bacteria, creating a barrier against the infection front; (c) attached to the walls of the pulp chamber, with a clear distinction between the connective tissue aggregate and the primary dentine; and (d) embedded within the inflamed pulpal stroma. Stained with Haematoxylin and Eosin. *Source:* Demant et al. (38)/Reproduced from John Wiley & Sons.

root-filled teeth are often associated with apical periodontitis. In addition, root-filled teeth are more often extracted than non-root-filled teeth (42–44).

Several outcomes interest the patient and the clinician (Table 4.2). One outcome would be that the pulp, even unintentionally, would be exposed during excavation, which would necessitate another treatment decision: either to go for a procedure such as pulp capping, partial or full pulpotomy or the more invasive treatment such as pulpectomy to avoid extraction.

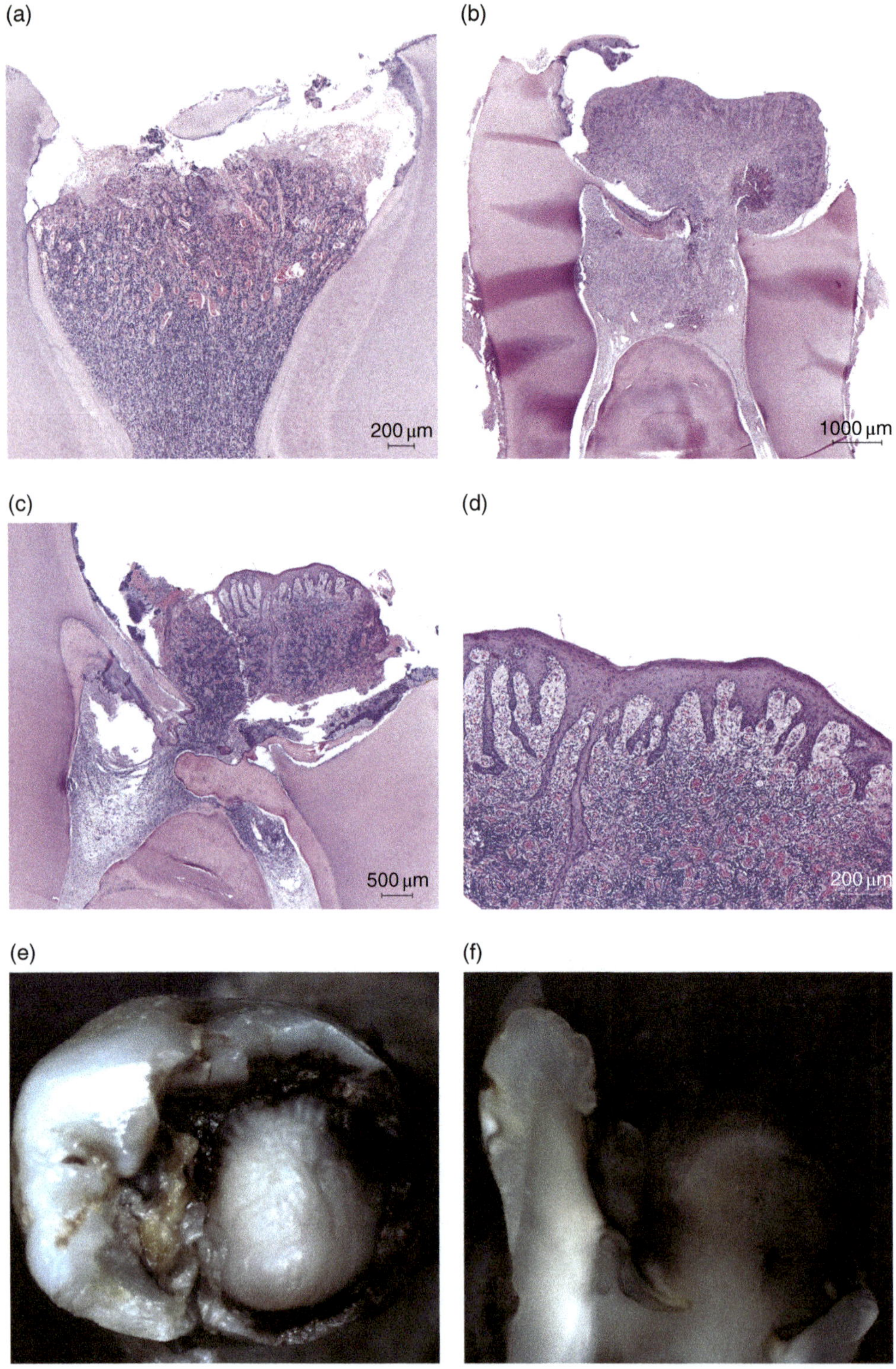

Figure 4.7 (a) Initial stages of polyps have highly vascular and inflamed tissue that barely protrudes from the pulp chamber, (b) to large polyps, (c) occasionally covered in a mature, stratified, squamous epithelium (detailed in d). (b, c) Biofilm is noted on the lateral borders of dentine and not on the surface of the polyps. (e) Stereo-macroscopic view of a large polyp protruding through the crown. (f) The macroscopic specimen shows the polyp penetrating the roof of the pulp chamber with lateral remnants of thin, dark, carious dentine; Haematoxylin and Eosin stain. *Source:* Demant et al. (34)/Reproduced from John Wiley & Sons.

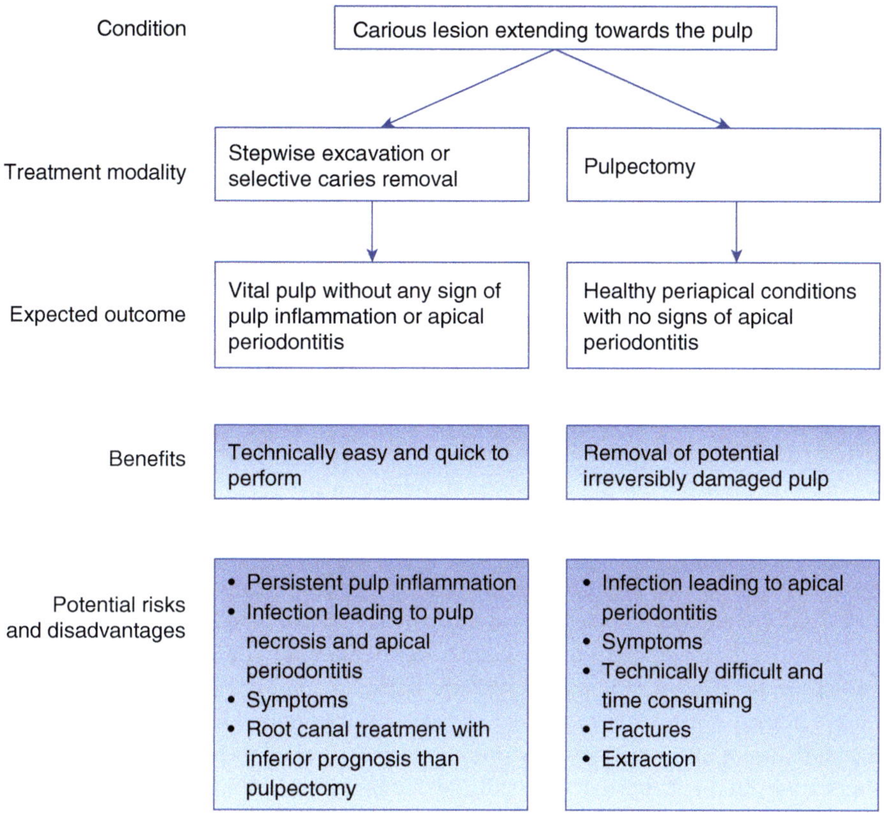

Figure 4.8 Not all treatments with stepwise excavation or selective caries removal are anticipated to be successful, and there are some potential risks and disadvantages. However, the benefits of the less invasive treatment of stepwise excavation or selective caries removal are substantial.

Table 4.2 Outcomes that should be checked after treatment of a deep caries lesion.

Outcome	Checked by
Pulp exposure during treatment	Visual inspection
Symptoms	Anamnesis
Pulp vitality	Sensate reaction to electrical and/or cold pulp test
Normal periapical conditions	Periapical radiograph
Restorative failure	Visual inspection, probing and bitewing radiograph

After the treatment has been performed, the desired outcome would be no symptoms, a vital pulp (usually checked by electrical and/or cold pulp tests) and normal periapical conditions – that is, no signs of periapical radiolucency on a periapical radiograph indicating necrosis of the pulp.

Other unwanted outcomes would be restorative failure, need for restoration replacement, or possible carious lesion progression. The integrity of the restoration is, from a biological view an important factor as the carious process is affected by the environment in which any bacteria reside. The principle of selective carious removal, either in one-stage, stepwise or indirect pulp capping, is that by carefully sealing the cavity, the environment will be different, and there will be a shift in the microbiome and residing microbes will change their behaviour so that they will no longer drive the carious lesion process further (45, 46).

These clinician-reported outcomes are what studies usually report, but from the patients′ perspective, there might be other outcomes which may be of importance (47).

Reported Outcome from Clinical Studies

As most outcomes of interest are related to the pulpal status, it is of importance to know the depth of the carious lesion and how the excavation procedure has been performed to be able to apply the results from clinical studies to clinical practice. Over the years, the amount of carious affected dental tissue that is considered to need to be removed has changed in teeth with deep lesions with a risk of pulp exposure. As introduced before, the trend has moved away from aggressive removal of carious tissue to hard dentine throughout the cavity (non-selective), to a more selective removal with only the periphery of the cavity being excavated to hard dentine (6, 48). This means that previous caries removal strategies to hard dentine in teeth with deep caries are considered overtreatment. Most published studies are conducted within secondary care settings, and thus, their results may be difficult to generalize and transfer to general dental practice settings. Comparisons of non-selective (complete) removal of carious tissue and selective removal (Table 4.3) show consistently that selective removal has a lower frequency of pulp exposures during excavation. After one year, there seems to be no difference between complete caries removal and any selective carious removal treatments regarding clinical and radiographic outcomes. When teeth with pulp exposures were excluded, any treatment modality showed a very high proportion of teeth with a successful outcome: normal clinical and radiographic conditions (49–53). One study with a five-year follow-up shows that stepwise excavation is more beneficial than non-selective (complete) caries removal (51).

Comparisons of selective carious removal in one-step and stepwise excavation (Table 4.4) show that the frequency of pulp exposure during stepwise exposure is greater than for selective carious removal in one step, most probably due to pulp exposures during the re-entry of the cavity. Regarding the other outcomes, vitality of the pulp and normal periapical conditions, there seems to be no difference at one year; both treatment modalities report high success rates (54, 55). One study with a five-year follow-up shows a higher cumulative success rate for selective carious removal in one step compared to stepwise excavation. It is worth noting that these poorer results for stepwise excavation may have been affected by many patients in this group failing to show up for the second appointment with re-entry and thus were left with a provisional restoration for a long period. One may also speculate that leaving cariously affected dentine in the preparation would jeopardize the longevity of the restoration. After five years, there was no difference in survival of the restorations placed after selective caries removal in one step to restorations placed after stepwise excavation; both composite and amalgam restorations performed equally well (58). Another point that could be addressed was the penetration depth of the carious lesions in the enrolled participants. The participants had relatively shallow lesions, and it could be speculated whether there was an indication to perform a two-step procedure.

Indirect pulp capping, a treatment considered to be more aggressive compared to one-step selective caries removal, has not been studied robustly in recent years. The clinical success has been reported to be about 72–94% after one to four years; however, no direct comparison was made to another vital pulp treatment (59–62).

Table 4.3 Randomized clinical studies comparing non-selective (complete) caries removal (CCR) to any selective carious removal (one step, stepwise or indirect pulp capping) and data on the setting, patient characteristics and the reported results.

Study	Setting	Patient/tooth characteristics	Dropouts	Reported results
Leksell et al. (49)	Sweden Six specialists in paediatrics	Posterior teeth in patients 6- to 16-year-olds Carious lesions judged on radiograph to lead to pulp exposure if CCR was performed	6 patients/ 7 molars were incomplete stepwise intervention, leaving 127 to be evaluated	Pulp exposure: 40% in CCR 18% in stepwise No difference; all of the 80 teeth with no pulp exposure showed normal clinical and radiographic conditions at 1 year
Orhan et al. (50)[a]	Turkey Outpatient clinic at a university	Permanent molars in patients up to 15 years Deep carious lesions judged on radiograph to lead to pulp exposure if CCR would be performed, i.e. three fourths or more of the dentine	60 teeth evaluated	Pulp exposure: 25% in CCR 5% in indirect pulp capping 6% in two-step indirect pulp capping No difference; all the 48 teeth with no pulp exposure showed normal clinical and radiographic conditions at 1 year
Bjørndal et al. (51)[b]	Denmark and Sweden Six centres; university and public dental clinics	Primary carious lesions in adults, mean age 29 years Carious lesions on radiograph involve 75% or more of the dentine	67 patients, leaving 239 to be evaluated	Pulp exposure: 36% in CCR 21% in stepwise Significant difference, in teeth with no pulp exposure, 46% in CCR and 60% in stepwise showed normal clinical and radiographic conditions at 5 years
Khokhar and Tewari (52)	India Postgraduate Institute	Molar teeth in patients 14–54-year-olds Carious lesions penetrating half or more of the dentine judged on radiograph	Four patients in CCR and 3 in one step, leaving 136 to be evaluated	Pulp exposure: 10% in CCR 0% in one step No difference in teeth with no pulp exposure: 98% in CCR and 93% in one-step selective carious removal showed normal clinical and radiographic conditions at 18 mo

[a] Original study of both primary and permanent teeth, the table shows data on permanent teeth. The author's definition of the two-step indirect pulp capping could be interpreted as a stepwise excavation or as a variation of the indirect pulp capping procedure.
[b] Shorter follow-up reported in (53).
Source: Adapted from Bjørndal et al. (53).

Table 4.4 Randomized clinical studies comparing selective carious removal one step to stepwise excavation and data on setting, patient characteristics and the reported results.

Study	Setting	Patient/tooth characteristics	Dropouts	Reported results
Maltz et al. (54)[a]	Brazil Public health services, etc.	Molars in patients with mean age of 17.17 ± 10.91; range 6–53 years More than half of the dentine thickness (radiograph)	42 were incomplete stepwise interventions. Large number of dropouts at different time intervals, leaving 229 teeth to be evaluated	Pulp exposure: 0% in one step 3% in stepwise Significant difference, 80% cumulative success in one step and 56% in stepwise in regard to vital pulp, normal periapical conditions, no symptoms at 5 years
Labib et al. (55)	Egypt Four dentists at university clinic	Premolars/molars in 18- to 47-year-old patients Occlusal/occlusal-proximal deep lesions penetrating more than 2/3 of the dentine judged on radiograph	7 teeth in one step and 8 in stepwise, leaving 106 to be evaluated	Pulp exposure: 0% in one step 8% in stepwise No difference, including teeth with pulp exposure: 89% in one step and 85% stepwise in regard to maintained pulp vitality and restoration integrity at 1 year

[a] Shorter follow-up reported in Maltz et al. (56, 57).

From longitudinal studies, based on data from registries, the survival of teeth which have been subjected to stepwise excavation was 72% after four years; in other words, the teeth have not been noted to have had root canal treatment or have been extracted. The only factor influencing this particular outcome is the age of the patient; older individuals seem to have a somewhat reduced chance of having a desirable outcome. The incidence of failure seems to be highest during the first 30 months; thereafter, the survival curve flattens, and the risk of failure is reduced (63).

Monitoring

Monitoring after an excavation procedure should be done based on the individual case and is influenced by the expected prognosis of the treatment and the probability of not detecting failure. In this regard, it is worth noting that the prognosis of root canal treatment is not worsened for a tooth with necrotic pulp compared with a vital pulp, as long as there is no periapical radiolucency (64). Signs of an unsuccessful caries excavation treatment, relating to the health of the pulp, could be any or a combination, connected to these conditions:

- Pain
- Loss of vitality
- Periapical radiolucency

For teeth with immature roots, there should also be radiological signs of continued root development (65).

Patients with symptoms following any type of carious-tissue removal in teeth with deep lesions should be cared for based on their symptoms. It is necessary to once more stress that there is an inherent difficulty in preoperatively assessing whether the pulp is reversibly inflamed, and therefore, the pulpal inflammatory status may progress to pulp necrosis and apical periodontitis. This process may, on many occasions, develop without any symptoms, and therefore, it is wise to monitor the vitality and the periapical conditions of these teeth with uncertain prognosis (65).

Evidence-based and Consensus Recommendations

Any decision on the type of treatment should ideally be made with knowledge of the evidence base for that particular therapy. As seen in Tables 4.3 and 4.4, there are only a few randomized clinical trials directly comparing one treatment to another available, and these types of studies are the foundation for any evidence-based recommendations. A randomized clinical trial will not automatically provide usable data for a recommendation; different types of biases will affect the value of the results, and when two randomized clinical trials come to different conclusions, the strength of any treatment recommendation will be hampered. In addition, it is uncommon with studies conducted in general dental practice settings where most of the treatments of deep caries lesions are performed, making the transfer of the results difficult. With few available studies, any posed recommendations are sometimes made with low-certainty evidence, which means that there is a substantial risk for new research altering the recommendation. This lack of studies affects the strength of recommendations made by organizations such as Cochrane, the International Caries Consensus Collaboration, the European Society of Endodontology, the American Association of Endodontists and stakeholders such as national organizations working with providing treatment recommendations. It is also evident that, due to the lack of evidence, these organizations come to somewhat different conclusions and recommendations (4, 6, 13, 66, 67).

Cochrane has stated in a report that the odds of failure, mainly due to pulp exposure, were higher for non-selective (complete) caries removal than stepwise excavation with moderate-certainty evidence. They also report that the odds of failure, mainly due to pulp exposure, may be higher for complete caries removal than selective caries removal in one step with very low-certainty evidence – in other words, complete caries removal should not be chosen over selective caries removal in one step or stepwise excavation for managing deep lesions (13). This recommendation is in line with what the International Caries Consensus Collaboration and the European Society of Endodontology propose (4, 6). The Caries Consensus Collaboration expresses their recommendation as 'In deeper lesions in teeth with still sensible (vital) pulps, preserving pulpal health should be prioritized over restoration success, while in shallow or moderately deep lesions, restoration longevity might be more important factor (strong recommendation)', in other words; in deeper carious lesions it is advisable to excavate to firm dentine (6). In the position statement from the American Association of Endodontists, it is obvious that they recommend a more invasive form of excavation as they recommend complete removal of infected and demineralized tissue in a deep carious lesion. This recommendation is based on the histological assessment of extracted teeth managed with selective excavation procedures showing pulpal inflammation and is diametrical to the other organizations (66, 68). The concern was based on the presence of bacteria in dentine but with a very limited observation period. Out of 12 teeth investigated, 8 were evaluated after 3 months, contrasting several years' of comparative clinical evidence as recently successfully reported on these less invasive approaches (13).

Uncertain and varied treatment recommendations lead to confusion. As a comparison, the national guidelines in some of the Nordic countries, although similar in demographics and organization of the public dental health services, propose different treatments for deep carious lesion. They all agree that non-selective caries removal should not be performed in teeth with deep carious lesions, though some advocate stepwise excavation, and others recommend stepwise or partial excavation in one step (66).

Any evidence-based treatment recommendation should be accompanied by some health-economic aspects. Although data is scarce, selective carious-tissue removal in one stage is reported as being more cost-effective than stepwise excavation when taking into account the risk for failure and costs that were not fully verified (13, 69, 70).

Epidemiology of Current Practice

Questionnaire studies have shown significant variation among dentists in their choice of treatments for deep carious lesions (71–74). In a multinational study including responses from dentists in France, Germany and Norway, most dentists opted for a non-selective carious removal strategy, which is now considered overtreatment (6). The dentists wrongly thought non-selective carious removal was needed to avoid the progression of the carious lesion. Unlike French and German dentists, most Norwegian dentists would perform stepwise excavation in a deep carious lesion (71). In the United Kingdom, a large proportion of clinicians working in primary care states prefer non-selective caries removal or selective caries removal in one stage. A smaller proportion prefer stepwise excavation when shown a bitewing radiograph of deep caries (74). In Finland, most dentists preferred either stepwise or selective caries removal in one step in asymptomatic teeth with deep lesions (73). However, the results from a questionnaire may differ from reality. From a retrospective radiographic study in Finland, it is evident that dentists did not adhere to their national current recommendations for less invasive methods, i.e. stepwise or selective caries removal in one step. Teenagers with deep carious lesions were most often treated with non-selective caries removal, followed by stepwise excavation (75).

These results underline the need to educate dentists regarding the possible benefits of performing selective caries removal treatments but also find effective ways to implement the concepts of minimally invasive caries removal strategies.

How Often Is Stepwise Excavation Performed?

One limiting factor for introducing and disseminating a treatment concept relates to economic issues. In many countries, various insurance or remuneration systems regulate and guide dentists on which dental treatments are advocated. Not all countries provide reimbursement for an extra visit when carrying out, e.g. a stepwise excavation procedure, as the case in the Nordic countries where there is reimbursement of stepwise excavation treatments (66). In other words, due to the reality of the economic resources given within an insurance-based agreement, less invasive carious removal strategies are not renumerated properly in many countries.

In Denmark, there is reimbursement for the extra procedure needed to perform a stepwise excavation. The number of stepwise excavations performed in adults has been steady over a 10-year period, whereas the number of root canal treatments has dropped. The number of extractions has remained more or less stable over the period, perhaps with a small increase (Figure 4.9).

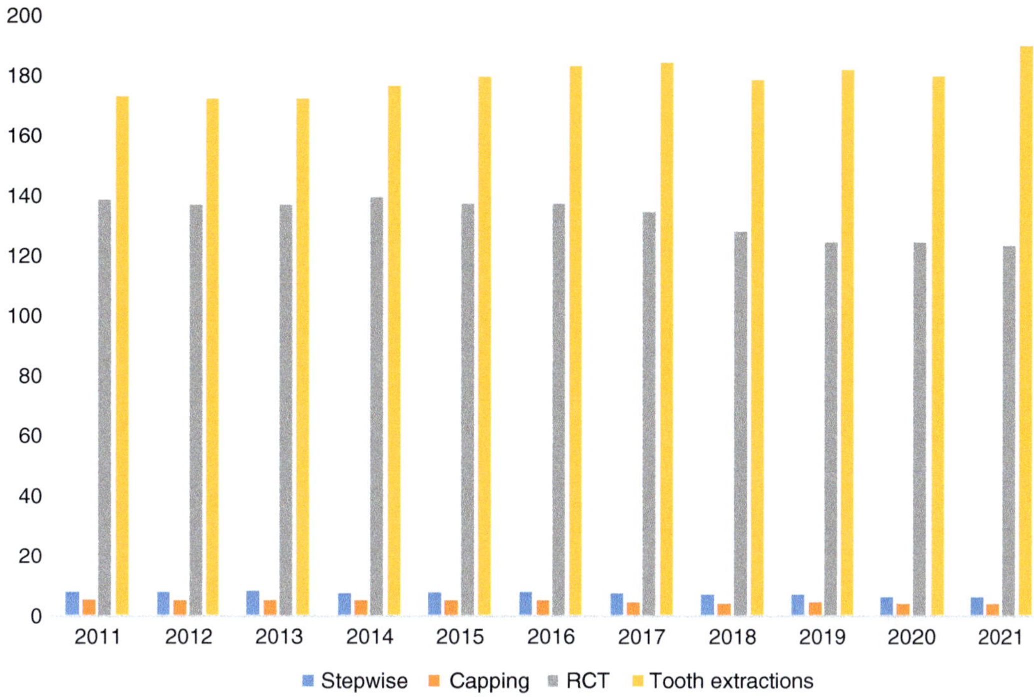

Figure 4.9 Number of registered treatments per 1000 patients. Stepwise excavations (blue), direct pulp capping (orange), root canal fillings (grey) and tooth extraction (orange) in the adult population during 2013–2021 in Denmark. The data on extractions also includes surgical removals, etc. *Source:* Strategy Analyse, Danish Dental Association, searched 23 April 2023.

Future

To obtain consistent and evidence-based recommendations on carious-tissue removal strategies in teeth with deep carious lesions, there are several issues that need to be addressed; some are tangible in the near future, and others are more challenging to solve.

First and foremost, there is a need to find ways to accurately assess the status of the pulp. Ideally, we would like to separate which pulps are inflamed but salvageable and those non-salvageable. If this could be determined with a high degree of certainty, the prognosis of any vital pulp treatment would be better and more accurate, as many of the unsuccessful treatments of deep carious lesions can be attributed to our inability to assess the pulpal status. So far, no diagnostic tests, biomarkers or sets of symptoms give conclusive guidance (5, 76). At this stage, the depth of the carious lesion seems to be a factor, which could be a good candidate to assess whether the pulp is savable, but this needs to be studied further in clinical trials. Is it the inner quarter of dentine, where there is a radiopaque zone between the carious lesion and dental pulp, which will form the threshold for teeth that are recommended as suitable for any type of selective caries removal? Deeper lesions than this seem to have microbes within the pulp space and profound inflammation, which could indicate an unsalvageable state (33, 34). Perhaps there are other factors, such as the progression rate of the lesion, colour and wetness of the dentine, which could provide information to the status of the pulp? Should a stepwise excavation approach be preferred in a rapidly progressing lesion (Figures 4.3 and 4.10), whereas selective caries removal in one stage is preferred in a more slowly progressing lesion? First stage in stepwise excavation arrests caries in the remaining dentine,

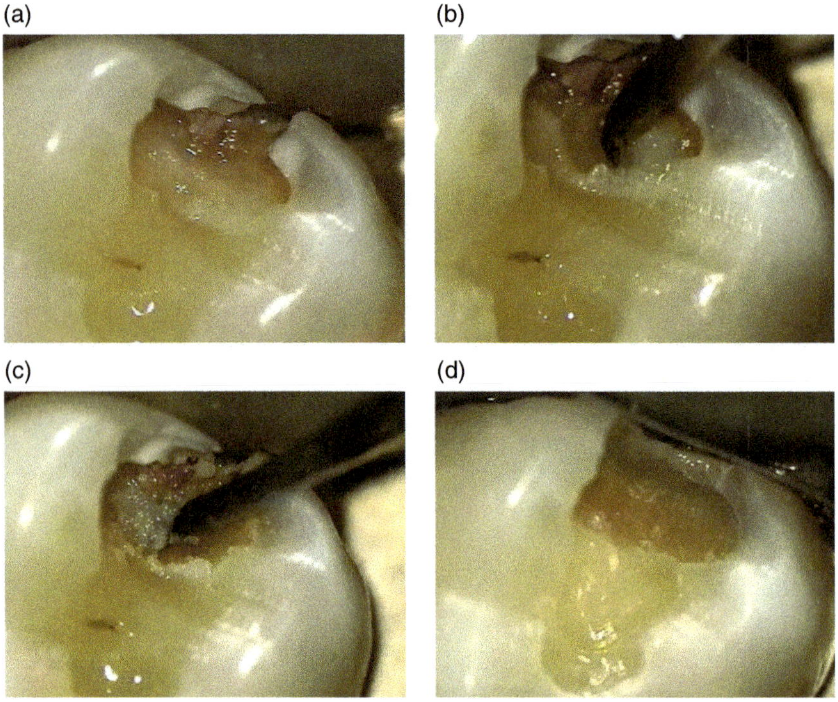

Figure 4.10 First stage of stepwise excavation of a tooth with an approximal lesion. The overlying enamel has been removed, revealing the carious dentine being light yellowish in colour, wet and extraordinarily soft, which are typical features of an active environment (a). The necrotic and disintegrated carious dentine is easily removed by hand excavator to soft dentine (b, c). The periphery of the cavity should be excavated to hard dentine in order to facilitate proper placement of a temporary restoration (d). *Source:* Lars Bjørndal (Book author).

which may not be needed in a more open and, thus, slowly progressing environment (Figure 4.3). Similarly, the patient's preferences could be decisive – patients dreading visiting a dental care facility and who often skip appointments should perhaps be better candidates for one-stage treatments.

Another important issue is the reporting of and, thus, the possibility to interpret the results of a study. For any study on deep caries excavation to be useful, there needs to be precise data on the carious lesion such as the depth, colour and consistency as well on the endpoint of excavation. Was the study aiming for excavation to soft, leathery, firm or hard dentine? Shortcomings in reporting what has been done lead to disparate results and heterogeneity. For instance, comparing the outcome from one study including teeth with caries lesions of approximately half the dentine thickness and employing a conservative excavation to leathery dentine will most likely terminate in very few pulp exposures as opposed to including teeth with more than ¾ of the dentine thickness and employing a radical excavation to hard dentine. Likewise, the pulpal status is different in teeth with different depths of the carious lesions, which would affect the outcome of pulp vitality and normal periapical conditions.

Patients and clinicians are interested in the prognosis of a treatment and not just the short-term prognosis. Studies with longer follow-ups than one year are needed. In the future, we need to know the 5- and 10-year outcomes after different treatments of the deep carious lesion and better understand the patients' perspectives. In anticipation of new research and based on the current evidence, minimally invasive approaches such as selective carious removal for the treatment of deep carious lesions are recommended.

References

1 Levin LG, Law AS, Holland GR, Abbott PV, Roda RS. Identify and define all diagnostic terms for pulpal health and disease states. *J Endod.* 2009;35(12):1645–57. https://doi.org/10.1016/j.joen.2009.09.032.

2 Bjørndal L, Laustsen MH, Reit C. Root canal treatment in Denmark is most often carried out in carious vital molar teeth and retreatments are rare. *Int Endod J.* 2006;39(10):785–90. https://doi.org/10.1111/j.1365-2591.2006.01149.x.

3 Wigsten E, Jonasson P, EndoReCo, Kvist T. Indications for root canal treatment in a Swedish county dental service: patient- and tooth-specific characteristics. *Int Endod J.* 2019;52(2):158–68. https://doi.org/10.1111/iej.12998.

4 Duncan HF, Galler KM, Tomson PL, Simon S, El-Karim I, Kundzina R, et al. European Society of Endodontology position statement: management of deep caries and the exposed pulp. *Int Endod J.* 2019;52(7):923–34. https://doi.org/10.1111/iej.13080.

5 Mejàre IA, Axelsson S, Davidson T, Frisk F, Hakeberg M, Kvist T, et al. Diagnosis of the condition of the dental pulp: a systematic review. *Int End J.* 2012;45(7):597–613. https://doi.org/10.1111/j.1365-2591.2012.02016.x.

6 Schwendicke F, Frencken JE, Bjørndal L, Maltz M, Manton DJ, Ricketts D, et al. Managing carious lesions: consensus recommendations on carious tissue removal. *Adv Dent Res.* 2016;28(2):58–67. https://doi.org/10.1177/0022034516639271.

7 Innes NP, Frencken JE, Bjørndal L, Maltz M, Manton DJ, Ricketts D, et al. Managing carious lesions: consensus recommendations on terminology. *Adv Dent Res.* 2016;28(2):49–57. https://doi.org/10.1177/0022034516639276.

8 Bjørndal L, Simon S, Tomson PL, Duncan HF. Management of deep caries and the exposed pulp. *Int Endod J.* 2019;52(7):949–73. https://doi.org/10.1111/iej.13128.

9 Ismail AI, Pitts NB, Tellez M, Authors of International Caries Classification and Management System (ICCMS), Banerjee A, Deery C, et al. The International Caries Classification and Management System (ICCMS™) an example of a caries management pathway. *BMC Oral Health.* 2015;15 Suppl 1(Suppl 1):S9. https://doi.org/10.1186/1472-6831-15-S1-S9.

10 Bjørndal L, Ramezanzade S. Chapter 3: Pathological features of coronal caries. *Monogr Oral Sci.* 2023;31:19–36. https://doi.org/10.1159/000530557.

11 Lim ZE, Duncan HF, Moorthy A, McReynolds D. Minimally invasive selective caries removal: a clinical guide. *Br Dent J.* 2023;234(4):233–40. https://doi.org/10.1038/s41415-023-5515-4.

12 Jurasic MM, Gillespie S, Sorbara P, Clarkson J, Ramsay C, Nyongesa D, et al. Deep caries removal strategies: findings from the national dental practice-based research network. *J Am Dent Assoc.* 2022;153(11):1078–1088.e7. https://doi.org/10.1016/j.adaj.2022.08.005.

13 Schwendicke F, Walsh T, Lamont T, Al-Yaseen W, Bjørndal L, Clarkson JE, et al. Interventions for treating cavitated or dentine carious lesions. *Cochrane Database Syst Rev.* 2021;7(7):CD013039. https://doi.org/10.1002/14651858.CD013039.pub2.

14 Jakovljevic A, Jaćimović J, Aminoshariae A, Fransson H. Effectiveness of vital pulp treatment in managing nontraumatic pulpitis associated with no or nonspontaneous pain: a systematic review. *Int Endod J.* 2022;2022:17. https://doi.org/10.1111/iej.13776.

15 Taha NA, Abuzaid AM, Khader YS. A randomized controlled clinical trial of pulpotomy versus root canal therapy in mature teeth with irreversible pulpitis: outcome, quality of life, and patients' satisfaction. *J Endod.* 2023;49(6):624–631.e2. https://doi.org/10.1016/j.joen.2023.04.001.

16 Jassal A, Nawal RR, Yadav S, Talwar S, Yadav S, Duncan HF. Outcome of partial and full pulpotomy in cariously exposed mature molars with symptoms indicative of irreversible pulpitis: a randomized controlled trial. *Int Endod J.* 2023;56(3):331–44. https://doi.org/10.1111/iej.13872.

17 Holmen L, Thylstrup A, Artun J. Clinical and histological features observed during arrestment of active enamel carious lesions in vivo. *Caries Res.* 1987;21(6):546–54. https://doi.org/10.1159/000261065.

18 Thylstrup A, Bruun C, Holmen L. In vivo caries models – mechanisms for caries initiation and arrestment. *Adv Dent Res.* 1994;8(2):144–57. https://doi.org/10.1177/08959374940080020401.

19 Bjørndal L, Thylstrup A. A structural analysis of approximal enamel caries lesions and subjacent dentin reactions. *Eur J Oral Sci.* 1995;103(1):25–31. https://doi.org/10.1111/j.1600-0722.1995.tb00006.x.

20 Brännström M, Lind PO. Pulpal response to early dental caries. *J Dent Res.* 1965;44(5):1045–50. https://doi.org/10.1177/00220345650440050701.

21 Bjørndal L, Darvann T, Thylstrup A. A quantitative light microscopic study of the odontoblast and subodontoblastic reactions to active and arrested enamel caries without cavitation. *Caries Res.* 1998;32(1):59–69. https://doi.org/10.1159/000016431.

22 Brännström M, Gola G, Nordenvall KJ, Torstenson B. Invasion of microorganisms and some structural changes in incipient enamel caries. A scanning electron microscopic investigation. *Caries Res.* 1980;14(5):276–84. https://doi.org/10.1159/000260465.

23 Parolo CC, Maltz M. Microbial contamination of noncavitated caries lesions: a scanning electron microscopic study. *Caries Res.* 2006;40(6):536–41. https://doi.org/10.1159/000095654.

24 Ekstrand KR, Bjørndal L. Structural analyses of plaque and caries in relation to the morphology of the groove-fossa system on erupting mandibular third molars. *Caries Res.* 1997;31(5):336–48. https://doi.org/10.1159/000262416.

25 Dige I, Grønkjær L, Nyvad B. Molecular studies of the structural ecology of natural occlusal caries. *Caries Res.* 2014;48(5):451–60. https://doi.org/10.1159/000357920.

26 Smith AJ, Duncan HF, Diogenes A, Simon S, Cooper PR. Exploiting the bioactive properties of the dentin-pulp complex in regenerative endodontics. *J Endod.* 2016;42(1):47–56. https://doi.org/10.1016/j.joen.2015.10.019.

27 Edwardsson S. Bacteriology of dentin caries. In: Thylstrup A, Leach SA, Qvist V (eds.) Dentine and Dentine Reactions in the Oral Cavity, IRL Press, Oxford, 1987, 95–102.

28 Fusayama T. Two layers of carious dentin; diagnosis and treatment. *Oper Dent.* 1979;4(2):63–70.

29 Fusayama T. *New Concepts in Operative Dentistry*, Quintessence Pub Co, Chicago, IL, 1980.

30 Ogawa K, Yamashita Y, Ichijo T, Fusayama T. The ultrastructure and hardness of the transparent layer of human carious dentin. *J Dent Res.* 1983;62(1):7–10. https://doi.org/10.1177/00220345830620011701.

31 Bjørndal L, Larsen T, Thylstrup A. A clinical and microbiological study of deep carious lesions during stepwise excavation using long treatment intervals. *Caries Res.* 1997;31(6):411–7. https://doi.org/10.1159/000262431.

32 Kleter GA. Discoloration of dental carious lesions (a review). *Arch Oral Biol.* 1998;43(8):629–32. https://doi.org/10.1016/s0003-9969(98)00048-x.

33 Reeves R, Stanley HR. The relationship of bacterial penetration and pulpal pathosis in carious teeth. *Oral Surg Oral Med Oral Pathol.* 1966;22(1):59–65. https://doi.org/10.1016/0030-4220(66)90143-5.

34 Demant S, Dabelsteen S, Bjørndal L. A macroscopic and histological analysis of radiographically well-defined deep and extremely deep carious lesions: carious lesion characteristics as indicators of the level of bacterial penetration and pulp response. *Int Endod J.* 2021;54(3):319–30. https://doi.org/10.1111/iej.13424.

35 Massler M. Pulpal reactions to dental caries. *Int Dent J.* 1967;17(2):441–60.

36 Nyvad B, Fejerskov O. Active and inactive root surface caries – structural entities? In: Thylstrup A, Leach SA, Qvist V (eds.) Dentine and Dentine Reactions in the Oral Cavity, IRL Press, Oxford, 1987, 165–79.

37 Schüpbach P, Guggenheim B, Lutz F. Human root caries: histopathology of advanced lesions. *Caries Res.* 1990;24(3):145–58. https://doi.org/10.1159/000261258.

38 Demant S, Schoenmaker T, van Erck SMG, Dabelsteen S, de Vries TJ, Bjørndal L. Intra-pulpal connective tissue formation and the advanced carious lesion: is chondrogenesis and heterotopic ossification a response to pulpal inflammation? *Int Endod J.* 2022;55(11):1212–24. https://doi.org/10.1111/iej.13821.

39 Dey D, Wheatley BM, Cholok D, Agarwal S, Yu PB, Levi B, et al. The traumatic bone: trauma-induced heterotopic ossification. *Transl Res.* 2017;186:95–111. https://doi.org/10.1016/j.trsl.2017.06.004.

40 Baume LJ. The biology of pulp and dentine. In: Myers HM (ed.) Monographs in Oral Science, vol. 8, Karger, Basel, 1980, 67–182.

41 Selden HS. Radiographic pulpal calcifications: normal or abnormal – a paradox. *J Endod.* 1991;17(1):34–7. https://doi.org/10.1016/S0099-2399(07)80159-2.

42 Tibúrcio-Machado CS, Michelon C, Zanatta FB, Gomes MS, Marin JA, Bier CA. The global prevalence of apical periodontitis: a systematic review and meta-analysis. *Int Endod J.* 2021;54(5):712–35. https://doi.org/10.1111/iej.13467.

43 Gesi A, Hakeberg M, Warfvinge J, Bergenholtz G. Incidence of periapical lesions and clinical symptoms after pulpectomy – a clinical and radiographic evaluation of 1-versus 2-session treatment. *Oral Surg Oral Med Oral Pathol Oral Radiol Endod.* 2006;101(3):379–88. https://doi.org/10.1016/j.tripleo.2005.05.073.

44 Eckerbom M, Magnusson T, Martinsson T. Reasons for and incidence of tooth mortality in a Swedish population. *Endod Dent Traumatol.* 1992;8(6):230–4. https://doi.org/10.1111/j.1600-9657.1992.tb00249.x.

45 Bowden GH, Hamilton IR. Environmental pH as a factor in the competition between strains of the oral streptococci *Streptococcus mutans*, *S. sanguis*, and "*S. mitior*" growing in continuous culture. *Can J Microbiol.* 1987;33(9):824–7. https://doi.org/10.1139/m87-143.

46 Bjørndal L, Larsen T. Changes in the cultivable flora in deep carious lesions following a stepwise excavation procedure. *Caries Res.* 2000;34(6):502–8. https://doi.org/10.1159/000016631.

47 Cushley S, Duncan HF, Lundy FT, Nagendrababu V, Clarke M, El Karim I. Outcomes reporting in systematic reviews on vital pulp treatment: a scoping review for the development of a core outcome set. *Int Endod J.* 2022;55(9):891–909. https://doi.org/10.1111/iej.13785.

48 Kidd EA. How 'clean' must a cavity be before restoration? *Caries Res.* 2004;38(3):305–13. https://doi.org/10.1159/000077770.

49 Leksell E, Ridell K, Cvek M, Mejàre I. Pulp exposure after stepwise versus direct complete excavation of deep carious lesions in young posterior permanent teeth. *Endod Dent Traumatol.* 1996;12(4):192–6. https://doi.org/10.1111/j.1600-9657.1996.tb00513.x.

50 Orhan AI, Oz FT, Orhan K. Pulp exposure occurrence and outcomes after 1- or 2-visit indirect pulp therapy vs complete caries removal in primary and permanent molars. *Pediatr Dent.* 2010;32(4):347–55.

51 Bjørndal L, Fransson H, Bruun G, Markvart M, Kjældgaard M, Näsman P, et al. Randomized clinical trials on deep carious lesions: 5-year follow-up. *J Dent Res.* 2017;96(7):747–53. https://doi.org/10.1177/0022034517702620.

52 Khokhar M, Tewari S. Outcomes of partial and complete caries excavation in permanent teeth: a 18 month clinical study. *Contemp Clin Dent.* 2018;9(3):468–73. https://doi.org/10.4103/ccd.ccd_344_18.

53 Bjørndal L, Reit C, Bruun G, Markvart M, Kjaeldgaard M, Näsman P, et al. Treatment of deep caries lesions in adults: randomized clinical trials comparing stepwise vs. direct complete excavation, and direct pulp capping vs. partial pulpotomy. *Eur J Oral Sci.* 2010;118(3):290–7. https://doi.org/10.1111/j.1600-0722.2010.00731.x.

54 Maltz M, Koppe B, Jardim JJ, Alves LS, de Paula LM, Yamaguti PM, et al. Partial caries removal in deep caries lesions: a 5-year multicenter randomized controlled trial. *Clin Oral Investig.* 2018;22(3):1337–43. https://doi.org/10.1007/s00784-017-2221-0.

55 Labib ME, Hassanein OE, Moussa M, Yassen A, Schwendicke F. Selective versus stepwise removal of deep carious lesions in permanent teeth: a randomised controlled trial from Egypt – an interim analysis. *BMJ Open.* 2019;9(9):e030957. https://doi.org/10.1136/bmjopen-2019-030957.

56 Maltz M, Garcia R, Jardim JJ, de Paula LM, Yamaguti PM, Moura MS, et al. Randomized trial of partial vs. stepwise caries removal: 3-year follow-up. *J Dent Res.* 2012;91(11):1026–31. https://doi.org/10.1177/0022034512460403.

57 Maltz M, Jardim JJ, Mestrinho HD, Yamaguti PM, Podestá K, Moura MS, et al. Partial removal of carious dentine: a multicenter randomized controlled trial and 18-month follow-up results. *Caries Res.* 2013;47(2):103–9. https://doi.org/10.1159/000344013.

58 Jardim JJ, Mestrinho HD, Koppe B, de Paula LM, Alves LS, Yamaguti PM, et al. Restorations after selective caries removal: 5-year randomized trial. *J Dent.* 2020;99:103416. https://doi.org/10.1016/j.jdent.2020.103416.

59 Hashem D, Mannocci F, Patel S, et al. Clinical and radiographic assessment of the efficacy of calcium silicate indirect pulp capping: a randomized controlled clinical trial. *J Dent Res.* 2015;94:562–8.

60 Hashem D, Mannocci F, Patel S, Manoharan A, Watson TF, Banerjee A. Evaluation of the efficacy of calcium silicate vs. glass ionomer cement indirect pulp capping and restoration assessment criteria: a randomised controlled clinical trial-2-year results. *Clin Oral Investig.* 2019;23(4):1931–9. https://doi.org/10.1007/s00784-018-2638-0.

61 Koc Vural U, Kiremitci A, Gokalp S. Which is the most effective biomaterial in indirect pulp capping? 4-year comparative randomized clinical trial. *Eur Oral Res.* 2022;56(1):35–41. https://doi.org/10.26650/eor.2022895748.

62 Rahman B, Goswami M. Comparative evaluation of indirect pulp therapy in young permanent teeth using biodentine and theracal: a randomized clinical trial. *J Clin Pediatr Dent.* 2021;45(3):158–64. https://doi.org/10.17796/1053-4625-45.3.3.

63 Alkademi H, Ahemdov N. Treatment outcome of stepwise caries removal in Sweden – a retrospective registry study. Master thesis. Faculty of Odontology, Malmö University, 2018. FULLTEXT01.pdf (diva-portal.org)

64 Rossi-Fedele G, Ng YL. Effectiveness of root canal treatment for vital pulps compared with necrotic pulps in the presence or absence of signs of periradicular pathosis: a systematic review and meta-analysis. *Int Endod J.* 2022. https://doi.org/10.1111/iej.13833. Advance online publication.

65 European Society of Endodontology. Quality guidelines for endodontic treatment: consensus report of the European Society of Endodontology. *Int Endod J.* 2006;39(12):921–30. https://doi.org/10.1111/j.1365-2591.2006.01180.x.

66 American Association of Endodontists. AAE position statement on vital pulp therapy. *J Endod.* 2021;47(9):1340–4. https://doi.org/10.1016/j.joen.2021.07.015.

67 Fransson H, Croft K, Stangvaltaite-Mouhat L, Bletsa A, Bjørndal L. Vital pulp treatments in teeth with deep carious lesions. *Tandläkartidningen.* 2023;2:56–62.

68 Ricucci D, Siqueira JF Jr, Rôças IN, Lipski M, Shiban A, Tay FR. Pulp and dentine responses to selective caries excavation: a histological and histobacteriological human study. *J Dent.* 2020;100:103430. https://doi.org/10.1016/j.jdent.2020.103430.

69 Schwendicke F, Stolpe M, Meyer-Lueckel H, Paris S, Dörfer CE. Cost-effectiveness of one- and two-step incomplete and complete excavations. *J Dent Res.* 2013;92(10):880–7. https://doi.org/10.1177/0022034513500792.

70 Savolainen N, Kvist T, Mannila J. Cost-effectiveness of partial versus stepwise caries removal of deep caries lesions – a decision-analytic approach. *Acta Odontol Scand.* 2023;81(4):311–8. https://doi.org/10.1080/00016357.2022.2143893.

71 Schwendicke F, Stangvaltaite L, Holmgren C, Maltz M, Finet M, Elhennawy K, et al. Dentists' attitudes and behaviour regarding deep carious lesion management: a multi-national survey. *Clin Oral Investig.* 2017;21(1):191–8. https://doi.org/10.1007/s00784-016-1776-5.

72 Crespo-Gallardo I, Hay-Levytska O, Martín-González J, Jiménez-Sánchez MC, Sánchez-Domínguez B, Segura-Egea JJ. Criteria and treatment decisions in the management of deep caries lesions: is there endodontic overtreatment? *J Clin Exp Dent.* 2018;10(8):e751–60. https://doi.org/10.4317/jced.55050.

73 Croft K, Kervanto-Seppälä S, Stangvaltaite L, Kerosuo E. Management of deep carious lesions and pulps exposed during carious tissue removal in adults: a questionnaire study among dentists in Finland. *Clin Oral Investig.* 2019;23(3):1271–80. https://doi.org/10.1007/s00784-018-2556-1.

74 Edwards D, Bailey O, Stone S, Duncan H. The management of deep caries in UK primary care: a nationwide questionnaire-based study. *Int Endod J.* 2021;54(10):1804–18. https://doi.org/10.1111/iej.13585.

75 Croft K, Kervanto-Seppälä S, Kerosuo E. Deep carious lesions and their management among Finnish adolescents: a retrospective radiographic study. *Clin Oral Investig.* 2022;26(11):6503–10. https://doi.org/10.1007/s00784-022-04599-3.

76 Donnermeyer D, Dammaschke T, Lipski M, Schäfer E. Effectiveness of diagnosing pulpitis: a systematic review. *Int Endod J.* 2022. https://doi.org/10.1111/iej.13762. Advance online publication.

5

Vital Pulp Treatment Modalities

Direct Pulp Capping

Till Dammaschke

Department of Periodontology and Operative Dentistry, University of Münster, Münster, Germany

Is Exposing the Pulp a Problem? An Introduction

As early as 1756, Philipp Pfaff (1713–1766; Royal Prussian Court Dentist to Frederick the Great) recognized that the vitality of the dental pulp could be preserved after exposure by providing it with a small cap made of thin gold foil (1). In the absence of suitable expertise for root canal preparation and obturation, interest in such treatment measures was high, and they were widely used, as the only alternative to maintaining pulp vitality was usually extraction of the tooth to relieve pain. In the following centuries, attempts were made to preserve pulp vitality under all circumstances, and as a result, a plethora of different materials and methods for direct pulp capping were propagated. Unfortunately, these methods were often not suitable for successfully maintaining pulp vitality and were usually doomed to failure (2). Therefore, in 1922, Hans-Hermann Rebel (1889–1967) formulated his doctrine: 'An exposed pulp is a lost organ' (3). Some years later, around 1930, Bernhard W. Hermann (1884–1954) introduced calcium hydroxide as an agent for maintaining pulp vitality and was able to prove histologically that vital pulp treatment (VPT) can be successfully performed using this material if the indication is correct (4, 5). Nevertheless, the doctrine formulated by Rebel a hundred years ago has persisted even today so that some dentists are of the opinion that exposure of the pulp tissue must be avoided at all costs, and it is, therefore, preferable to leave carious dentine in the cavity beneath the filling. Furthermore, many possess the opinion that – if pulp exposure does occur – vital extirpation and root canal treatment are unavoidable.

Both doctrines have been proven not to be true. It is now known that the principle of wound healing at the pulp is no different from that of other tissues of the body. Wound healing is always the programmed response of the host to an injury. The goal is to regenerate or repair the tissue (6). Thus, there has been an encouraging renaissance of interest in VPT. The purpose of direct pulp capping is to protect the pulp tissue and stimulate new hard tissue formation through an appropriate wound dressing. This should preserve the vitality of the tooth (7, 8).

It is well known that teeth can be preserved in the long term by adequately performing root canal treatment. For example, several years ago, the so-called 'Toronto study' showed that in teeth with apical lesions, the success rate four to six years after root canal treatment was 79% and without initial apical lesions (e.g. after vital extirpation) 93% (9). However, one problem with root canal-treated teeth is that a non-vital tooth can be loaded with more than twice the masticatory force compared

Vital Pulp Treatment, First Edition. Edited by Henry F. Duncan and Ikhlas A. El-Karim.

with a vital tooth before the proprioceptors respond (10, 11). This means that root canal-treated teeth do not register foreign bodies in food, for example, until they bite down harder, which in the long term can lead to mechanical overload and fracture of the tooth. Other problems that can occur after root canal treatment include increased susceptibility to caries due to increased plaque accumulation and altered microflora (12) and tooth discolouration (13). Root canal treatment may also prove to be more complex than initially anticipated, which may affect the success of the treatment. If the initial root canal treatment is unsuccessful, a more complex procedure (re-treatment or apicectomy) may be required to save the tooth (14, 15).

In contrast, direct pulp capping is a non-invasive, comparatively simple technique that can be performed with a significantly lower expenditure of time than root canal treatment, does not entail costly restorations and is, therefore, cost-effective (16). In addition, the vital pulp offers the best protection against the invasion of microorganisms into the root canal system. When correctly indicated and performed, direct pulp capping is associated with high success rates comparable with root canal treatment (14, 15).

Management of Traumatic and Iatrogenic Pulp Exposures

The pulp can either be exposed during caries excavation or as a consequence of trauma. In the case of dental trauma, the enamel and dentine can be fractured by the application of force, so that the pulp tissue is exposed (Figure 5.1). These so-called 'complicated' crown fractures predominantly affect caries- and restoration-free teeth of juvenile patients. Therefore, the dentine around the exposure area is free of microbial colonization (17–19). The same applies when the pulp is exposed by the removal of sound dentine during operative procedures, the so-called iatrogenic exposure of the dental pulp (20). In both cases, the prognosis of direct pulp capping can be considered good, since the existence of a 'healthy' pulp that has not been damaged by caries and is therefore capable of regeneration can be assumed (18, 19). In the case of trauma with additional dislocation injuries, however, the situation may be aggravated by the fact that the blood supply and thus the defence capability of the pulp tissue of the fractured tooth is compromised (21).

Preparation of cavities or crowns could also lead to an exposure of dentinal tubules, so direct access for bacterial toxins to the pulp is created without exposing the pulp tissue itself (20). In

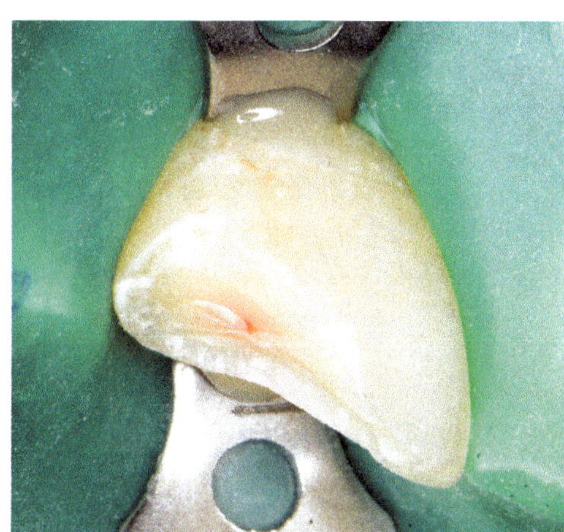

Figure 5.1 Tooth 21 with a complicated crown fracture after trauma, resulting in exposure of the pulp. The prognosis of direct pulp capping can be considered good, since the tooth is caries-free and there were no microorganisms in the dentine and near the pulp before the trauma.

adolescents, an additional complication is that the dentine-pulp complex is even more susceptible to microbial contamination due to the presence of very wide dentinal tubules (17).

If saliva and, thus, microorganisms from the oral cavity penetrate the portion of the crown pulp exposed by trauma or iatrogenically, the pulp tissue must be considered microbially contaminated. The depth of this contamination correlates with the duration of exposure of the pulp tissue to the oral cavity. The longer the exposed area remains unattended, the deeper the microorganisms penetrate into the pulp tissue. Therefore, in both cases, i.e. after traumatic as well as iatrogenic exposure of the pulp, VPT must be performed as quickly as possible (17).

It is known from animal experiments that traumatic or iatrogenic pulp exposure leads to superficial alterations in the pulp tissue (22), but the microbial contamination after an exposure time of 2 hours to a maximum of 24 hours can be classified as low, so direct pulp capping is still possible (23, 24). In the case of a longer pulp exposure time of up to seven days, an infection or inflammation to a depth of approximately 2 mm can be assumed (18, 19). In this case, direct pulp capping is no longer indicated. Instead, a partial or complete pulpotomy must be performed (see Chapter 8. Vital Pulp Treatment for Traumatic Dental Injuries). In general, however, partial pulpotomy after trauma has a higher certainty of success than direct pulp capping and is, therefore, to be favoured in these cases.

With regard to tooth survival, higher success rates are generally reported in the literature for direct pulp capping in these teeth compared with carious teeth, since there has presumably been no or only minimal contamination of the pulp tissue with microorganisms prior to capping (17, 25). Thus, iatrogenic exposure of the pulp in caries-free dentine or after tooth trauma provides ideal conditions for VPT in most cases and should not be reserved only for children and adolescents (18, 19).

In contrast, caries invasion of the pulp leads to microbial infection of the pulp, resulting in pulp inflammation (26). As a result, the pulp has a reduced capacity to respond and heal compared with mechanical exposure, where there is no pre-existing inflammation (25).

Indications for Direct Pulp Capping

The basic prerequisite for successful VPT is vital pulp tissue that is capable of regeneration. The problem is that the exact condition of the pulp is difficult to determine clinically (27). In most cases, a textbook distinction is made between reversible and irreversible pulpitis. This clinical diagnosis is based on objective but also subjective findings. According to the definition, in reversible pulpitis, the inflammation is assumed to subside and the pulp should return to normal. In irreversible pulpitis, the vital pulp has a high level of inflammation that is not compatible with healing (28).

Clinically, reversible pulpitis is characterized by pain that is tied to a stimulus. The painful tooth can be localized by the patient, and the sensibility test is positive (29). Histologically, there are moderate signs of inflammation, migrated lymphocytes and plasma cells, hyperaemia, a decrease in cell count, odontoblasts appear flatter and most importantly, no or hardly any bacteria in the pulp chamber. In contrast, in irreversible pulpitis, irritation stimulated, sustained pain or even spontaneous pain, pain on heat, with the offending tooth not clearly locatable by the patient. The sensibility test is positive, which makes diagnosis difficult for the dentist. Histologically, there are signs of inflammation with polymorphonuclear neutrophilic granulocytes, micro-abscesses and even partial necrosis caused by bacteria that have already invaded the pulp chamber (30).

The presence of microorganisms in the pulp tissue is decisive for whether pulpitis can heal (reversible) or not (irreversible). However, this cannot be readily determined clinically, as irreversible pulpitis can be clinically asymptomatic in 14–60% of cases (29, 31). Thus, in pulpitis, the histologic findings frequently deviate from the clinical picture. Thus, in 15.6% of cases, the clinical and histological diagnosis do not coincide (30). In other histological examinations, a discrepancy between clinical and histological findings could even be shown in 60–80% of cases, i.e. pulpal changes were clinically underestimated ('hypodiagnosis') (32, 33).

The clinical classification of the symptoms into reversible and irreversible pulpitis, therefore, says little about the actual regenerative capacity of the tissue and is therefore increasingly questioned (27). It merely facilitates the treatment decision for the practitioner, as a schematic approach can be taken (7).

Spontaneous pain or even pain in response to a stimulus (e.g. in the sensibility test) does not provide a reliable indication of the condition of the pulp. Even with irreversible pulpitis, a patient does not necessarily respond to a cold or heat test with pain. Pain does not correlate with the extent of inflammation, is always subjective and cannot be detected histologically (34).

If the pulp tissue is exposed during treatment, the bleeding of the tissue can be used for diagnostic purposes. The extent of the pulp haemorrhage can be considered a more reliable diagnostic method than the sensibility test and pain symptoms. If the pulp tissue is free of inflammation or if only superficial inflammation has occurred as a result of the caries, the pulp bleeding is weak. If, on the other hand, microorganisms or bacterial toxins have already penetrated the pulp and the inflammatory reaction extends deeper into the tissue, the pulp bleeding is more severe. The extent of bleeding may, therefore, reflect the degree of pulp inflammation. Prolonged or severe bleeding is indicative of irreversible pulpitis. Therefore, pulp tissue with severe or persistent haemorrhage has been reported to have a significantly worse chance of healing (35–38). But, not all studies have shown this, e.g. Careddu and Duncan could proof that prolonged bleeding time (as well as preoperative tenderness to percussion) was not an indicator of higher failure rates (39).

In clinical studies, haemostasis was achieved within six minutes after partial or total pulpotomy in 84% of cases in teeth with symptoms of irreversible pulpitis, and the pulp was vital after capping (40, 41). Clinically, it should, therefore, be possible to control pulp haemorrhage within approximately five minutes (7), although it must be emphasized that scientific evidence as to the prolonged bleeding time above which the pulp must be considered unsuitable for vital preservation is still lacking (27). Several studies reported successful VPT even after bleeding times of up to 25 minutes (42, 43).

The exact correlation between haemorrhage and pulp inflammation is still unclear. However, it can be concluded that in a healthy, uninfected pulp, pulp haemorrhage stops on its own or can be easily controlled, whereas in an inflamed pulp, profuse haemorrhage should be expected (35–38) (Figure 5.2a,b).

Factors Affecting the Outcomes of Direct Pulp Capping

Patient Age

Patient age *per se* is not a contraindication for direct pulp capping. In patients of advancing age, the regenerative power of the pulp tissue seems to decrease (8, 17) as pulp volume, vascularity, immune defence and functional repair mechanisms decrease (44, 45). However, in principle, direct pulp

(a) (b)

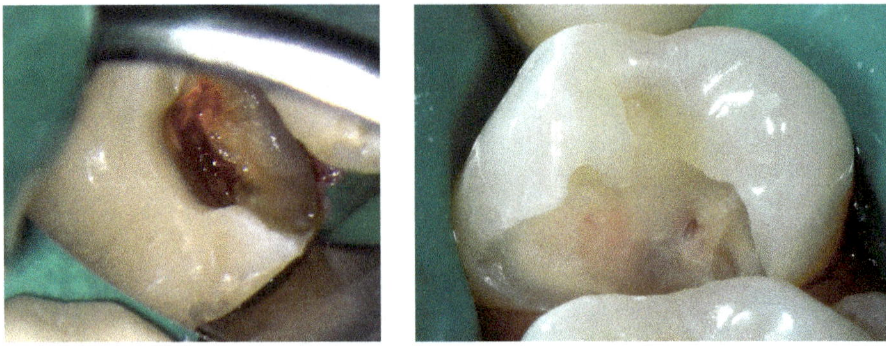

Figure 5.2 (a) Pronounced bleeding from the pulp tissue exposed over a small area is an indication that microorganisms have invaded the pulp. Instead of direct capping, partial pulpotomy may be indicated in this case. (b) Correct haemostasis after exposure of the pulp tissue with NaOCl 3%. This is a proxy measure that no microorganisms have penetrated the tissue and that there is, therefore, a high probability of being able to preserve the pulp vitality by direct capping.

(a) (b)

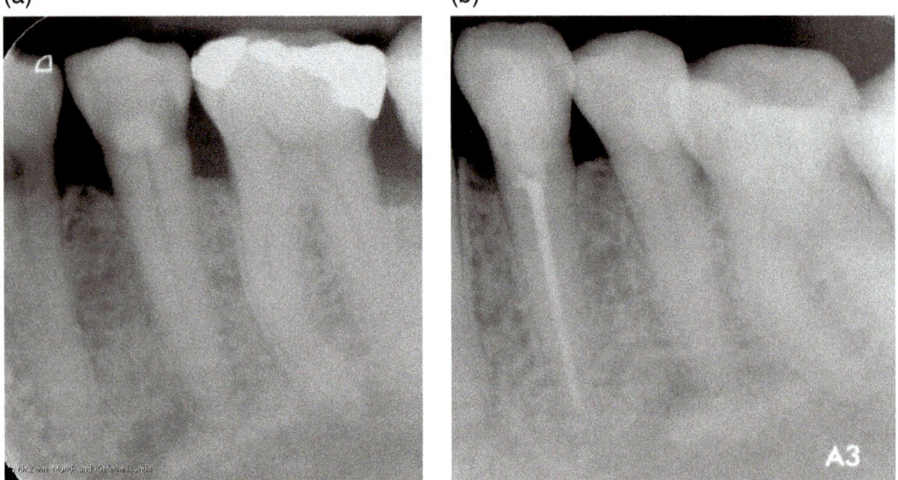

Figure 5.3 (a) Preoperative radiograph of a 77-year-old patient shows caries distal to Tooth 35. Exposure of the pulp occurred during caries excavation. The patient's age does not contraindicate an attempt at vital preservation. (b) Radiograph of the Tooth 35 five years after direct capping with a hydraulic calcium silicate cement (Biodentine). No pathological changes could be detected apically on Tooth 35. The patient, now 82 years old, was symptom-free and the tooth was unremarkable in the sensitivity and percussion tests. Tooth 34 had to undergo root canal treatment in the meantime.

capping can be successfully performed in older patients (Figure 5.3a,b). However, the chronological age of the patient does not necessarily correlate with the healing capacity of the pulp. Rather, the biological age of the tissue is relevant, i.e. the history of a tooth during its functional period. Teeth with a history of trauma, extensive restorations, or intrapulpal mineralization tend to have a worse prognosis than teeth with a primary carious defect (8, 17) (Figure 5.4).

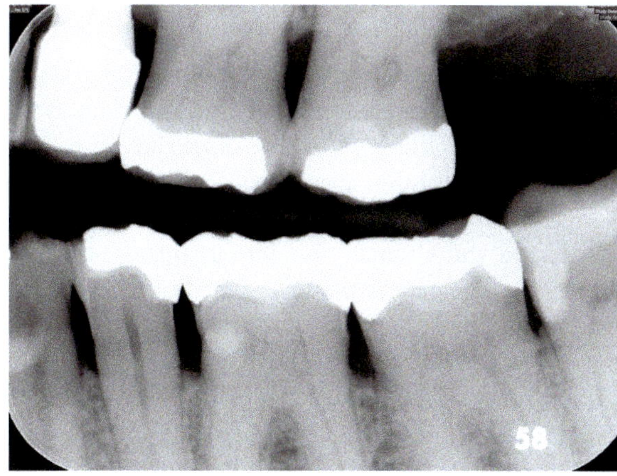

Figure 5.4 The intrapulpal hard tissue formations on the molar teeth may indicate pre-damage of the pulp, as the tissue reacts to inflammation with mineralization. This is caused by the extensive restorations with presumably preceding caries. The regenerative capacity of the pulp may then be limited – regardless of the age of the patient.

Exposure Size

It is known from many studies that the exposure size has no influence on the success of direct pulp capping. The requirement that the exposure area of the pulp chamber should be a maximum 1 mm^2 in size cannot be sustained today. When treating the pulp after trauma or partial pulpotomy, the pulp tissue is exposed over a large area. Nevertheless, direct pulp capping can be successful as long as infection of the tissue with microorganisms can be avoided (8, 17) (Figure 5.5). However, it should be kept in mind that if the pulp is exposed over a large area during caries excavation, large-scale penetration of bacteria into the dentine has probably also occurred. This extensive contamination of the tissue may reduce the chances of success of direct pulp capping. If necessary, a partial pulpotomy can be performed in this case (see Chapter 6. Vital Pulp Treatment Modalities: Pulpotomy – Partial and Complete).

Location of the Pulp Exposure

The position of the pulp exposure has been discussed as a factor influencing the prognosis of direct pulp capping. However, presumably, the location of the cavity (occlusal or incisal versus cervical or lateral) does not influence the success of direct pulp capping. Nor do there appear to be significant differences in prognosis for specific tooth groups (anterior, premolars, molars) or jaws (maxillary or mandibular) (8, 17).

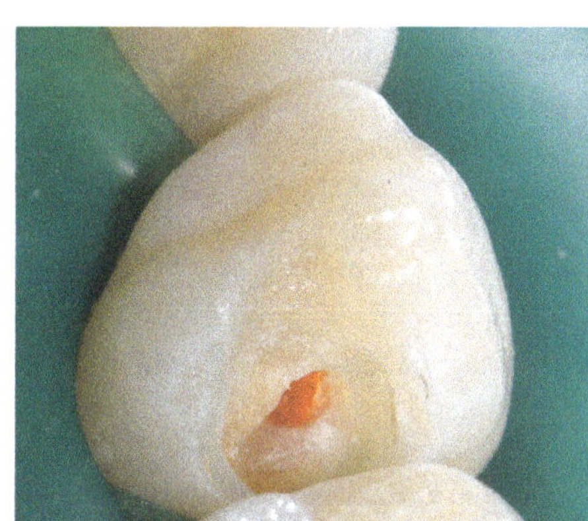

Figure 5.5 If the pulp tissue is not inflamed, the size of the pulp exposure has no influence on the success of direct pulp capping.

Microorganisms

Only a non-inflamed, bacteria-free pulp can maintain vitality in the long term, i.e. in the absence of microbial infections, human dental pulp shows a proven regenerative capacity when directly capped with calcium hydroxide suspension or hydraulic calcium silicate cement (HCSC) (7, 8). Microorganisms and their metabolites play a crucial role in the development of pathogenic pulpal changes and periapical diseases. Kakehashi et al. demonstrated in a histological study of germ-free rats that in the absence of microorganisms, the pulp has the regenerative power to close an exposure site by hard tissue regeneration, even in the absence of capping material or final restoration. The presence or absence of microorganisms is the determining factor in the healing of exposed pulp tissue (46).

Due to the protected location of bacteria in the dentinal tubules during the carious process, phagocytosis (killing of microorganisms) by defence cells from the bloodstream does not occur until the pulp tissue is in direct contact with the caries (47–49). This is a major problem with direct pulp capping because pulp tissue infected with microorganisms loses its regenerative capacity (50)

It does not even have to be the microorganisms directly that cause inflammation of the pulp tissue. It is sufficient that metabolic products produced by the bacteria, so-called endotoxins, such as lipopolysaccharides and lipoteichoic acid, diffuse into the pulp via dentinal tubules to cause an inflammatory reaction (51–54). Therefore, to exclude pulp infection during or after direct pulp capping, treatment should always be performed with sterile instruments under dental dam application. The caries should be completely excavated and the cavity disinfected and definitively restored with a bacteria-proof restoration (7, 8).

Caries Excavation

With regard to the preservation of the vitality of the pulp, the therapy of deep, caries-altered dentine has been the subject of controversial discussion for decades. The recommended therapeutic spectrum ranges from leaving the carious dentine largely intact to complete excavation into the caries-free dentine. The following different and partly contradictory concepts can be distinguished: Ultraconservative caries excavation, selective caries excavation, two-stage incomplete caries excavation, two-stage complete caries excavation and complete caries excavation (55, 56).

With the exception of two-stage and complete caries excavation, all other excavation concepts deliberately leave dentinal caries in place close to the pulp. Thus (in the spirit of Rebel (3)), avoiding pulp exposure is the prime objective. The idea behind this is to apply a tight adhesive seal over the remaining carious dentine and thus cut off the caries bacteria from access to fermentable carbohydrates (substrate). The bacteria are said to 'starve' under the filling without a substrate supply. Recently, therefore, the so-called 'selective caries excavation' has been recommended as an alternative to complete caries excavation (55, 56). The pros and cons of different concepts of caries excavation are not the focus of this chapter on direct pulp capping. However, the following considerations should be kept in mind: In addition to cariogenic bacteria, which metabolize carbohydrates from food, certain anaerobic asaccharolytic bacteria, which use nitrogenous substrates for energy, also occur in infected dentine. Proteins and glycoproteins from demineralized collagen and tissue fluid from the dentinal tubules serve as food. These anaerobic asaccharolytic bacteria, therefore, do not require a substrate supply from 'outside' and can remain active even under dense, dentine-adhesive fillings. The degradation products of these microorganisms can then lead to chronic inflammation of the pulp tissue (57–60).

Bacteria left in the dentine always pose a risk of caries recurrence and, even after the microorganisms have died, form a reservoir of endotoxins. They can maintain inflammatory processes in the pulp (61). Endotoxins readily diffuse through 0.5 mm thick dentine (51). Endotoxins that have penetrated the pulp release inflammatory mediators from odontoblasts and macrophages, leading to chronic inflammation of the pulp tissue (54). Therefore, even inactive caries histologically lead to changes in the pulp tissue (62). Consequently, histologically, chronic pulp inflammation may occur after 'selective caries excavation'. Due to the bacterial infection, ideal healing is not to be expected. However, the teeth are clinically asymptomatic and react inconspicuously to a sensibility test. Patients' clinical responses to the sensibility test may not correlate with histologic findings (63–65). Therefore, merely considering the absence of clinical symptoms after 'selective caries excavation' as a treatment success is too short-sighted. Only histological analysis can assess the actual condition of the dental pulp tissue after 'selective caries excavation' (26, 27). Such histological studies prove that the pulp remains free of inflammation in the long term after 'selective caries excavation' has been lacking. Therefore, these clinical results of 'selective caries excavation' should be interpreted with caution. A direct comparison of 'selective caries excavation' with complete excavation and subsequent capping of the pulp showed that 'selective caries excavation' histologically leads to chronic inflammation of the pulp in 68–100% of cases and thus to a failure of the treatment. In contrast, complete caries excavation followed by indirect or direct pulp capping with calcium hydroxide resulted in histological failure in only 7–33%. In all cases, patients were clinically symptom-free throughout the follow-up period of three months to five years (63, 64). Accordingly, a higher probability of success of 'selective caries excavation' compared with VPT after pulp exposure cannot be established (7). Hence, the current statement of the American Association of Endodontists (AAE) on VPT calls for complete caries removal and the elimination of all infected tissues (66). Thus, to prevent bacterial contamination of the pulp, the goal of caries excavation should be to completely remove the infected dentine – even at the risk of exposing the pulp tissue – and to directly cap the pulp with biocompatible and potentially bioactive materials (e.g. HCSC).

Haemostasis and Cavity Disinfection

As already mentioned, adequate haemostasis must be ensured if pulp tissue is exposed. Pulp haemorrhage should be easily controlled. Increased bleeding may indicate a higher degree of inflammation in the pulp, leading to a reduced ability to repair (26). In addition to pulp diagnostics, it is also important that the capping material be applied directly onto the exposed pulp tissue. No blood residue should remain between the wound dressing and the pulp tissue. A blood coagulum restricts the formation of hard tissue and thus pulp healing, since a blood coagulum is a breeding ground for possibly remaining pathogenic microorganisms. In addition, chemotactic inflammatory mediators are released into the pulp tissue, which leads to a chronic inflammatory state of the pulp and not to healing (67, 68).

A third reason for effective haemostasis is that the moisture and contamination of the dentine near the exposed site due to bleeding may make it more difficult to get a pulp-capping material to adhere to dentine. If the capping material does not adhere properly to the dentine, leaks occur and microorganisms can migrate into the pulp (26).

Haemostasis can ideally be performed together with cavity disinfection. Traditionally, hydrogen peroxide (H_2O_2) was often used to clean the cavity after caries excavation. It acts as a peroxidase on tissue catalases, releasing nascent oxygen. H_2O_2 has a little corrosive or toxic effect on pulp tissue, shows good haemostasis in exposed pulp and mechanical cleaning effects due to foaming in contact with blood. However, the disinfecting effect of H_2O_2 is mostly overestimated and may not be sufficient for cavity disinfection in the context of caries excavation (8). Histologically, it has been found that after haemostasis with H_2O_2, emphysema formation may occur in the pulp, which has a negative effect on healing (69).

Sodium hypochlorite (NaOCl) at a concentration of about 3% seems to be much more suitable in this case. NaOCl is effective in haemostasis, has a disinfecting effect on dentine surfaces, and removes blood, fibrin and biofilm residues from dentine surfaces, as well as dentine chips and damaged pulp cells from the superficial pulp tissue. NaOCl has a non-toxic effect on pulp tissue and does not appear to interfere with the healing of the exposed pulp. It is even possible that the high pH of NaOCl is beneficial to pulp healing. NaOCl at concentrations below 2.5% is probably not sufficiently effective in terms of disinfection and haemostasis. Concentrations above 5%, on the other hand, may be too aggressive and thus damaging to the tissue (8).

Nevertheless, a histological study showed that after rinsing for 15 minutes with 5 ml NaOCl 5.25%, dissolution effects occurred on the vital pulp tissue, but these were limited to the superficial three to five cell layers. There were no changes in deeper pulp areas and no changes in the dentine. Presumably, the perfused pulp tissue buffers the effect of NaOCl (70). Due to this superficial tissue-dissolving effect, a kind of 'chemical amputation' of the pulp probably occurs, whereby irreversibly damaged pulp cells are removed (71). Therefore, a randomized clinical trial clearly demonstrated that the use of NaOCl for cavity disinfection significantly improves success rates in direct pulp capping. In 84 patients, the pulp was exposed during complete caries excavation. After irrigation of the pulp wound with either isotonic saline (0.9% NaCl) or NaOCl (2.5%) and direct pulp capping with MTA, survival rates after one year were only 55% in the saline group but 89% in the NaOCl group (71).

Conversely, it could be disadvantageous that NaOCl negatively influences the adhesion of dentine adhesives and composite resins to dentine. However, the reported data is inconsistent in this respect. For some dentine adhesives, dentine pretreatment with NaOCl has no significant effect on the adhesion of the resin-based composite restoration (72). To be on the safe side, the cavity should be rinsed again with water before definitive adhesive restoration (7, 8).

Chlorhexidine digluconate (CHX) at a concentration of 2% is a possible alternative to NaOCl (73). Histologically, there was no significant difference in pulp healing and pulp tissue morphology after haemostasis with NaOCl (0.5–5.25%) and CHX (2%) in direct pulp capping. Both solutions showed no negative effects on the pulp tissue (74, 75). However, in general, the disinfecting effect of CHX 2% on carious dentine is lower than that of NaOCl (76). Therefore, CHX mouth rinsing solutions in a concentration of 0.1–0.2% should not be used here, as they are neither sufficiently antimicrobial nor sufficiently haemostatic.

In paediatric dentistry, ferric sulphate has been recommended for arresting pulp haemorrhage on deciduous teeth. In permanent teeth, these haemostatic agents such as ferric sulphate, aluminium chloride and other materials are not indicated because they would 'mask' the true inflammatory state of the pulp due to their high effectiveness in stopping bleeding (77). One might thus be tempted to directly cap a pulp that is irreversibly inflamed. Moreover, these substances are tissue-damaging and may interfere with wound healing (78). Thus, after haemostasis with ferric sulphate, postoperative discomfort was significantly more common after direct pulp capping (26).

Selection of the Pulp Capping Material

Calcium hydroxide suspensions have been considered the universal standard material for maintaining pulp vitality since the first publications by B. W. Hermann around 1930 (4, 5). The desirable properties of calcium hydroxide include an initial high alkaline pH, which is responsible for stimulating cells and enzymes of the pulp. It neutralizes both the low pH acids produced by cariogenic bacteria and bacterial toxins, inhibits macrophages and, thus, inflammation, exhibits antibacterial properties and promotes defence mechanisms and pulp tissue repair. The disadvantages of calcium hydroxide include poor sealing to dentine, mechanical instability and resorption over time (79). The slow decay of calcium hydroxide after hard tissue formation may lead to microleakage and allow slow penetration of microorganisms through defects (80). Tunnel defects have been demonstrated in the hard tissue formed after direct pulp capping with calcium hydroxide, through which bacteria and their toxins may then secondarily enter the pulp (81).

In order to compensate for the disadvantages of aqueous calcium hydroxide suspensions, in the 1960s, other delivery forms of calcium hydroxide such as hard setting cement (calcium salicylate ester cement; e.g. Dycal, Dentsply Sirona or Kerr Life, Kerr Dental) were developed. In contrast to aqueous calcium hydroxide suspension, hard-setting calcium hydroxide cements offer a better seal of the dentine-pulp complex. But, these preparations show a lower release of hydroxyl ions, resulting in a lower pH value and a significantly weaker antimicrobial effect (79, 82). In addition, hard-setting calcium salicylate ester cement dissolves under the overlaying restoration in the long term (79, 83) and, therefore, does not provide the necessary permanent support for the main filling (84). Hard tissue formation under calcium salicylate ester cement develops more slowly and is less uniform. Hard tissue regeneration is, therefore, weaker compared to aqueous calcium hydroxide suspensions. In addition, inflammation occurs more frequently (68, 85, 86). Some additives necessary for the setting of calcium hydroxide cements may possibly have a toxic effect on the pulp (86). Hence, salicylate ester-based hard-setting calcium hydroxide cement cannot be recommended as a first-choice agent for direct pulp capping (7, 8, 17).

HCSCs consist of a cement powder mixed with water. The main components of the powder are tri- and/or dicalcium silicate, which are also found in Portland cement. During hydration, i.e. when the cement sets, calcium hydroxide is formed, i.e. calcium and hydroxyl ions are released (87). Identical to calcium hydroxide preparations, calcium ions have a positive effect on pulp cell regeneration. HCSC, therefore, stimulates the mitotic index of pulp cells (88). Hydroxyl ions contribute to a sustained alkaline pH (89, 90) and stimulate the release of growth factors and cytokines from the surrounding dentine, which also amounts to the formation of reparative hard tissue (91). In addition to calcium hydroxide, silicon is released during the HCSC setting (92). The exact function of silicon in hard tissue formation is unclear, but it probably plays a role in the early stages of mineralization (93) and contributes to the induction of hard tissue formation (94). Furthermore, silicon can remineralize demineralized dentine *in vitro* (95). Another key advantage of HCSCs in pulp capping is that they interfere with the modulation of inflammatory and pain mediators at the molecular level. Application of HCSC to the exposed pulp tissue results in decreased vascularization and vasodilation, as well as decreased recruitment of inflammatory cells. As a result, tissue pressure within the pulp decreases, and so does the pain response. Therefore, after pulp capping, both inflammatory responses and pain are suppressed. This has a positive effect on the healing process and the patient´s well-being after treatment (96).

The setting properties of HCSCs are not affected by the presence of tissue fluids or blood. They are, therefore, also referred to as 'hydraulic' cement, as they set in contact with both air and water (87). HCSC forms a tight bond to the dentine. The small particle size of HCSC allows penetration of these cement particles into the dentinal tubules (97), which produces adhesion to dentine comparable to that of glass ionomer cement (98). In combination with the alkaline pH, this also helps to trap residual cariogenic bacteria at the transition from dentine to HCSC, thus preventing bacterial advancement, caries progression and persistent pulp damage (99).

Upon contact with calcium- and phosphate-containing (body) fluids, these cements exhibit hydroxyapatite-like crystal formation on their surfaces (100, 101). Osteoblasts, cementoblasts, periodontal ligament cells and (in the case of capping) pulp cells, therefore, deposit directly on the HCSC surface, as the material is recognized as 'non-foreign', which explains the biocompatibility of these cement (102).

Overall, all data available to date indicate that HCSC is a biocompatible, non-cytotoxic material that promotes an antibacterial environment and surface morphology favourable for the reparative formation of hard tissue. HCSC stimulates the release of dentine matrix components necessary for hard tissue repair and regeneration in mechanically exposed healthy and partially inflamed pulps (7, 103). However, odontoblast-like cells and the formation of dentine or dentine-like tissue could not be detected after direct pulp capping with an HCSC (RetroMTA; BioMTA, Daejeon, Korea). Therefore, the newly formed hard tissue was not 'regular dentine' and does not appear to be the product of the differentiation of pulp cells into odontoblasts (104). This observation is identical to the results after direct pulp capping with calcium hydroxide (105). Therefore, hard tissue formation after direct pulp capping appears to be dystrophic intrapulpal mineralization in response to therapy (104, 105).

The advantages of these HCSCs compared to the typically used calcium hydroxide products are the higher mechanical strength, the lower solubility and the better sealing of the dentine. Disadvantages of calcium hydroxide are avoided when using HCSC: dissolution of the capping material as well as mechanical instability and, thus, long-term protection against bacterial microleakage. HCSCs appear very promising in pulp vitality preservation. Recent studies seem to support their potential and extended use in maintaining pulp vitality (8, 103).

ProRoot MTA (Tulsa/Dentsply, Tulsa, OK, USA) was the first HCSC to be introduced into dentistry in the mid-1990s. One disadvantage of ProRoot MTA is that it can cause discolouration of the tooth. This can be particularly problematic in the pulp capping of anterior teeth after trauma (106). The discolouration is due to heavy metals contained in the MTA, such as bismuth oxide (used as a radiographic contrast agent) (107, 108) or iron (109). The discolouration is mainly caused by the oxidation of these metals after contact with NaOCl or the uptake of blood components (109, 110). Other HCSCs contain less or small amounts of heavy metals and their potential to discolour teeth is minimal. HCSCs with zirconia, zirconia, or tantalum oxide as the radiographic contrast agent are particularly stable in colour (106).

Since the introduction of ProRoot MTA, a variety of new HCSCs have been developed, such as Biodentine (Septodont, St. Maur-des Fossés, France) (111). Thus, more than 40 different HCSCs are currently commercially available internationally. Studies have demonstrated physicochemical and bioinductive properties comparable to MTA, indicating a promising application in vital maintenance (111, 112). In general, HCSCs are superior to all calcium hydroxide products in maintaining pulp vitality, with no significant differences between the various HCSCs in terms of mode of action (113).

In contrast to HCSC and calcium hydroxide, all light-, dual- or auto-curing materials containing monomers such as dentine adhesives or composite resins are not suitable for pulp capping. This also applies to composite resins where calcium hydroxide, Portland cement or calcium silicate has been added as a filler (7, 8, 17). (For further details, see Chapter 7. Vital Pulp Treatment: Material Selection.)

Definitive Restoration

In order to reliably prevent (re)contamination of the dentine-pulp complex, the cavity must be restored with a bacteria-proof, definitive filling in the same treatment appointment after direct pulp capping. Ideally, this should be done with a dentine-adhesive and resin-based composite

Box 5.1 Prerequisite for Successful Direct Pulp Capping

Vital pulp treatment (VPT) can only be successful if bacterial infection of the pulp can be reliably excluded before, during and after therapy (7, 8). Therefore, the following must be observed for successful direct pulp capping:

- The tooth should be free of symptoms or should show only mild symptoms of reversible pulpitis beforehand.
- There should be no signs and symptoms indicative of 'irreversible pulpitis' present.
- Dental dam and controlled draining from treatment in the pulp-near dentine third.
- Reduce microbes by using sterile instruments.
- Complete caries excavation.
- Bleeding from the exposed pulp can be controlled without difficulty.
- Disinfecting the cavity and sufficient haemostasis with approx. 3% NaOCl (or 2% CHX).
- Antibacterial wound dressing (ideally HCSC).
- Bacteria-proof final restoration (adhesive composite resin filling) in the same treatment session.
- Patient age, size and location of pulp exposure, and tooth type have no significant effect on success (17).

In all other cases, pulpotomy may be indicated in some circumstances to preserve tooth vitality (see Chapter 6. Vital Pulp Treatment Modalities: Pulpotomy – Partial and Complete). However, a dental dam and a well-placed, sealing coronal restoration in the same treatment session are still mandatory.

restoration. If the cavity is only restored with a temporary material (such as glass ionomer cement) after direct pulp capping, the success rate of VPT decreases significantly (14, 114). If a bacteria-proof, definitive filling is not possible in the same treatment session, this argues against the attempt to preserve pulp vitality (7, 8) (Box 5.1).

Contraindications for Direct Pulp Capping

If the previously listed points cannot be observed, direct pulp capping should be avoided. Another contraindication is the lack of retention for the capping material (wound dressing), e.g. when the pulp is exposed during crown preparation. Repeated, extended restorations close to the pulp from pretreatments can also be expected to limit the possibility of pulp regeneration. The same applies to radiologically visible intrapulpal changes such as denticles or pulp stones. This is usually an indication that the pulp is probably damaged and healing reduced. In the case of periodontal-endodontic lesions and radiologically visible apical changes, VPT is contraindicated, since, in these cases, extensive infection of the pulp tissue must always be expected (8, 17).

The characteristics of a healthy pulp wound ideally include elastic, blood-filled tissue surrounded by caries-free, healthy dentine. However, if yellowish discoloured or even necrotic pulp tissue is present, direct pulp capping is contraindicated. In this case, removal of infected, acutely inflamed or necrotic pulp tissue (partial pulpotomy) or, if necessary, complete pulpotomy (removal of the entire coronal pulp) may be considered as the last possible vital pulp-preserving measure (8, 64) (see Chapter 6. Vital Pulp Treatment Modalities: Pulpotomy – Partial and Complete) (Boxes 5.2 and 5.3).

Box 5.2 Contraindications for Direct Pulp Capping

- Spontaneous pain
- Severe prolonged bleeding or discharge of serous or purulent exudate from the pulp
- Necrotic pulp tissue
- Existing periradicular changes
- Periodontally damaged teeth
- Radiologically recognizable intrapulpal mineralization
- Lack of retention for a wound dressing (e.g. during crown preparation)
- Lack of retention for an immediate definitive bacteria-proof restoration
- Unable to apply dental dam
- Repeated extensive restorations in close proximity to the pulp (=> high biological age of the pulp)

Box 5.3 The Procedure and Clinical Protocol of Direct Pulp Capping

1) After local anaesthesia, the tooth is isolated under a dental dam and the clinical crown is disinfected with NaOCl (2.5–5%), CHX (2%) or alcohol (70%). The primary preparation is completed with diamond burs in a high-speed contra-angle handpiece under constant water cooling.
2) A complete caries excavation is performed with bud burs in a low-speed handpiece supplemented by hand instruments if necessary. Optical magnification and illumination are strongly recommended for this purpose. Shortly before reaching the pulp chamber, a new, sterile instrument should be used in order to minimize the possible spread of microorganisms, e.g. infected dentine chips.
3) The cavity and the exposure area are cleaned with NaOCl 2.5–5%. Pulp bleeding can be staunched with a NaOCl-soaked cotton pellet under moderate pressure. (CHX 2% can be used as an alternative to NaOCl.) A pulp bleeding should be staunched within approx. five minutes. If pulp haemorrhage cannot be stopped after approx. five minutes, an attempt can be made to perform a partial or complete pulpotomy and, after successful haemostasis and assessment of the tissue condition, to cap the resected pulp or root pulp. All infected tissue must be removed. If sufficient haemostasis is not achieved even after a complete pulpotomy, a pulpectomy (vital extirpation) must be performed.
4) If no bleeding occurs after pulp exposure, the area must be examined for necrotic tissue. If present, the necrotic pulp tissue is removed with a diamond instrument at high speed under permanent water cooling until perfused tissue is exposed.
5) HCSC (or calcium hydroxide suspension) is prepared according to the manufacturer's instructions.
6) Using a suitable instrument, the HCSC is applied to the exposed pulp in a thickness of approx. 1.5 mm, including part of the surrounding dentine. A sufficient dentine margin must be left free of cement for the dentine-adhesive restoration. Calcium hydroxide suspension, on the other hand, is only applied over a small area in the region of the pulp exposure and must be provided with a subbase (e.g. phosphate cement and glass ionomer cement) before application of a definitive restorative material.

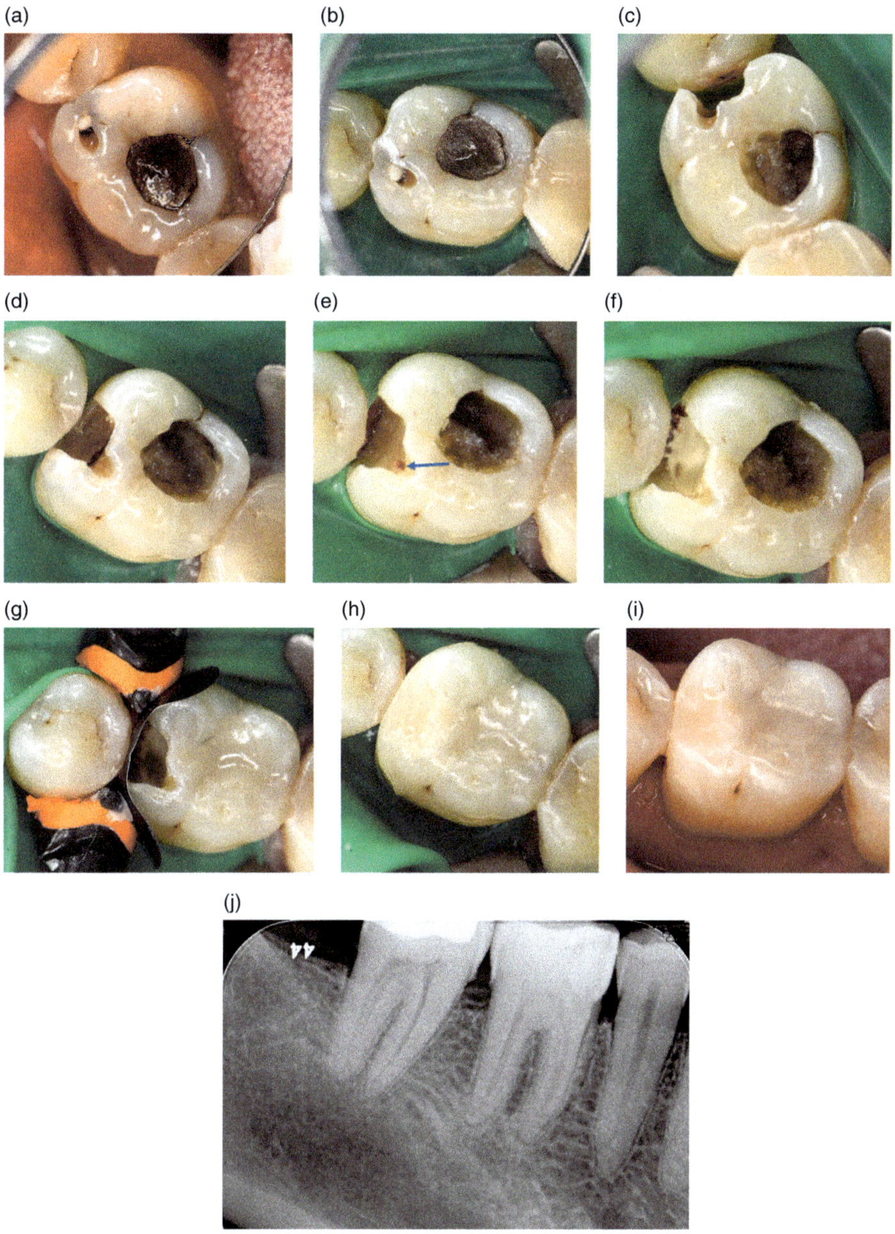

Figure 5.6 (a) A 62-year-old patient presents for filling therapy with an approximal caries on Tooth 46 mesially. (b) Tooth 46 was placed under a dental dam for controlled (absolute) drainage. (c) After disinfection of the tooth with alcohol (70%), a primary preparation of the mesial box was made and the old amalgam filling was removed occlusally. (d) Incomplete caries excavation in the mesial box and complete caries excavation occlusally. (e) Complete excavation of proximal caries mesially on Tooth 46 resulted in exposure of the pulp chamber (blue arrow). Haemostasis and cavity disinfection was performed with NaOCl (3%). Since the pulp bleeding was easy to stop, it can be assumed that the tissue is not inflamed. Discoloured but hard dentine is not bacterially colonized and therefore does not pose a problem for vitality maintenance and can be left in the cavity. (f) A calcium silicate cement (Biodentine, Septodont) was selected for direct pulp capping and placed as a subbase with cement pluggers under slight pressure in the cavity against the parapulpal cavity wall. (g) To bridge the initial setting time of Biodentine (approx. 15 minutes), the occlusal cavity was first provided with a composite filling and a matrix (Composi-Tight 3D, Garrison) and wedge were placed. (h) After the Biodentine had set for 15 minutes, the cavity was definitively restored with composite (Estelite, Tokuyama) using a self-etching dentine adhesive (Optibond XTR, Kerr). The use of a self-etching dentine adhesive is advantageous as there is no risk of washing out the freshly placed Biodentine when removing the etching gel. (i) Finished and polished composite restoration. (j) The radiograph, taken one year after direct pulp capping, showed no pathological changes apically on Tooth 46. The tooth was unremarkable in the sensibility and percussion tests. The patient reported being completely symptom-free both immediately after treatment and one year later.

7) Etching with a phosphoric acid gel and rinsing with water is not possible at this stage, as the HCSC would be washed away. Therefore, the setting time of HCSC (at least 15 minutes, depending on the preparation) should be observed.
8) Alternatively, the HCSC can be covered after application with a small amount of a light-curing flowable compomer, a resin-reinforced glass ionomer cement (RMGI), a self-etching, self-adhesive flowable composite resin or a flowable composite resin in combination with a self-etching dentine adhesive. The HCSC (or calcium hydroxide suspension) must be completely covered.
9) The cavity is then definitively restored adhesively with a dentine bonding agent and composite resin in the same appointment (use according to manufacturer's instructions).
10) The sensibility of the pulp should be checked with a cold test at the next appointment (Figure 5.6a–j).

Source: Adapted from (8).

Evidence-based Outcomes of Direct Pulp Capping

Outcome of Direct Pulp Capping After Deep Caries Excavation

Success rates for VPT vary widely in the literature, especially for direct pulp capping of carious teeth. One review reported success rates ranging from 64% to 97% over the different follow-up periods (115). Early clinical failures (within days or weeks) are multifactorial but certainly, correlate with inaccurate pulp diagnosis or inadequate identification and removal of carious dentine and necrotic pulp tissue. Inaccurate pulp diagnosis may underestimate the inflammatory state of the pulp, leading to irreversible pulpitis and pulp necrosis with postoperative pain (8).

Although conditions for VPT appear less favourable during excavation of deep caries than after iatrogenic pulp exposure or trauma injury, high success rates are still possible, e.g. Ricucci et al. reported success rate of direct pulp capping with calcium hydroxide in 225 teeth from 148 patients was 100%, 95%, 95%, 86% and 89% at 1, 5, 10, 20 and 35 years follow-up examination, respectively (116). Logically, the histological success remains unclear.

An evaluation of 14 clinical studies with over 2300 cases of calcium hydroxide pulp capping even showed success rates of up to 90% when performed by experienced clinicians (25). More realistic results are probably weighted and pooled success rates of direct pulp capping calculated by Aguilar and Linsuwanont as 87.5%, 95.4%, 87.7% and 72.9% after 6 months to 1 year, 1–2 years, 2–3 years and more than 3 years, respectively (117). Assuming correct indication and technical execution, the success rate of direct pulp capping with calcium hydroxide in carious teeth can be 70.1% (±10.1%) in the long term, according to a meta-analysis (118).

HCSC has been recommended for direct pulp capping to increase success rates (103). Various clinical studies have shown that after application of HCSC, success rates are roughly estimated to be 10% higher than with calcium hydroxide, averaging around 80% (114, 119–122).

In recent years, several meta-studies have been published comparing the success rates of both capping materials. Generally, direct pulp capping with HCSC was shown to result in higher clinical success rates (117, 123–127), with lower pulp inflammatory response and more pronounced hard tissue regeneration (123, 124).

Current pooled success rates differed by material and follow-up. For calcium hydroxide, the success rate was 74% at 6 months, 65% at 1 year, 59% at 2–3 years and 56% at 4–5 years. The success rate of MTA at the same time points was 91%, 86%, 84% and 81%. The success rate of Biodentine was 96% at 6 months, 86% at 1 year and 86% at 2–3 years. These meta-analyses showed that HCSC were generally more successful than calcium hydroxide at 1 year and at 2–3 years (127). Also, a GRADE analysis showed that in permanent teeth, the risk of failure was significantly lower when an HCSC was used instead of calcium hydroxide for direct pulp capping (128). There was no significant difference in success rates between the different HCSCs (125–127).

Unfortunately, the actual health status or pathology of the pulp cannot be determined from clinical signs, symptoms or radiographic appearance. The actual, i.e. histological, condition of the pulp remains unclear because all currently available clinical tests are unable to do so. Only histological analysis can assess the actual condition of the dental pulp tissue after direct pulp capping (26, 27). Histologically, the success rate for direct pulp capping is therefore, basically lower than the clinical one, at 66% (64).

Regarding hard tissue regeneration after direct pulp capping, however, it should be noted that the completeness and thickness of hard tissue regeneration are not clearly positively correlated with clinical success. From a clinical perspective, the most important outcome is the long-term pulp vitality and the absence of clinical symptoms (124).

Outcome of Direct Pulp Capping After Dental Trauma

VPT after dental trauma offers a high degree of certainty of success, provided that the pulp is not pre-damaged or the blood supply is not compromised by an accompanying dislocation injury. For direct pulp capping with calcium hydroxide, treatment success is reported to be 54–90% (129–131). When HCSC is used, the chances of success are probably higher.

For the most part, however, direct pulp capping after trauma is recommended only for small-area pulpal exposures treated shortly after injury. In the majority of cases, a partial pulpotomy is preferable, especially when the pulp is widely exposed, and treatment cannot be performed within the first hours after trauma (18, 19). In addition, partial pulpotomy has a higher certainty of success. In the literature, success rates of 86–100% are reported here, even when using calcium hydroxide (131–134) (see Chapter 8. Vital Pulp Treatment for Traumatic Dental Injuries).

However, it is important to note, both for direct pulp capping in the context of caries excavation and after trauma, that the overall success rates reported in the individual studies are very heterogeneous and have minimal commonality in terms of evaluation methods and the follow-up period. Apart from the recording of the parameter 'pain', there is a lack of patient-related data. Therefore, a consensus should be sought and a core outcome set should be developed to achieve an improvement in the success rates of direct pulp capping and other treatments to maintain pulp vitality (135).

Future Developments in Direct Pulp Capping

According to the current state of knowledge, direct pulp capping is indicated for teeth that are asymptomatic or, at most, show symptoms of reversible pulpitis. In comparison, the evidence for VPT in teeth with 'irreversible pulpitis' is still comparatively low; in particular, clinical studies with long-term examination periods are lacking (136). Nevertheless, based on the data available to date, partial and complete pulpotomy can be regarded as a valid treatment option for 'irreversible pulpitis' and may be considered as an alternative to vital extirpation and root canal treatment (15). Therefore, it seems possible that in the future, there will be a general shift from direct pulp capping to pulpotomy in order to prophylactically remove infected pulp tissue before capping.

While VPT is indicated in 'reversible pulpitis', the diagnosis of 'irreversible pulpitis' often leads to pulpectomy and initiation of root canal treatment (137). Recently, therefore, an attempt was made to establish an extended diagnostic scheme (138). According to this, a distinction can be made between initial, mild, moderate and severe pulpitis. Treatment options for initial and mild pulpitis are indirect or direct pulp capping, and for moderate pulpitis, partial or complete pulpotomy. In contrast, for severe pulpitis, complete pulpotomy or, in the case of persistent pulp haemorrhage, vital extirpation is indicated (138). Thus, the proposed new classification could lead to more frequent preservation of pulp vitality, as it seems to be beneficial in cases where VPT is considered as a treatment option (139).

Another important tool for successful direct pulp capping would be the development of a chairside immediate test for inflammatory mediators. With the help of such a test, it should be possible to immediately examine blood from the pulp exposure site and decide whether direct pulp capping, a partial or complete pulpotomy is indicated – or whether it is better to perform a vital extirpation (136). This is because even before the cellular immune response is activated, the molecular immune response releases inflammatory mediators such as cytokines (IL-1, IL-2, IL-6, IL-8, TNF-β and others) (140, 141). These molecules, expressed in the early stages of pulpal inflammation, can serve as markers for the diagnosis of inflammatory changes in the pulp tissue (140, 142). Recent studies show that elevated levels of biomarkers from dentine fluid, pulp blood, gingival crevicular fluid and periapical fluid correlate with different stages of pulpal inflammation (140–142). Thus, molecular-based diagnosis may have the potential to improve clinical diagnosis of true pulp disease (136, 141).

Further development of existing pulp capping materials would also be desirable. HCSC seem to work very well on the pulp, but they are sometimes poorly handled, and the processing time is significantly too long and should be significantly shortened. The addition of anti-inflammatories or drugs that promote reparative processes would also be an improvement (143). The bond of the HCSC to the dentine on the one hand (98) and to lining materials or the final restoration on the other hand (144) should also be improved. In order to ensure a worldwide use of HCSC in direct pulp capping, low-cost HCSCs are desirable.

Together with our advances in pulp biology and dental materials, changes in treatment protocols that promote VPT and survival will ultimately contribute to improved dental health for all patients. A paradigm shift away from root canal treatment and VPT is certainly conceivable in the future. The publication of S3-level treatment guides for direct pulp capping and other VPTs is therefore desirable to provide clinicians with evidence-based treatment guidelines in order to judiciously implement these therapies (136).

Conclusions

An exposed pulp is anything but a lost organ. In the absence of microorganisms, human dental pulp shows exceptional regenerative capacity when capped with materials indicated for VPT. HCSC and traditional calcium hydroxide suspensions clearly promote pulp tissue regeneration, with HCSC such as MTA or Biodentine being the better alternatives to aqueous calcium hydroxide suspensions due to their material advantages in terms of stability and insolubility. The success rates of direct pulp capping are independent of the age of the patient and the size of the pulp exposure. In contrast, remaining caries, microorganisms and monomers from restorative materials negatively influence success, as these lead to tissue inflammation. To protect against microorganisms, therefore, dental dams should always be placed in the pulp-near dentine third from the time of treatment and a careful caries excavation with cavity disinfection should be carried out. A definitive, bacteria-proof restoration of the cavity must be carried out in the same session as the capping. If these conditions are observed and HCSC is used, success rates of approx. 80% for direct pulp capping is quite realistic, even if the pulp is exposed during caries excavation.

References

1 Pfaff P. *Abhandlung von den Zähnen des menschlichen Körpers und deren Krankheiten*, Haude und Spener, Berlin, 1756.
2 Dammaschke T. The history of direct pulp capping. *J Hist Dent.* 2008;56:9–23.
3 Rebel H-H. Über die Ausheilung der freigelegten Pulpa. *Dtsch Zahnheilkd.* 1922;55:3–83.
4 Hermann B. Ein weiterer Beitrag zur Frage der Pulpenbehandlung. *Zahnärztl Rundsch.* 1928;37:1327–76.
5 Hermann BW. Dentinobliteration der Wurzelkanäle nach der Behandlung mit Kalzium. *Zahnärztl Rundsch.* 1930;39:888–99.
6 Duncan HF, Cooper PR, Smith AJ. Dissecting dentine-pulp injury and wound healing responses: consequences for regenerative endodontics. *Int Endod J.* 2019;52:261–6.
7 Dammaschke T, Galler K, Krastl G. Current recommendations for vital pulp treatment. *Dtsch Zahnärztl Z Int.* 2019;1:43–52.
8 Bogen G, Dammaschke T, Chandler N. Vital pulp therapy. In: Berman LH, Hargreaves KM (eds.) Cohen's Pathways of the Pulp, 12th Ed., Elsevier, St. Louis, MO, 2021, 902–38.
9 Farzaneh M, Abitol S, Lawrence HP, Friedman S. Treatment outcome in endodontics – the Toronto study. Phase II: initial treatment. *J Endod.* 2004;30:302–9.
10 Randow K, Glantz PO. On cantilever loading of vital and non-vital teeth. An experimental clinical study. *Acta Odontol Scand.* 1986;44:271–7.
11 Awawdeh L, Hemaidat K, Al-Omari W. Higher maximal occlusal bite force in endodontically treated teeth versus vital contralateral counterparts. *J Endod.* 2017;43:871–5.
12 Merdad K, Sonbul H, Bukhary S, Reit C, Birkhed D. Caries susceptibility of endodontically versus nonendodontically treated teeth. *J Endod.* 2011;37:139–42.
13 Krastl G, Allgayer N, Lenherr P, Filippi A, Taneja P, Weiger R. Tooth discoloration induced by endodontic materials: a literature review. *Dent Traumatol.* 2013;29:2–7.
14 Dammaschke T, Leidinger J, Schäfer E. Long-term evaluation of direct pulp capping – treatment outcomes over an average period of 6.1 years. *Clin Oral Investig.* 2010;14:559–67.
15 Krastl G, Galler K, Dammaschke T, Schäfer E. Is pulpotomy a valid treatment option for irreversible pulpitis? *Dtsch Zahnärztl Z Int.* 2021;2:80–7.
16 Hørsted-Bindslev P, Bergenholtz G. Vital pulp therapies. In: Bergenholtz G, Hørsted-Bindslev P, Erik-Reit C (eds.) Textbook of Endodontology, Blackwell Munksgaard, Oxford, 2003, 66–91.
17 Schäfer E, Dammaschke T. Probleme bei der Vitalerhaltung der Pulpa. In: Hülsmann M, Schäfer E (eds.) Probleme in der Endodontie. Prävention, Identifikation und Management, 2nd Ed., Quintessenz, Berlin, 2019, 37–48.
18 Krastl G, Weiger R, Filippi A, Van Waes H, Ebeleseder K, Ree M, et al. Endodontic management of traumatized permanent teeth: a comprehensive review. *Int Endod J.* 2021;54:1221–45.
19 Krastl G, Weiger R, Ebeleseder K, Galler K. Present status and future directions: endodontic management of traumatic injuries to permanent teeth. *Int Endod J.* 2022;55(Suppl 4):1003–19.
20 Bergenholtz G. Iatrogenic injury to the pulp in dental procedures: aspects of pathogenesis, management and preventive measures. *Int Dent J.* 1991;41:99–110.

21 Robertson A, Andreasen FM, Andreasen JO, Noren JG. Long-term prognosis of crown-fractured permanent incisors. The effect of stage of root development and associated luxation injury. *Int J Paediatr Dent.* 2000;10:191–9.

22 Cox CF, Bergenholtz G, Fitzgerald M, Heys DR, Heys RJ, Avery JK, et al. Capping of the dental pulp mechanically exposed to the oral microflora – a 5 week observation of wound healing in the monkey. *J Oral Pathol.* 1982;11:327–39.

23 Cvek M, Cleaton-Jones PE, Austin JC, Andreasen JO. Pulp reactions to exposure after experimental crown fractures or grinding in adult monkeys. *J Endod.* 1982;8:391–7.

24 Heide S, Mjör IA. Pulp reactions to experimental exposures in young permanent monkey teeth. *Int Endod J.* 1983;16:11–9.

25 Baume L, Holz J. Long-term clinical assessment of direct pulp capping. *Int Dent J.* 1981;31:251–60.

26 Hilton TJ. Keys to clinical success with pulp capping: a review of the literature. *Oper Dent.* 2009;34:615–25.

27 Donnermeyer D, Dammaschke T, Lipski M, Schäfer E. Effectiveness of diagnosing pulpitis: a systematic review. *Int Endod J.* 2023;56(Suppl. 3):296–325.

28 American Association of Endodontists. *Glossary of Endodontic Terms*, 10th Ed., American Association of Endodontists, Chicago, IL, 2020. https://www.aae.org/specialty/clinical-resources/glossary-endodontic-terms/.

29 Seltzer S, Bender IB, Ziontz M. The dynamics of pulpal inflammation: correlations between diagnostic data and actual histologic findings in the pulp. *Oral Surg Oral Med Oral Pathol.* 1963;16:869–77.

30 Ricucci D, Loghin S, Siqueira JF Jr. Correlation between clinical and histologic pulp diagnoses. *J Endod.* 2014;40:1932–9.

31 Michaelson PL, Holland GR. Is pulpitis painful? *Int Endod J.* 2002;35:829–32.

32 Barańska-Gachowska M, Zaleski W, Waszkiewicz-Gołoś H. Clinical diagnosis and the histological findings in dental pulp. *Pol Med J.* 1969;8:712–24.

33 Barańska-Gachowska M, Waszkiewicz-Gołoś H. Diagnostic significance of clinical manifestations in evaluation of the stage of dental pulp in the light of histological examinations. *Pol Med J.* 1969;8:725–35.

34 Lin LM, Ricucci D, Saoud TM, Sigurdsson A, Kahler B. Vital pulp therapy of mature permanent teeth with irreversible pulpitis from the perspective of pulp biology. *Aust Endod J.* 2020;46:154–66.

35 Langeland K. Management of the inflamed pulp associated with deep carious lesion. *J Endod.* 1981;7:169–81.

36 Matsuo T, Nakanishi T, Shimizu H, Ebisu S. A clinical study of direct pulp capping applied to carious-exposed pulps. *J Endod.* 1996;22:551–6.

37 Christensen GJ. Pulp capping 1998. *J Am Dent Assoc.* 1998;129:1297–9.

38 Kang CM, Sun Y, Song JS, Pang N-S, Roh B-D, Lee C-Y, et al. A randomized controlled trial of various MTA materials for partial pulpotomy in permanent teeth. *J Dent.* 2017;60:8–13.

39 Careddu R, Duncan HF. A prospective clinical study investigating the effectiveness of partial pulpotomy after relating preoperative symptoms to a new and established classification of pulpitis. *Int Endod J.* 2021;54:2156–72.

40 Taha NA, Khazali MA. Partial pulpotomy in mature permanent teeth with clinical signs indicative of irreversible pulpitis: a randomized clinical trial. *J Endod.* 2017;43:1417–21.

41 Taha NA, Abdelkhader SZ. Outcome of full pulpotomy using Biodentine in adult patients with symptoms indicative of irreversible pulpitis. *Int Endod J.* 2018;51:819–28.

42 Cao Y, Bogen G, Lim J, Shon WJ, Kang MK. Bioceramic materials and the changing concepts in vital pulp therapy. *J Calif Dent Assoc.* 2016;44:278–90.

43 Qudeimat MA, Alyahya A, Hasan AA, Barrieshi-Nusair KM. Mineral trioxide aggregate pulpotomy for permanent molars with clinical signs indicative of irreversible pulpitis: a preliminary study. *Int Endod J.* 2017;50:126–34.

44 Murray PE, Stanley HR, Matthews JB, Sloan AJ, Smith AJ. Age-related odontometric changes of human teeth. *Oral Surg Oral Med Oral Pathol Oral Radiol Endod.* 2002;93:474–82.

45 Goodis HE, Kahn A, Simon S. Aging and the pulp. In: Hargreaves K, Goodis HE, Tay F (eds.) Seltzer and Bender's Dental Pulp, 2nd Ed., Quintessence, Hanover Park, IL, 2012, 421–46.

46 Kakehashi S, Stanley HR, Fitzgerald RJ. The effects of surgical exposure of dental pulps in germ-free and conventional laboratory rats. *Oral Surg Oral Med Oral Pathol.* 1965;20:340–9.

47 Hahn CL, Liewehr FR. Relationships between caries bacteria, host responses, and clinical signs and symptoms of pulpitis. *J Endod.* 2007;33:213–9.

48 Hahn CL, Liewehr FR. Innate immune responses of the dental pulp to caries. *J Endod.* 2007;33:643–51.

49 Hahn CL, Liewehr FR. Update on the adaptive immune responses of the dental pulp. *J Endod.* 2007;33:773–81.

50 Ricucci D, Siqueira JF Jr. Vital pulp therapy. In: Ricucci D, Siqueira JF Jr (eds.) Endodontology – An Integrated Biological and Clinical View, Quintessence, London, 2013, 67–106.

51 Nissan R, Segal H, Pashley D, Stevens R, Trowbridge H. Ability of bacterial endotoxin to diffuse through human dentin. *J Endod.* 1995;21:62–4.

52 Love RM. Bacterial adhesins – their role in tubule invasion and endodontic disease. *Aust Endod J.* 2002;28:25–8.

53 Love RM, Jenkinson HF. Invasion of dentinal tubules by oral bacteria. *Crit Rev Oral Biol Med.* 2002;13:171–83.

54 Schweikl H, Buchalla W, Krifka S. Cell responses to cariogenic microorganisms and dental resin materials – crosstalk at the dentin-pulp interface? *Dent Mater.* 2017;33:514–24.

55 Buchalla W, Frankenberger R, Galler K, Krastl G, Kunzelmann K-H, Paris S, et al. Aktuelle Empfehlungen zur Kariesexkavation. Wissenschaftliche Mitteilung der Deutschen Gesellschaft für Zahnerhaltung (DGZ). *Dtsch Zahnärztl Z.* 2017;72:484–94.

56 European Society of Endodontology (ESE) developed by, Duncan HF, Galler KM, Tomson PL, Simon S, El-Karim I, et al. European Society of Endodontology position statement: management of deep caries and the exposed pulp. *Int Endod J.* 2019;52:923–34.

57 Paddick JS, Brailsford SR, Kidd EA, Beighton D. Phenotypic and genotypic selection of microbiota surviving under dental restorations. *Appl Environ Microbiol.* 2005;71:2467–72.

58 Lima KC, Coelho LT, Pinheiro IV, Rôças IN, Siqueira JF Jr. Microbiota of dentinal caries as assessed by reverse-capture checkerboard analysis. *Caries Res.* 2011;45:21–30.

59 Rôças IN, Lima KC, Assuncao IV, Gomes PN, Bracks IV, Siqueira JF Jr. Advanced caries microbiota in teeth with irreversible pulpitis. *J Endod.* 2015;41:1450–5.

60 Rôças IN, Alves FR, Rachid CT, Lima KC, Assunção IV, Gomes PN, et al. Microbiome of deep dentinal caries lesions in teeth with symptomatic irreversible pulpitis. *PLoS One.* 2016;11:e0154653.

61 Cooper PR, Takahashi Y, Graham LW, Simon S, Imazato S, Smith AJ. Inflammation-regeneration interplay in the dentine-pulp complex. *J Dent.* 2010;38:687–97.

62 Kuwabara RK, Massler M. Pulpal reactions to active and arrested carious lesions. *J Dent Child.* 1966;33:190–204.

63 Wang U. Die indirekte Pulpaüberkappung mit Calxyl im Vergleich zur sogenannten "natürlichen Pulpaüberkappung" – Klinische und histologische Untersuchung. *SSO Schweiz Monatsschr Zahnheilkd.* 1953;63:1135–75.

64 Ricucci D, Siqueira JF Jr, Li Y, Tay FR. Vital pulp therapy: histopathology and histobacteriology-based guidelines to treat teeth with deep caries and pulp exposure. *J Dent.* 2019;86:41–52.

65 Ricucci D, Siqueira JF Jr, Rôças IN, Lipski M, Shiban A, Tay FR. Pulp and dentine responses to selective caries excavation: a histological and histobacteriological human study. *J Dent.* 2020;100:103430.

66 American Association of Endodontists. AAE position statement on vital pulp therapy. *J Endod.* 2021;47:1340–4.

67 Schröder U. Evaluation of healing following experimental pulpotomy of intact human teeth and capping with calcium hydroxide. *Odontol Rev.* 1972;23:329–40.

68 Schröder U. Effects of calcium hydroxide-containing pulp-capping agents on pulp cell migration, proliferation, and differentiation. *J Dent Res.* 1985;64(4):541–8.

69 Gängler P. Die Reaktionen des Pulpa-Dentin-Systems auf Medikamente. *Stomatol DDR.* 1976;26:327–30.

70 Rosenfeld EF, James GA, Burch BS. Vital pulp tissue response to sodium hypochlorite. *J Endod.* 1978;4:140–6.

71 Ballal NV, Duncan HF, Wiedemeier DB, Rai N, Jalan P, Bhat V, et al. MMP-9 levels and NaOCl lavage in randomized trial on direct pulp capping. *J Dent Res.* 2022;101:414–9.

72 Colombo M, Beltrami R, Chiesa M, Poggio C, Scribante A. Shear bond strength of one-step self-etch adhesives to dentin: evaluation of NaOCl pretreatment. *J Clin Exp Dent.* 2018;10:e127–33.

73 Boushell LW, Walter R. Fundamentals of tooth preparation. In: Ritter AV, Boushell LW, Walter R (eds.) Sturdevant's Art and Science of Operative Dentistry, 7th Ed., Elsevier, St. Louis, MO, 2019, 120–35.

74 Silva AF, Tarquinio SB, Demarco FF, Piva E, Rivero ER. The influence of haemostatic agents on healing of healthy human dental pulp tissue capped with calcium hydroxide. *Int Endod J.* 2006;39:309–16.

75 Bal C, Alacam A, Tuzuner T, Tirali RE, Baris E. Effects of antiseptics on pulpal healing under calcium hydroxide pulp capping: a pilot study. *Eur J Dent.* 2011;5:265–722.

76 Hamed SJ, Al-Yasiri IK, Nibrass TA, Al-Feron MA. Antibacterial activity of calcium hydroxide combined with chlorohexidine or sodium hypochlorite against gram positive and gram negative bacteria. *J Nat Sci Res.* 2014;4:55–61.

77 Zanini M, Hennequin M, Cousson PY. Which procedures and materials could be applied for full pulpotomy in permanent mature teeth? A systematic review. *Acta Odontol Scand.* 2019;77:541–51.

78 Lemon RR, Steele PJ, Jeansonne BG. Ferric sulfate hemostasis: effect on osseous wound healing. Left in situ for maximum exposure. *J Endod.* 1993;19:170–3.

79 Staehle HJ. *Calciumhydroxid in der Zahnheilkunde*, Hanser, 1990.

80 Mohammadi Z, Dummer PMH. Properties and applications of calcium hydroxide in endodontics and dental traumatology. *Int Endod J.* 2011;44:697–730.

81 Cox CF, Sübay RK, Ostro E, Suzuki S, Suzuki SH. Tunnel defects in dentin bridges: their formation following direct pulp capping. *Oper Dent.* 1996;21:4–11.

82 Fisher FJ, McCabe JF. Calcium hydroxide base materials: an investigation into the relationship between chemical structure and antibacterial properties. *Br Dent J.* 1978;144:341–4.

83 Barnes IE, Kidd EA. Disappearing dycal. *Br Dent J.* 1979;147:111.

84 Motsch A. Die Unterfüllung – eine kritische Diskussion der verschiedenen Zemente und Präparate. In: Akademie Praxis und Wissenschaft in der DGZMK (ed.) Neue Füllungsmaterialien: Indikation und Verarbeitung, Hanser, 1990, 35–65.

85 Phaneuf RA, Frankl SN, Ruben MP. A comparative histological evaluation of three commercial calcium hydroxide preparations on the human primary dental pulp. *J Dent Child.* 1968;35:61–76.

86 Liard-Dumtschin D, Holz J, Baume LJ. Le coiffage pulpaire direct – essai biologique sur 8 produits. *Schweiz Monatsschr Zahnmed.* 1984;94:4–22.

87 Berzins DW. Chemical properties of MTA. In: Torabinejad M (ed.) Mineral Trioxide Aggregate. Properties and Clinical Applications, Wiley Blackwell, 2014, 17–36.

88 Dammaschke T, Stratmann U, Wolff P, Sagheri D, Schäfer E. Direct pulp capping with mineral trioxide aggregate: an immunohistological comparison with calcium hydroxide in rodents. *J Endod.* 2010;36:814–9.

89 Fridland M, Rosado R. MTA solubility: a long term study. *J Endod.* 2005;31:376–9.

90 Camilleri J. Characterization of hydration products of mineral trioxide aggregate. *Int Endod J.* 2008;41:408–17.

91 Koh ET, Torabinejad M, Pitt Ford TR, Brady K, McDonald F. Mineral trioxide aggregate stimulates a biological response in human osteoblasts. *J Biomed Mater Res.* 1997;37:432–9.

92 Camilleri J, Kralj P, Veber M, Sinagra E. Characterization and analyses of acid-extractable and leached trace elements in dental cements. *Int Endod J.* 2012;45:737–43.

93 Carlisle EM. Silicon: a possible factor in bone calcification. *Science.* 1970;176:279–80.

94 Han L, Okiji T. Uptake of calcium and silicon released from calcium silicate-based endodontic materials into root canal dentine. *Int Endod J.* 2011;44:1081–7.

95 Saito T, Toyooka H, Ito S, Crenshaw MA. In vitro study of remineralization of dentin: effects of ions on mineral induction by decalcified dentin matrix. *Caries Res.* 2003;37:445–9.

96 Lundy FT, Giraud T, El Karim IA, About I. Biodentine™ in inflammation and pain control. In: About I (ed.) Biodentine™ – Properties and Clinical Application, Springer, Cham, 2022, 51–66.

97 Atmeh AR, Chong EZ, Richard G, Festy F, Watson TF. Dentin-cement interfacial interaction: calcium silicates and polyalkenoates. *J Dent Res.* 2012;91:454–9.

98 Kaup M, Dammann CH, Schäfer E, Dammaschke T. Shear bond strength of Biodentine, ProRoot MTA, glass ionomer cement and composite resin on human dentine ex vivo. *Head Face Med.* 2015;11:14.

99 Yoo JS, Chang SW, Oh SR, Perinpanayagam H, Lim SM, Yoo YJ, et al. Bacterial entombment by intratubular mineralization following orthograde mineral trioxide aggregate obturation: a scanning electron microscopy study. *Int J Oral Sci.* 2014;6:227–32.

100 Gandolfi MG, van Lunduyt K, Taddei P, Modena E, Van Meerbeek B, Prati C. Environmental scanning electron microscopy connected with energy dispersive X-ray analysis and Raman techniques to study ProRoot mineral trioxide aggregate and calcium silicate cements in wet conditions and in real time. *J Endod.* 2010;36:851–7.

101 Kaup M, Schäfer E, Dammaschke T. An in vitro study of different material properties of Biodentine compared to ProRoot MTA. *Head Face Med.* 2015;11:16.

102 Torabinejad M, Parirokh M. Mineral trioxide aggregate: a comprehensive literature review – part II: leakage and biocompatibility investigations. *J Endod.* 2010;36:190–202.

103 Dammaschke T, Camp JH, Bogen G. MTA in vital pulp therapy. In: Torabinejad M (ed.) Mineral Trioxide Aggregate – Properties and Clinical Applications, Wiley Blackwell, Ames, IA, 2014, 71–110.

104 Dammaschke T, Nowicka A, Lipski M, Ricucci D. Histological evaluation of hard tissue formation after direct pulp capping with a fast-setting mineral trioxide aggregate (RetroMTA) in humans. *Clin Oral Investig.* 2019;23:4289–99.

105 Ricucci D, Loghin S, Lin LM, Spångberg LSW, Tay FR. Is hard tissue formation in the dental pulp after the death of the primary odontoblasts a regenerative or a reparative process? *J Dent.* 2014;42:1156–70.

106 Możyńska J, Metlerski M, Lipski M, Nowicka A. Tooth discoloration induced by different calcium silicate-based cements: a systematic review of in vitro studies. *J Endod.* 2017;43:1593–601.

107 Berger T, Baratz AZ, Gutmann JL. In vitro investigations into the etiology of mineral trioxide tooth staining. *J Conserv Dent.* 2014;17:526–30.

108 Dettwiler CA, Walter M, Zaugg LK, Lenherr P, Weiger R, Krastl G. In vitro assessment of the tooth staining potential of endodontic materials in a bovine tooth model. *Dent Traumatol.* 2016;32:480–7.

109 Shokouhinejad N, Nekoofar MH, Pirmoazen S, Shamshiri AR, Dummer PMH. Evaluation and comparison of occurrence of tooth discoloration after the application of various calcium silicate-based cements: an ex vivo study. *J Endod.* 2016;42:140–4.

110 Lenherr P, Allgayer N, Weiger R, Filippi A, Krastl G. Tooth discoloration induced by endodontic materials: a laboratory study. *Int Endod J.* 2012;45:942–9.

111 About I. Recent trends in tricalcium silicates for vital pulp therapy. *Curr Oral Health Rep.* 2018;5:178–85.

112 Parirokh M, Torabinejad M, Dummer PMH. Mineral trioxide aggregate and other bioactive endodontic cements: an updated overview – part I: vital pulp therapy. *Int Endod J.* 2018;51:177–205.

113 Camilleri J, Atmeh A, Li X, Meschi N. Present status and future directions: hydraulic materials for endodontic use. *Int Endod J.* 2022;55(Suppl 3):710–77.

114 Harms CS, Schäfer E, Dammaschke T. Clinical evaluation of direct pulp capping using a calcium silicate cement – treatment outcomes over an average period of 2.3 years. *Clin Oral Investig.* 2019;23:3491–9.

115 Leong DJX, Yap AU. Vital pulp therapy in carious pulp-exposed permanent teeth: an umbrella review. *Clin Oral Investig.* 2021;25:6743–56.

116 Ricucci D, Rôças IN, Alves FRF, Cabello PH, Siqueira JF Jr. Outcome of direct pulp capping using calcium hydroxide: a long-term retrospective study. *J Endod.* 2023;49:45–54.

117 Aguilar P, Linsuwanont P. Vital pulp therapy in vital permanent teeth with cariously exposed pulp: a systematic review. *J Endod.* 2011;37:581–7.

118 Gulabivala K, Ng Y-L. Outcomes of endodontic therapy. In: Rotstein I, Ingle JI (eds.) Ingle's Endodontics, 7th Ed., PMPH USA, Shelton, CT, 2019, 1019–66.

119 Hilton TJ, Ferracane JL, Mancl L. Northwest practice-based research collaborative in evidence-based dentistry (NWP). Comparison of CaOH with MTA for direct pulp capping: a PBRN randomized clinical trial. *J Dent Res.* 2013;92(7 Suppl):16S–22S.

120 Mente J, Hufnagel S, Leo M, Michel A, Gehrig H, Panagidis D, et al. Treatment outcome of mineral trioxide aggregate or calcium hydroxide direct pulp capping: long-term results. *J Endod.* 2014;40:1746–51.

121 Kundzina R, Stangvaltaite L, Eriksen HM, Kerosuo E. Capping carious exposures in adults: a randomized controlled trial investigating mineral trioxide aggregate versus calcium hydroxide. *Int Endod J.* 2017;50:924–32.

122 Lipski M, Nowicka A, Kot K, Postek-Stefańska L, Wysoczańska-Jankowicz I, Borkowski L, et al. Factors affecting the outcomes of direct pulp capping using Biodentine. *Clin Oral Investig.* 2018;22:2021–9.

123 Li Z, Cao L, Fan M, Xu Q. Direct pulp capping with calcium hydroxide or mineral trioxide aggregate: a meta-analysis. *J Endod.* 2015;41:1412–7.

124 Zhu C, Ju B, Ni R. Clinical outcome of direct pulp capping with MTA or calcium hydroxide: a systematic review and meta-analysis. *Int J Clin Exp Med.* 2015;8:17055–60.

125 Paula AB, Laranjo M, Marto CM, Paulo S, Abrantes AM, Casalta-Lopes J, et al. Direct pulp capping: what is the most effective therapy? Systematic review and meta-analysis. *J Evid Based Dent Pract.* 2018;18:298–314.

126 Matsuura T, Ziauddin SM, Kawata-Matsuura VKS, Sugimoto K, Yamada S, Yoshimura A. Long-term clinical and radiographic evaluation of the effectiveness of direct pulp capping materials: a meta-analysis. *Dent Mater J.* 2021;40:1–7.

127 Cushley S, Duncan HF, Lappin MJ, Chua P, Elamin AD, Clarke M, et al. Efficacy of direct pulp capping for management of cariously exposed pulps in permanent teeth: a systematic review and meta-analysis. *Int Endod J.* 2021;54:556–71.

128 Schwendicke F, Brouwer F, Schwendicke A, Paris S. Different materials for direct pulp capping: systematic review and meta-analysis and trial sequential analysis. *Clin Oral Investig.* 2016;20:1121–32.

129 Fuks AB, Bielak S, Chosak A. Clinical and radiographic assessment of direct pulp capping and pulpotomy in young permanent teeth. *Pediatr Dent.* 1982;4:240–4.

130 Ravn JJ. Follow-up study of permanent incisors with complicated crown fractures after acute trauma. *Scand J Dent Res.* 1982;90:363–72.

131 Hecova H, Tzigkounakis V, Merglova V, Netolicky J. A retrospective study of 889 injured permanent teeth. *Dent Traumatol.* 2010;26:466–75.

132 Cvek M. Partial pulpotomy in crown-fractured incisors – results 3 - 15 years after trauma. *Acta Stomatol Croat.* 1993;27:167–73.

133 Alqaderi H, Lee CT, Borzangy S, Pagonis TC. Coronal pulpotomy for cariously exposed permanent posterior teeth with closed apices: a systematic review and meta-analysis. *J Dent.* 2016;44:1–7.

134 Wang G, Wang C, Qin M. Pulp prognosis following conservative pulp treatment in teeth with complicated crown fractures – a retrospective study. *Dent Traumatol.* 2017;33:255–60.

135 Cushley S, Duncan HF, Lundy FT, Nagendrababu V, Clarke M, El Karim I. Outcomes reporting in systematic reviews on vital pulp treatment: a scoping review for the development of a core outcome set. *Int Endod J.* 2022;55:891–909.

136 Duncan HF. Present status and future directions – vital pulp treatment and pulp preservation strategies. *Int Endod J.* 2022;55(Suppl 3):497–511.

137 Schäfer E, Bürklein S, Hülsmann M. Probleme der Diagnostik. In: Hülsmann M, Schäfer E (eds.) Probleme in der Endodontie. Prävention, Identifikation und Management, 2nd Ed., Quintessence, Berlin, 2019, 1–36.

138 Wolters WJ, Duncan HF, Tomson PL, Karim IE, McKenna G, Dorri M, et al. Minimally invasive endodontics: a new diagnostic system for assessing pulpitis and subsequent treatment needs. *Int Endod J.* 2017;50:825–9.

139 Richert R, Ducret M, Alliot-Licht B, Bekhouche M, Gobert S, Farges JC. A critical analysis of research methods and experimental models to study pulpitis. *Int Endod J.* 2022;55:14–36.

140 Rechenberg DK, Galicia JC, Peters OA. Biological markers for pulpal inflammation: a systematic review. *PLoS One.* 2016;11:e0167289.

141 Zanini M, Meyer E, Simon S. Pulp inflammation diagnosis from clinical to inflammatory mediators: a systematic review. *J Endod.* 2017;43:1033–51.

142 Hirsch V, Wolgin M, Mitronin AV, Kielbassa AM. Inflammatory cytokines in normal and irreversibly inflamed pulps: a systematic review. *Arch Oral Biol.* 2017;82:38–46.

143 Al-Natour B, Rankin R, McKenna R, McMillan H, Zhang SD, About I, et al. Identification and validation of novel biomarkers and therapeutics for pulpitis using connectivity mapping. *Int Endod J.* 2021;54:1571–80.

144 Schmidt A, Schäfer E, Dammaschke T. Shear bond strength of lining materials to calcium-silicate cements at different time intervals. *J Adhes Dent.* 2017;19:129–35.

6

Vital Pulp Treatment Modalities

Pulpotomy – Partial and Complete

Roberto Careddu[1], Mark Lappin[2], Henry F. Duncan[1], and Ikhlas A. El-Karim[2]

[1] *Division of Restorative Dentistry and Periodontology, Dublin Dental University Hospital, Trinity College Dublin, Dublin, Ireland*
[2] *Department of Restorative Dentistry, School of Medicine, Dentistry and Biomedical Sciences, Queen's University Belfast, Belfast, Northern Ireland, UK*

Introduction

The dental pulp is a highly vascular and innervated connective tissue that forms an interconnected structure with dentine known as dentine-pulp complex. Microbial insult is the main cause of pulpal injury, but other irritants including trauma, chemicals and iatrogenic damage caused by overheating, can lead to pulpitis (1). The pulp responds to injurious stimuli by mounting a protective inflammatory response characterized by the release of inflammatory mediators to control the infection. The presence of a mixed bacterial biofilm that becomes increasingly anaerobic as the infection becomes established causes a cascade of inflammatory reactions that are evident long before bacteria come into direct contact with the pulp tissue (2). Bacteria infiltration of the pulp stimulates first a localized acute response that, if not treated, assumes chronic features and eventually culminates in necrosis (3). However, if the irritant is removed and the tooth properly restored, this protective inflammatory response can be modulated to initiate healing and a repair process with subsequent tertiary dentine formation that forms a protective barrier to seal the pulp from further damage (4, 5).

The intensity and duration of the stimuli play a role in the pulp response to injury. For instance, low-grade traumatic or microbial irritation of the dental pulp will lead to activation of primary odontoblasts and upregulation of secretory activity in the form of reactionary dentine formation; however, severe injury associated with deep caries and bacterial invasion of the pulp usually results in death of odontoblasts. However, if an environment inductive of healing is created, these can be replaced with odontoblast-like cells to produce reparative dentine (4). Unlike deep caries, severe injury caused by trauma, as in luxation or avulsion injuries, is often accompanied by the distribution of the blood of the tooth, leading to irreversible damage and ultimately pulpal necrosis. A traumatic event such as a complicated coronal fracture can expose healthy pulp to microorganisms and lead to pulpitis and localized infection and a protective and reparative inflammatory response, as described above, provided the blood supply to the tooth remains intact.

The ability of the dental pulp to heal following injury is well documented in studies that laid the scientific foundation for pulp preservation therapies (2, 4, 6). The need to maintain pulp vitality is

Vital Pulp Treatment, First Edition. Edited by Henry F. Duncan and Ikhlas A. El-Karim.

not new, with pulp capping procedures documented as early as 1756 with many different materials being advocated as potential pulp capping agents (7). Over the years, pulpotomy and pulp capping procedures have been carried out empirically by clinicians with little consensus on protocols and indications (8). As a result of unpredictable outcomes, allied to poor clinical technique, suggestions were made to limit vital pulp treatment (VPT) to deciduous teeth or immature permanent teeth (9). An exception was made for teeth with an iatrogenic or 'sterile exposure' in which a traumatic event exposed the pulp in the absence of caries, and the tooth was treated immediately after. Specifically, the presence of symptomatology or bacterial infection was considered a negative prognostic factor that required root canal treatment (9).

In recent years, advances in pulp biology have improved our understanding of the healing and regenerative capabilities of dental pulp and the advent of the hydraulic calcium silicate cement, has led to a change of scope of VPT with a shift from only treatment for deciduous and immature teeth to a possible viable alternative for root canal treatment for permanent teeth. An emerging body of evidence suggests a success rate for pulpotomy similar to that of root canal treatment (RCT) in teeth with symptomatic irreversible pulpitis (10, 11). Consequently, both the European Society of Endodontology (ESE) and the American Association of Endodontists (AAE) introduced guidance encouraging preserving the vitality of the pulp and recognizing pulpotomy as an option that should be considered in the decision-making process for the treatment of deep carious lesions or pulp exposures in mature permanent teeth (12, 13).

Definitions

There are a range of VPTs available; however, whenever the pulp is exposed directly due to bacterial infiltration or severely traumatized, the most appropriate management is to remove part of the affected pulp with a partial or complete pulpotomy. The ESE position statement on the management of deep caries and exposed pulp (13) defined pulpotomies as follows:

i) A partial pulpotomy is a clinical procedure in which a small portion of the coronal pulp is in direct contact with the affected area after pulp exposure is removed, followed by the application of a biomaterial directly onto the remaining pulp tissue prior to placement of a permanent restoration.
ii) A full (or complete) pulpotomy involves the complete removal of the coronal pulp and the application of a biomaterial directly onto the pulp tissue at the level of the root canal orifice(s), prior to placement of a permanent restoration.

Indications

Definitive Treatment for Asymptomatic Cariously Exposed Pulp

In teeth with moderate or deep caries lesions (lesion extend to the inner quarter of dentine) but with zone of hard or firm dentine between the caries lesion and the pulp, removal of caries using selective caries removal (14, 15) and placement of a restoration is sufficient to reverse pulp inflammation. Selective caries removal reduces the risk of pulp exposure and therefore recommended by the ESE for the management of deep caries (13). If, however, non-selective caries removal approach is used and the pulp is exposed, direct pulp capping or pulpotomy under enhanced disinfection protocols and use of a hydraulic calcium silicate cement is recommended (13). A high success rate for direct pulp capping of the cariously exposed pulp with symptoms of reversible pulpitis using Mineral Trioxide Aggregate (MTA) or Biodentine has been reported (16). Similarly, more than 90% success rate for full coronal pulpotomy as definitive treatment for cariously exposed pulps with signs and symptoms of reversible pulpitis was reported in a systematic review (17). Compared with root canal treatment, complete pulpotomy, was also shown to have the same success rate for teeth with cariously exposed pulp and symptoms of reversible pulpitis (18).

Partial pulpotomy is also a successful alternative for the cariously exposed pulp (19). In this systematic review, the meta-analysis indicated a 92% (CI: 0.83–0.97) two-year success rate for partial pulpotomy; however, the preoperative pulpal status was identified as a significant factor, with studies including teeth with the diagnosis of irreversible pulpitis displaying significantly lower results.

Unlike the situation of deep caries mentioned above, caries can also penetrate the entire thickness of the dentine in what is defined as extremely deep caries (5). In this scenario, pulp exposure is inevitable with invasion of pulp space by pathogenic bacteria and therefore, selective caries removal and placement of restoration is not appropriate even if the tooth presents with clinical symptoms suggestive of reversible pulpitis (5). This is an example of the limitations of our exiting pulpal diagnostic methods where there is clear lack of correlation between symptoms and the pathological status of the cariously exposed pulp. The AAE classification defined such pathology as chronic irreversible pulpitis (20), and therefore root canal treatment was recommended. Studies, however, reporting specifically on the depth of caries and in particular that used the recently introduced terminology of extremely deep caries (5) are still lacking and urgently warranted.

In summary, teeth with deep caries, extending to the inner third of dentine with clear radiographic evidence of dentine and absence of symptoms indicating more than reversible pulpitis, selective caries removal to avoid pulp exposure is recommended (13). If in such teeth asymptomatic exposure occurs during caries removal VPT in the form of direct pulp capping or pulpotomy is suggested. Pulpotomy is also indicated for cases with extremely deep caries where exposure is inevitable. Pulpotomy should be performed under an enhanced disinfection protocol (rubber dam and wound lavage with 2.5% sodium hypochlorite), and a hydraulic calcium silicate cement is used as pulp capping material. The decision to perform direct pulp capping or partial/complete pulpotomy depends on direct inspection and the ability to control pulpal bleeding during the operative procedure.

Definitive Treatment for Symptomatic Irreversible Pulpitis

Irreversible pulpitis (IRP) is a clinical diagnosis that indicates an inflamed pulp that is incapable of healing and for which root canal treatment is indicated (20). Accumulating evidence, however, suggests that preservation of at least part of irreversibly inflamed pulp is feasible, putting into question the terminology of irreversible damage.

Several studies including retrospective and prospective studies have shown a high success rate for partial as well as full pulpotomy as definitive treatments for teeth with signs and symptoms suggestive of IRP. In a systematic review including only studies that reported on symptomatic irreversible pulpitis, Cushley et al. showed 95% clinical and radiographic success for full pulpotomy at 12-month which falls to 88% at three years. When compared to root canal treatment, full pulpotomy has a similar success rate in one randomized control trial, comparing the two treatments for teeth with symptoms of irreversible pulpitis (21). A recent systematic review reported no difference in postoperative pain between pulpotomy and root canal treatment in teeth with symptomatic irreversible pulpitis (22).

In another recent meta-analysis by Ather et al. in 2022, an overall success of 86% [95% CI: 0.76–0.92]; $I^2 = 81.9\%$) for full pulpotomy for teeth with IRP was reported (23). Notably, the success was shown to be higher in teeth with asymptomatic (91%) compared to symptomatic irreversible pulpitis (84%) and the same for the open (96%) versus closed apex (83%) in permanent teeth. It should be noted here that cases of asymptomatic irreversible pulpitis are those with extremely deep caries mentioned above and, based on the outcome of this review, should be treated with pulpotomy rather than root canal treatment.

Partial pulpotomy has also been investigated as the definitive treatment for teeth with deep caries and signs and symptoms of irreversible pulpitis. Taha et al. reported a higher two-year success rate for partial pulpotomy using MTA compared with calcium hydroxide in teeth with symptomatic IRP (24). Subsequent studies using hydraulic calcium silicate cement conformed to good outcomes for partial pulpotomy (25, 26). However, when compared to full pulpotomy, the success of partial pulpotomy was lower, but the difference was not statistically significant (25, 26). This would suggest that the two procedures could be considered as definitive treatment for teeth with symptomatic IRP. Partial pulpotomy offers the advantage of being a more conservative procedure in which much of the coronal pulp is preserved; however, the technique may be more sensitive to perform than full pulpotomy, a factor that may need to be considered during the treatment planning for such cases (13).

In summary, in permanent teeth with deep caries and signs and symptoms of IRP, full pulpotomy is suggested as an alternative to root canal treatment. Evidence from emerging studies suggested a comparable success rate for partial and complete pulpotomy for irreversible pulpitis. These procedures should be carried out under enhanced protocol, with disinfection, magnification and use of hydraulic calcium silicate cement to ensure high success.

Definitive Treatment for Traumatically Exposed Pulp

Unlike carious exposure, traumatic injuries to the dental pulp are not contaminated wounds and therefore the success of VPTs such as pulpotomy is likely to be high. Traumatic injuries often occur in children with immature or young permanent teeth (27) in which the maintenance of pulp vitality is of importance to ensure root development and to avoid subsequent complicated endodontic treatment. VPTs can therefore present a number of advances over conventional endodontic procedures for traumatized teeth. In fact, Cvek 1978 first introduced partial pulpotomy for the management of traumatized teeth. The technique involves the removal of coronal pulp tissue adjacent to a pulp exposure following coronal tooth fracture. By preserving pulpal tissue, the potential for continued root development is maintained in immature permanent teeth as well as enabling healing of the radicular pulp tissue. High success rates of between 87.5 and 100% were reported for Cvek pulpotomy, and the process can readily be applied to both mature and immature teeth. Data from a systematic review on the outcome of partial pulpotomy for traumatized permanent anterior teeth showed 89% (95% confidence interval 86–91), indicating that partial pulpotomy may be considered a reliable, definitive treatment option for asymptomatic traumatized permanent anterior teeth with exposed pulp rather than full pulpotomy (28).

A high success rate has also been reported for both partial and complete pulpotomy complicated crown fractures. An overall success range ranging from 75% to 96% was reported (29), suggesting the utility of this treatment over conventional direct pulp capping, which was shown to be associated with lower success (30). A large body of evidence demonstrated a high incidence of pulp necrosis following direct pulp capping in cases of complicated crown fractures (31, 32).

Subsequently, clinical guidelines issued by the ESE and the International Association of Dental Traumatology (IADT) currently indicate that pulp exposure in traumatized mature and immature permanent teeth should be treated by a VPT (33, 34). The ESE recommend VPT, preferably with non-staining hydraulic calcium silicate cement as capping material, but they suggest favourable results can also be achieved with calcium hydroxide. The ESE and IADT suggest partial pulpotomy as the preferred treatment, particularly for large exposures and cases with treatment delay. Direct pulp capping was only suggested for minor exposures treated within the first hours after trauma. In case of questionable pulp healing following severe injury with concomitant luxation injury, ESE 2021 suggest root canal treatment over VPT.

In summary, in managing the traumatically exposed pulp, partial pulpotomy is recommended for large exposures and cases with treatment. Direct pulp capping is indicated for minor exposures treated within the first hours after trauma. Pulpectomy and root canal treatment are considered in cases of questionable pulp healing as in concomitant luxation injuries.

Other Indications

Pulpotomy procedures have shown promising results in the management of severely furcation-involved molars requiring vital root resection. As an alternative to conventional endodontics, pulpotomy procedures were performed on 15 maxillary molars with class II and class II furcation defects using hydraulic calcium silicate-based cement. Four weeks following these procedures, affected roots were resected by periodontal microsurgery (35). The results showed that the function and vitality of the treated molars were maintained in 100% of cases after a mean follow-up period of 4.9 years. All resected teeth showed reduced probing depths, stable clinical attachment and radiographic bone levels. This offers a great advantage over root canal treatment, which has been reported to negatively impact on the survival of periodontally involved molars with complications such as root fractures been cited as leading failures in these cases (36).

Pulpotomy has traditionally been used as a temporary or emergency treatment for pain relief for teeth with symptomatic irreversible pulpitis. The procedure often offers effective pain relief similar to pulpectomy (37, 38). Pulpotomy may be preferred as it requires significantly less time and is a simple technique that effectively relieves symptoms.

In multi-rooted teeth with partial pulp necrosis, a successful combination of root canal treatment and pulpotomy was reported (39). In these teeth, conventional root canal treatment was performed in roots with non-vital pulp and apical periodontitis, while pulpotomy was performed in roots with vital pulp, suggesting that in advanced cases of irreversible pulpitis, VPT can still be used to preserve pulp tissue in the same tooth as necrotic tissue was removed.

Contraindications

There are general contraindications for restorative treatment that could automatically apply to pulpotomy including, poor oral hygiene, uncontrolled caries, periodontal disease, unrestorable tooth and teeth that cannot be adequately isolated. Contraindications that are procedure-specific are not common and include the inability to control pulpal bleeding, the presence of necrotic pulp/lack of bleeding and the need to post and core restoration. Teeth exhibiting spontaneous pain, continuous uncontrollable pulp bleeding or the presence of necrotic tissue in the pulp chamber are generally not predictable candidates for partial pulpotomy (40). Traumatic dental injuries that affect the pulpal blood supply should be carefully considered as negative prognostic factor for pulpotomy and if evident would be a contraindication for VPT.

The Procedure

Microbial contamination of the pulp wound is one of the major negative prognostic factors for VPT. In the case of cariously exposed pulp, the use of an enhanced protocol to limit the contamination, maximize technical precision and improve the tissue response is recommended (5, 13). Reported variation in the success of pulp capping after carious exposure (41, 42), led to a classification of pulp exposure based on presence (class II) or absence (Class I) of bacterial contamination (43). In the case of carious exposure (class II), the classification reinforces the need for an enhanced approach, which is not as critical if the pulp is traumatically exposed (Class I). Class II exposure is usually seen in teeth with deep and extremely deep caries where bacteria contamination and severe inflammation are usually evident where VPT with partial or full pulpotomy rather than direct pulp capping is recommended (5). Here, an enhanced protocol, which uses an antiseptic technique, antibacterial lavage, magnification for careful carious tissue removal and the use of a hydraulic calcium silicate cement (HCSC), is recommended (5, 13).

Aseptic Operatory Field

Meticulously controlled isolation of the tooth is essential to ensure a high-quality endodontic treatment in general and VPT. It is paramount to use not only a dental dam throughout all the stages of the treatment but also to maintain the operatory field as aseptic as possible by using sterile instruments and antimicrobial irrigating solutions such as sodium hypochlorite (NaOCl) (13). The isolation of several teeth may be preferred as it improves visibility and facilitates better space for instruments and direct application of the water coolant to the pulp tissue. Ligatures and inversion of the dental dam can be helpful, and liquid dam should be used to ensure a tight seal with the tooth (44) (Figure 6.1). The isolated area, including tooth/teeth and clamps, should be routinely disinfected to decrease the bacterial contamination. Different protocols have been proposed, including swabbing the area with hydrogen peroxide, followed by chlorhexidine, iodine or NaOCl (45, 46). Although, several methods have been shown to be effective in decreasing bacterial load, NaOCl decontamination appears to be effective in causing damage to bacterial DNA (47). It is fundamental to repeat the decontamination of the operatory field after the removal of old restorations and caries as this can readily contaminate areas that were previously cleaned (46) (Figure 6.2).

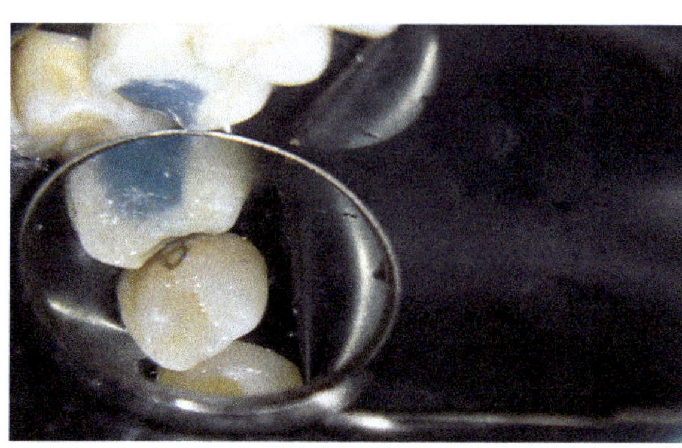

Figure 6.1 Isolation of several teeth allows better visibility. The rubber dam is inverted or blocked with ligatures to ensure a tight seal.

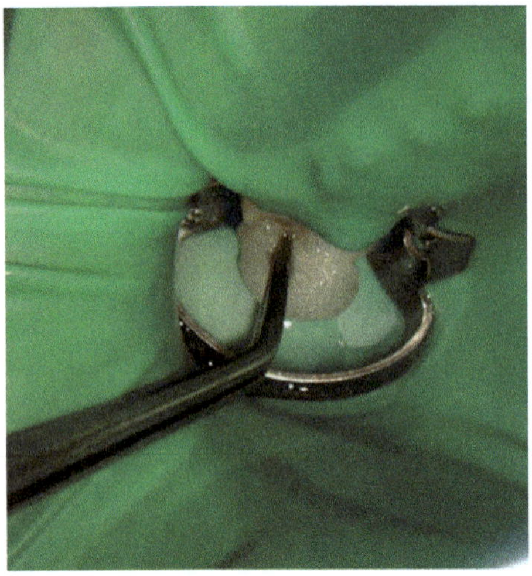

Figure 6.2 The tooth, clamp and rubber dam are decontaminated by swabbing a disinfectant-soaked cotton pallet.

Magnification and Caries Detection

The use of magnification systems is recommended in endodontics as it improves visibility, illumination of the operative field as well as operator ergonomics. The increased vision during an enhanced class II pulp capping is useful throughout the treatment and ideally should be used throughout the entire treatment as it ensures better vision during the non-selective caries removal, the subsequent management of exposed pulp tissue and finally verifies the placement of the restorative material (48). In general, partial pulpotomies are technically demanding procedures. As a result, practitioners without access to magnification may prefer to carry out a full coronal pulpotomy as it is easier to manipulate the pulp at the level of the orifice (13). Magnification loupes and microscopes can be efficiently used; however, the second offers better magnification and illumination albeit at greater expense. Complete and correct removal of all the carious tissue is essential after pulp exposure and is enhanced by increasing the visibility and caries detectors. Different methods are available to check the presence of remaining decay are available, from fluorescence lamps to caries detectors dye (42, 48) (Figure 6.3).

Bleeding Control and Antibacterial Lavage

Inflamed dental pulp usually bleed during pulpotomy procedures, and effective control of bleeding and the avoidance of blood clot formation between the capping material and the pulp tissue is essential for successful treatment outcome. There is, however, a lack of consensus regarding how

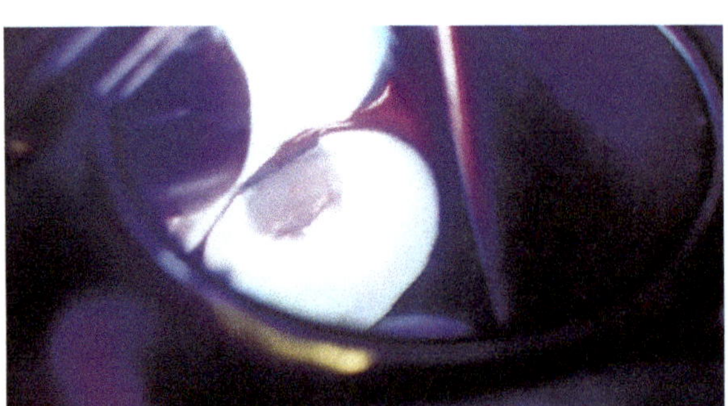

Figure 6.3 Immunofluorescence lamps can be useful in detecting the residual affected tissue after non-selective caries removal.

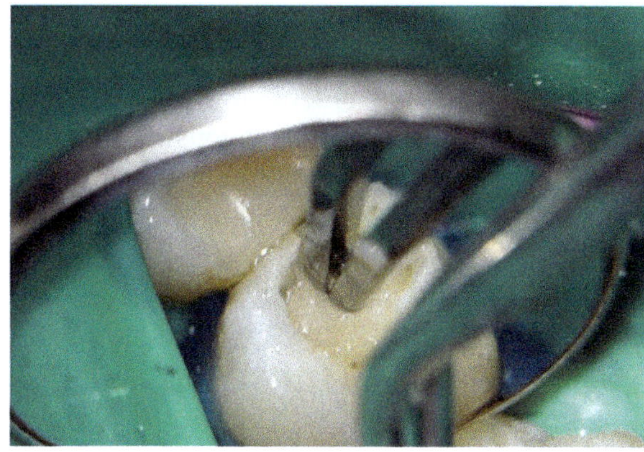

Figure 6.4 Bleeding control is achieved by pressing a cotton pallet soaked in NaOCl against the pulp.

best to manage the exposed pulp and control of haemorrhage, being no exception (8, 49). Over the years, many agents have been used to arrest bleeding, including NaOCl (0.5–5, 25%), saline solution, chlorhexidine (0.2–2%), water, ethanol (75%) and anaesthetic solution (42, 48, 50–52). The ESE position statement (2019) on managing deep carious lesions recommended using either sodium hypochlorite or chlorhexidine. The rationale behind using these two agents is the ability to achieve haemostasis while disinfecting the area, which is fundamental in class II pulpotomies due to the exposure of the pulp and infection (13). The most popular lavage is NaOCl; however, there is still a need for further, well-designed studies to assess if there is a significant improvement in the quality of treatment when sodium hypochlorite is used (53). One recent randomized control trial indicated decreased pain (54) and improved success after one year when the exposed pulp was rinsed with NaOCl rather than saline in a pulp capping study (55). The arrest of bleeding should be achieved in five minutes after gently pressing a NaOCl-soaked sterile cotton pallet against the pulp; however, if haemostasis is not achieved during this time, further pulp removal may be necessary (5, 13) (Figure 6.4).

Capping Materials

The ideal material for VPT should possess a number of characteristics including maintaining pulpal vitality, stimulating the hard tissue bridge formation, releasing fluoride, being bactericidal/bacteriostatic, adhering to both dentine and restorative materials, being insoluble, being able to resist high forces, offering a good bacterial seal, being radiopaque and being able to be sterilized (56).

For many years, calcium hydroxide has been considered the material of choice for pulp capping (7). Indeed, this material has characteristics suitable for VPT, and even though its mechanism of action is still partially unknown, it promotes the formation of a hard tissue bridge (57). Despite its popularity, this material does not appear to be the best choice when it comes to VPT as it has been demonstrated that hydraulic calcium silicate cements (HCSCs) outperform this material both histologically and clinically (24, 58–61). Calcium hydroxide materials are soluble, and they do not predictably promote the formation of a continuous hard tissue bridge (58). Since the introduction of MTA in the 1990s (62), hydraulic calcium silicate cements have become the gold standard for conservative management of exposed pulp.

MTA has multiple indications in endodontics due to its high biocompatibility and bioactivity, excellent long-term seal, hydrophilic setting properties and good radiopacity. However, the material also has some limitations, with the presence of bismuth oxide as a radiopacifier resulting in an increase in setting times and tooth discolouration, while the handling of the material is also not user-friendly (56). In order to overcome the limitations of the material, other HCSCs were introduced with different formulations that modified characteristics including setting time, handling and discolouration potential while keeping similar biocompatibility and bioactive properties (63–66). Despite similarities in action, there are different formulations of HCSC:

- *Powder and liquid hand mixed.* The classic MTA formulation consists of a liquid and powder that are manually mixed until the formation of a 'sand-like' consistency that is then applied onto the pulp tissue (Figure 6.5a–c). Common brands include; ProRoot MTA (Denstply Sirona, Ballaigues, Switzerland) and Angelus MTA (Angelus, Londrina, Brazil). These materials have a relatively long setting time and according to the manufacturer's instructions a moist cotton pellet should be placed over them before restoring the tooth with a temporary filling at the first visit, before placing the permanent restoration after verifying final set at a subsequent visit. They are becoming less popular as VPT materials because of the difficult handling, long setting time and the fact that many of them induce discolouration (56).
- *Powder and liquid capsules.* The most common example is Biodentine (Septodont, Sant-Maur-des-Fossés, France), a popular product for VPT (Figure 6.6a). The powder and liquid are in a capsule and produce a material of consistent viscosity that has been proven to be reliable as VPT material (67–69). Although Biodentine is marketed as a setting in 12 minutes, clinical studies have reported longer setting times, even up to 45 minutes (48). The manufacturers suggest that Biodentine can also be used to fill the entire cavity and as a temporary filling material and can

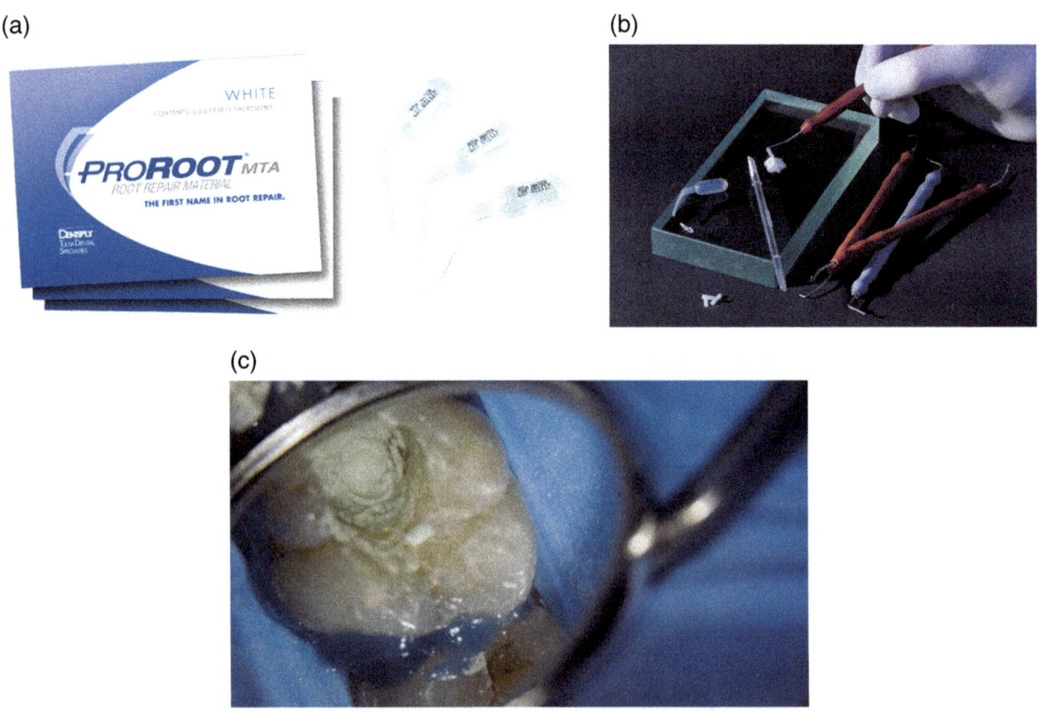

Figure 6.5 (a) ProRoot was one of the first HCSCs available, (b) hand mixing of MTA until reaching a 'sand-like' consistency, (c) sand-like consistency MTA is gently applied over the pulp. *Source:* (a) Dentsply Sirona.

(a) (b)

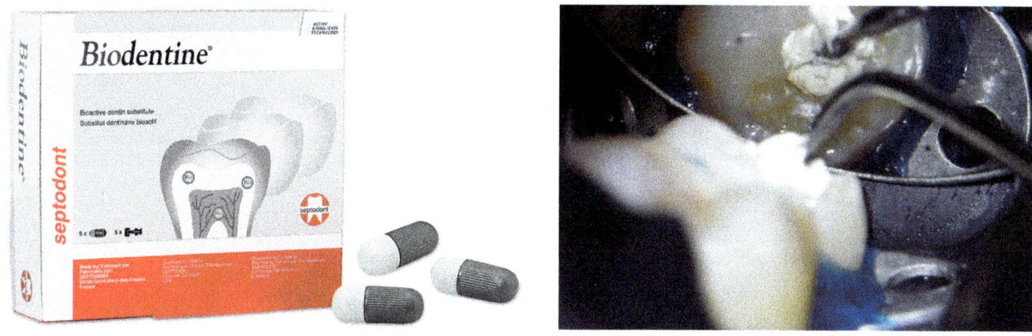

Figure 6.6 (a). Biodentine is capsulated where a liquid is added before mixing in an amalgamator mixer. (b). The creamy-like material is brought into the cavity with an amalgam plugger or other suitable instrument. All the cavity can be filled with Biodentine used as temporary filling. *Source:* (a) Septodont Holding.

(a) (b)

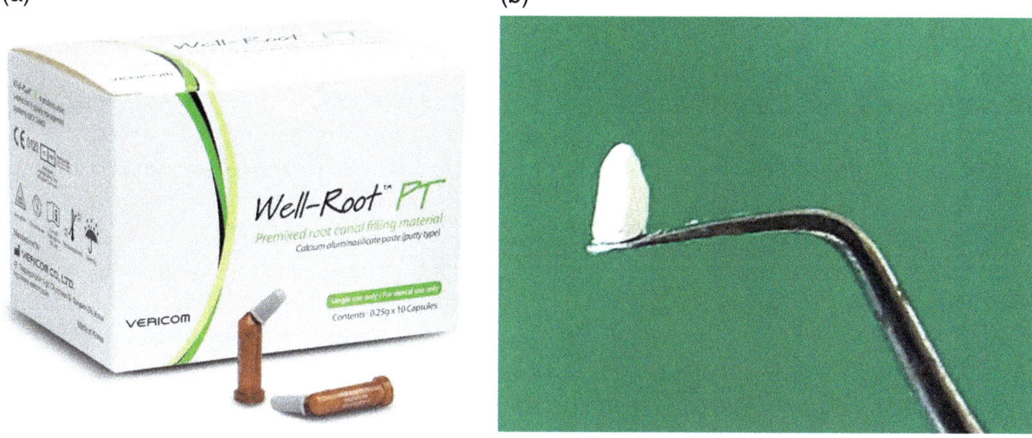

Figure 6.7 (a). Well root PT is a premixed putty HCSC that comes ready mixed in capsules. (b). The putty formulation makes the material very easy to manipulate clinically. *Source:* (a) NewDental/VERICOM CO., LTD.

last up to six months (Figure 6.6b). Notably, and problematically the radiopacity is below ISO standards, which makes difficult to distinguish the material from dentine and filling materials on the radiograph.

- *Premixed*. Premixed HCSCs come in putty formulation, with common products including; Totalfill Putty (FKG, La Chaux-de-Fonds, Switzerland) and Well Root PT (Vericom, Anyang, South Korea) (Figure 6.7a). Their consistency and the handling make them very easy to manipulate, carry and apply (Figure 6.7b). Setting times; however, can vary between the different brands (70).
- *Light cured*. Theracal (BISCO, Schaumburg, USA) is an example here (Figure 6.8). It is a flowable premixed material that can be light-cured directly after application, increasing its practicality for immediate restoration. However, it is resin-based, and studies have reported poor results compared with other HCSCs and a poorer pulpal response to this material (71–73).

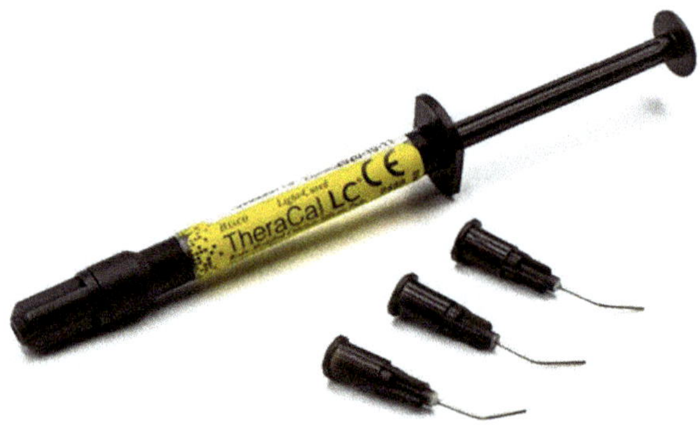

Figure 6.8 Theracal is a light-cured bioactive material.

Clinical Protocol

Armamentarium

In summary, the enhanced protocol is recommended for the management of the infected and exposed pulp and requires the following armamentarium:

- Magnification: Ideally, a microscope as it allows optimal vision and illumination. Magnification loupes can be a valid alternative.
- Dental dam: has to be correctly positioned, ensuring tight moisture control and asepsis.
- Disinfection agent for the dental field: NaOCl is the best disinfectant to use, however CHX has also be advocated by some investigators.
- Sterile cotton wool pellets:
- Sterile high-speed burs: it is necessary to have two sets of burs, one for caries removal and another one for pulpotomy procedure. Both of them have to be sterile, but it is important to not contaminate the burs used for pulpotomy with decayed tissue and make sure that they are sharp and new.
- Decay detectors: fluorescence lamp or decay dye.
- Sharp excavator: to remove the affected tissue that can be found over the pulp in order to decrease the risk of accidental exposure.
- Application tools: For carrying the hydraulic calcium silicate cements and adapting them to the wound, they may vary according to the type of material used.

Assessment and Anaesthesia

Partial and full pulpotomy share a very similar operative protocol, differing only in the volume of pulp tissue removed. Although pulpotomy procedures have been promoted as being technically easier to carry out compared with root canal treatment, they are actually technically demanding and require meticulous execution (13). Dealing with vital pulp tissues requires focus, particularly with regard to the maintenance of a clean operatory field, careful manipulation of pulp tissue and ensuring a high-quality seal of the post-endodontic restoration.

VPT procedures should not be carried out without a proper preoperative assessment and plan, as the outcome of the therapy is influenced by a correct diagnosis (48). Detailed pain history, particularly previous pain experience and presence or absence of spontaneous pain, should be ascertained. Sensibility tests with heat and cold should be performed, followed by a radiographic assessment to check for periapical radiolucency and the extension of caries. The first can be

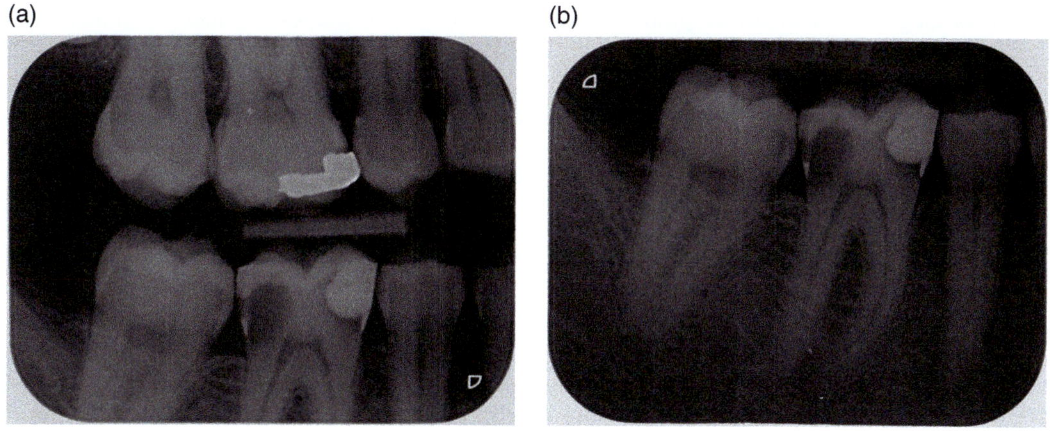

Figure 6.9 (a) and (b) It is recommended to assess the tooth for both apical pathology and extension of caries. Bitewings (a) is the best way to assess caries depth, while a periapical radiograph (b) is required to assess the periapical area.

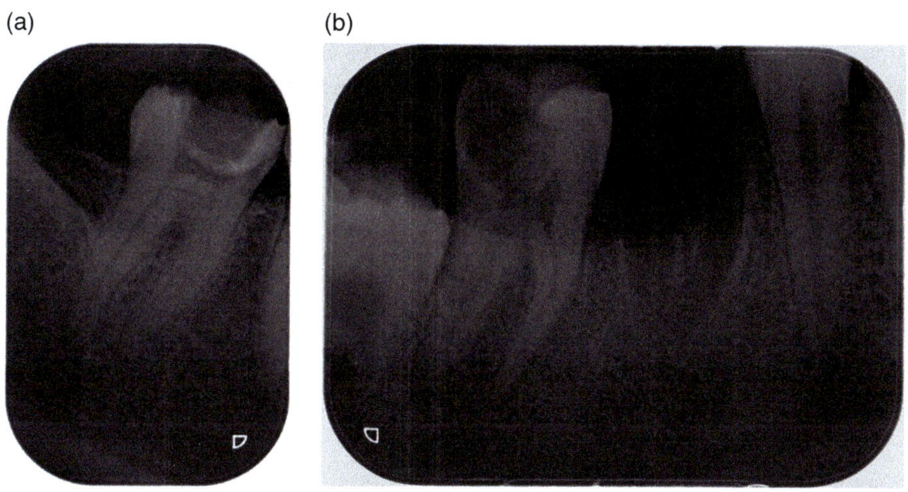

Figure 6.10 (a) and (b) Deep lesion. Even though the cavity is deep, a radiopaque layer can be clearly seen between the cavity and the pulp. Extremely deep lesion. The caries lesion extends into the full depth of dentine and appears in contact with the pulp tissue. Pulp exposure is unavoidable.

assessed with a periapical x-ray, while the second should be checked with an intraoral bitewing x-ray as it has been shown to be the more reliable test for interproximal caries detection (74) (Figure 6.9a,b). It is crucial to know the extent of caries as there is a difference between deep (Figure 6.10a) and extremely deep carious lesions (Figure 6.10b) with regard to bacteria penetration and the severity of pulpal inflammation (75, 76).

The classification of pulpitis into the dichotomous clinical diagnoses, reversible and irreversible pulpitis, has been challenged due to the fact that cases deemed as irreversible pulpitis can actually be treated successfully with VPT (24, 75–78). As a result, a new classification that divides the pulp status in initial, mild, moderate and severe pulpitis has been proposed and subsequently used to classify cases preoperatively before partial pulpotomy (48) (see Chapter 3). Results demonstrated that cases diagnosed with severe pulpitis and treated by partial pulpotomy had a significantly poorer success rate after one year (48, 79).

Pulp exposure and subsequent management require adequate anaesthesia. The procedure may take a considerable amount of time, so the presence of adrenaline is critical to maintain the analgesic effect. A 2% lignocaine with adrenaline 1:80,000 solution appears to be sufficient to perform VPT, although some authors report the use of 4% articaine with adrenaline 1:100,000 (24, 48, 78, 80). Both local infiltrations and nerve blocks can be used; however, an intra-pulpal injection should be avoided due to the risk of damaging the pulp tissue.

Pre-VPT Preparatory Procedures

Pre-VPT preparatory procedures are performed in order to allow working in a completely isolated and aseptic field. It is important to focus on limiting the potential of contamination as well as optimizing marginal seal.

Depending on the clinical scenario, different preparatory steps may be required:

a) The tooth has 'sound' proximal walls (i.e. class I cavity), and the pulpotomy can be completed immediately without the need for extensive preparation of the site (Figure 6.11a,b).
b) Interproximal defects are present and may extend subgingivally (Figure 6.12a); in this case, a pre-VPT restoration may be required (Figure 6.12b,c). The need for this stage is guided by the ability to isolate the area effectively: if the tooth can be completely isolated and it is clear that after non-selective caries removal, the operative area will not be contaminated by saliva or blood, there is no need to carry this out. However, if isolation is challenging or compromised, a pre-VPT stage is recommended, as a marginal seal is important for the success of the treatment.

If necessary, gingivectomy or crown lengthening procedures can be performed during this phase. After careful assessment (Figure 6.13a,b), the carious dentine is grossly removed from the entire cavity, and non-selective caries removal on the cavity margins (Figure 6.13c), avoiding pulp exposure if possible. The tooth is then isolated with a dental dam, and after the margin is caries-free, a resin-based composite (RBC) restoration can be placed (Figure 6.13d,e). As this stage aims to improve the marginal seal prior to dental dam placement, the volume of RBC placed should be

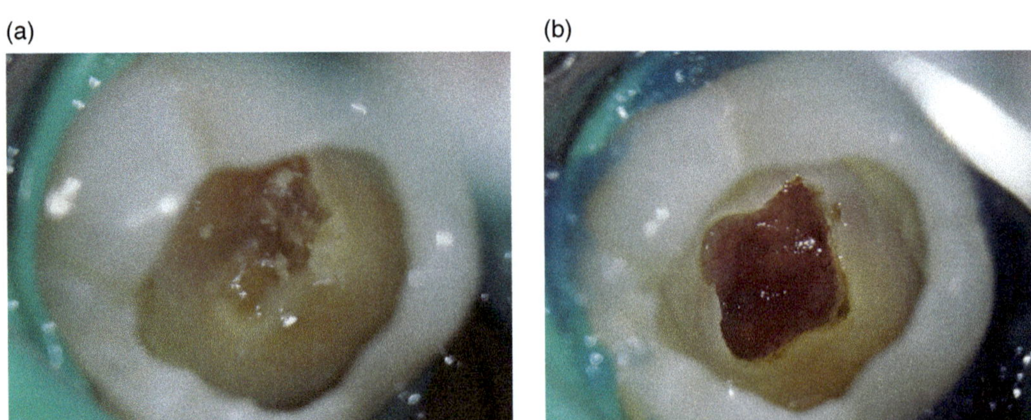

Figure 6.11 (a) Deep occlusal cavity with 'sound' walls. (b) Pulpotomy performed without previous build up procedures.

(a) (b) (c)

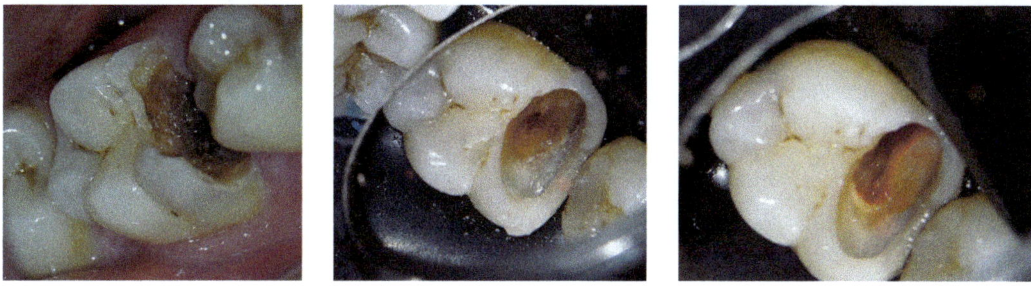

Figure 6.12 (a) Deep mesial cavity with loss of interproximal wall. (b) The mesial margin is rebuilt with composite before the exposure. (c) The pulpotomy is performed.

minimized. Often, in order to achieve a seal, it is necessary to modify the standard matrices or use a multiple matrix system (e.g. matrix in matrix technique) (Figure 6.13d). The use of matrices may damage the dam, which should be carefully inspected after the completion of the pre-VPT: If the dam displays any minimal tears, it should be replaced, while if it is still offering good isolation, it can be disinfected (Figure 6.13e,f). It is always advisable to check radiographically that the margins of the restoration are adequate (Figure 6.13g,h).

Caries Removal

Non-selective (complete) removal of all carious dentine is essential. Complete elimination of all affected dentine has the advantage of decreasing bacterial contamination while offering a better substrate for adhesion (81). Tactile feedback on caries removal should be supplemented with caries detectors when required, as they can be useful in assisting the removal of the affected tissue without over-removal of healthy dentine (82). The pulp should only be exposed if the caries penetrates the pulp chamber; therefore, it is important to be careful when in close proximity to the pulp in order to avoid accidental exposure. After removal of the softened carious dentine from the peripheral areas with a water-cooled bur, a sharp, sterile hand excavator can be used over the pulpal aspect of the cavity (Figure 6.14a). If the pulp is exposed and more affected tissue is present, it should be completely removed, ensuring that the burs are very well cooled and carious dentine chips are not pushed into the pulp tissue (Figure 6.14b). Depending on the size of the exposure and degree of bleeding, a small partial pulpotomy (e.g. the removal of a pulp horn) can be performed, or alternatively, the entire pulp chamber's roof can be removed as part of a full pulpotomy procedure in cases where bleeding cannot be adequately controlled, suggesting a need for removal of more inflamed pulp tissues. All these procedures cause some degree of pulpal contamination with bacteria, so a precise aseptic is critical. At this stage, a second disinfection of tooth, dental dam and clamp should be performed (46).

Pulp Tissue Removal (Pulpotomy)

Visualizing the exposed pulp tissue may be helpful when deciding the volume of pulp tissue to be removed (81). When pulpal inflammation is present, bleeding can be copious and rinsing with NaOCl can help to visualize the extent of the exposure and reduce bacterial load in the pulp (55). At this stage, all carious tissue should be removed using a fresh, sterile bur in a fast handpiece; for optimum control, a red-ring contra-angle can be used. It is critical to perform a 'clean' surgical cut

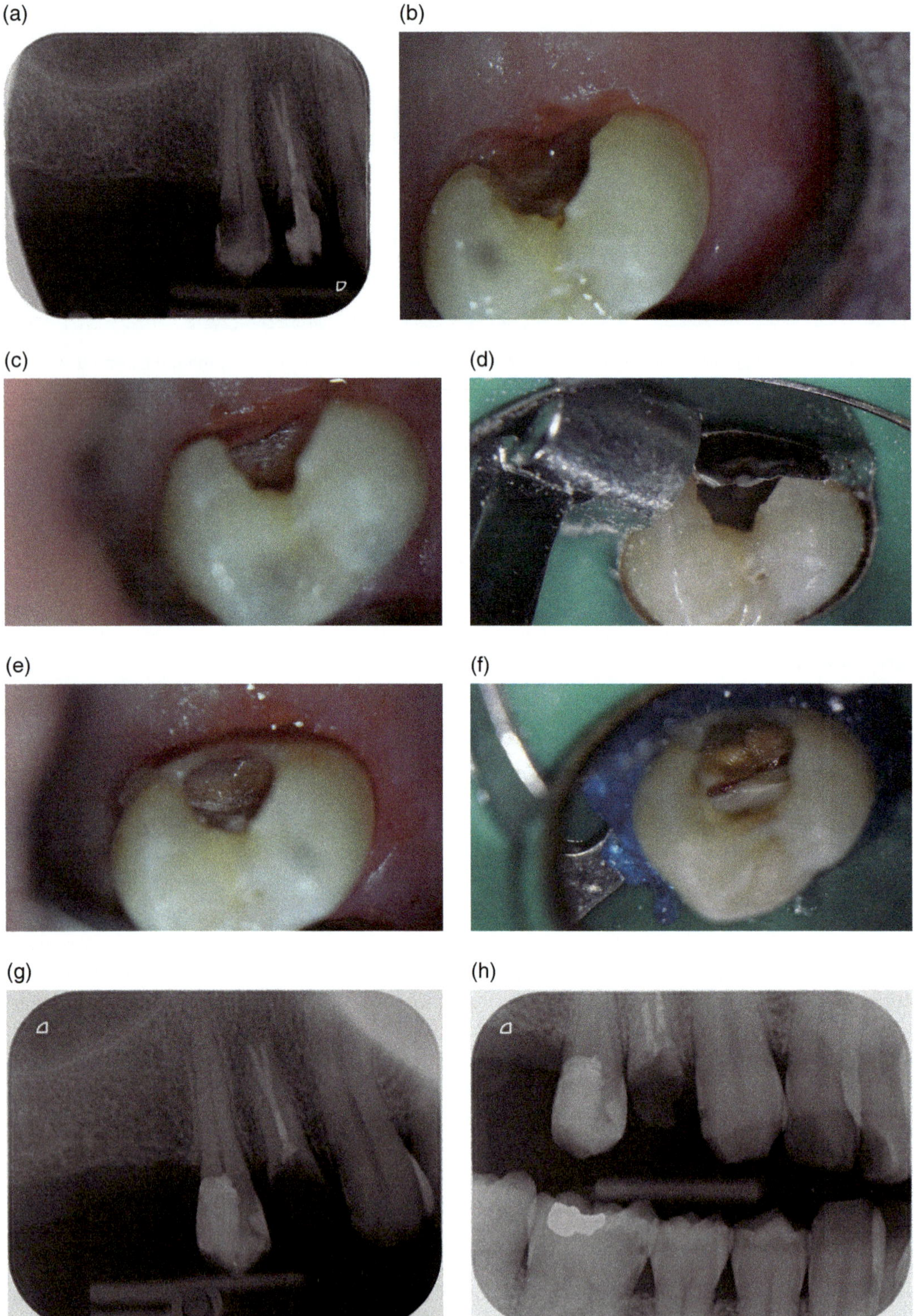

Figure 6.13 (a) Extremely deep carious cavity on tooth 1.5. The tooth was vital, and a VPT has been planned. (b) Caries extend to/or below gingival. (c) Caries were grossly removed before rubber dam placement. (d) After placing the dental dam, a clean margin was obtained, and a 'matrix in matrix' solution was used to ensure a good seal of the RBC. (e) The Pre-VPT RBC restoration was created, and the dental dam was replaced due to damage. (f) The partial pulpotomy is completed. (g and h) The quality of VPT and restoration is checked with bitewings and periapical X-ray.

(a) (b)

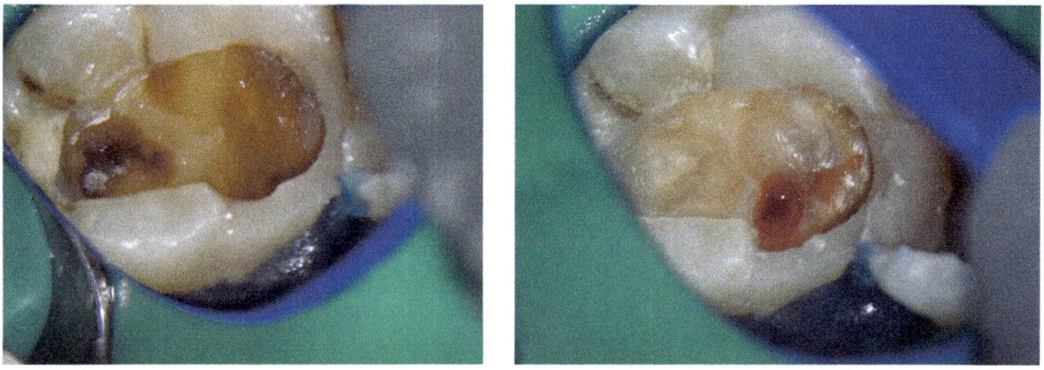

Figure 6.14 (a) After gross carious tissue removal, affected, soft tissue is still present in the pulp chamber area. (b) After gross non-selective caries removal, the pulp is exposed.

(a) (b)

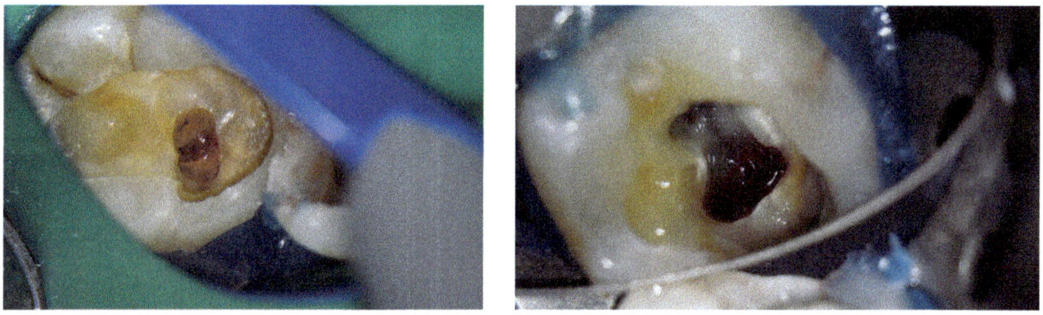

Figure 6.15 (a) In a partial pulpotomy procedures 2–3 mm of pulp tissue are removed. (b) In a full coronal pulpotomy: the pulp tissue is removed up to the orifices.

without leaving pulp tissue in areas such as pulp horns, where it can get necrotic and cause the failure of the procedure. In this phase, a copious and correct delivery of water coolant is crucial and should be used intermittently to allow the water to reach it. In a partial pulpotomy, usually, 2–3 mm of pulp is removed (Figure 6.15a), while whenever a full pulpotomy is required, the bur is used to remove all the pulp tissue to the root canal orifices (13) (Figure 6.15b).

Achieving Haemostasis

Bleeding control is of fundamental importance in VPT, as it allows both the visual inspection of the pulp and the effective placement of a pulp-capping biomaterial. Uncontrollable haemorrhage after several minutes, even in the presence of pressure and NaOCl application, indicates that further tissue removal is required. For example, if after partial pulpotomy bleeding remains, more pulp should be removed and a full pulpotomy carried out. If bleeding cannot be arrested at the root canal orifices, a root canal treatment is indicated (13). Although several irrigants including saline, water, local anaesthetic and ethanol have been used for this purpose (53), NaOCl is the most used agent and has recently been shown in 2% concentration, at least with pulp capping to significantly

(a)

(b) (c)

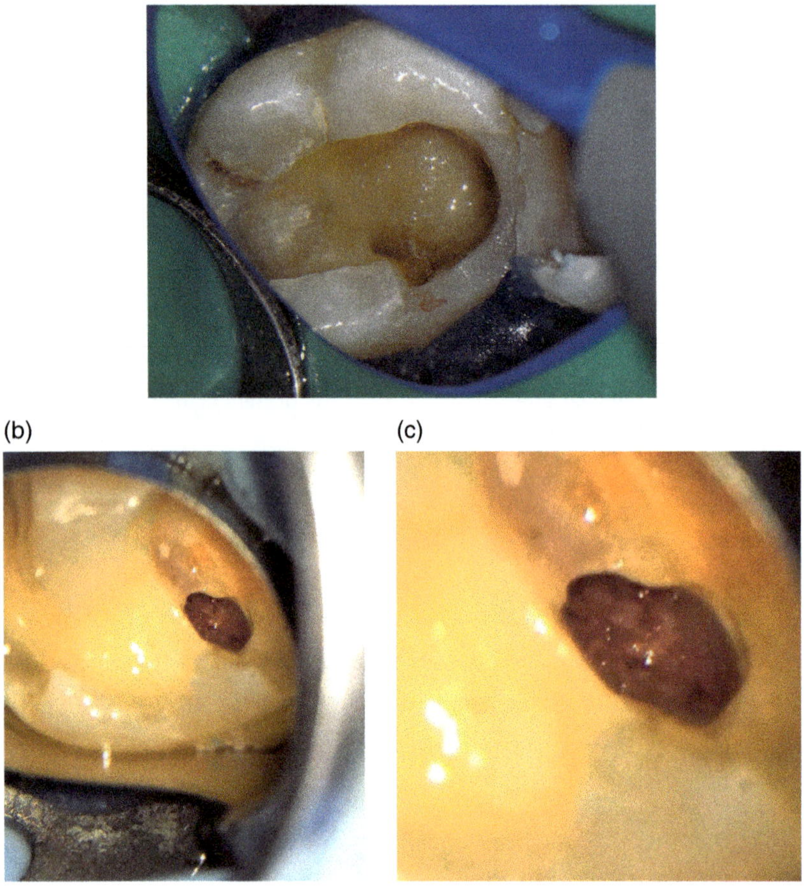

Figure 6.16 (a) Cotton pellets soaked in NaOCl pressed against the pulp tissue are an effective way to stop the bleeding while disinfecting. (b) and (c) Aspect of the pulp after partial pulpotomy and successful bleeding control.

reduce postoperative pain and increase the success of pulp capping procedures after one year (55). Whether NaOCl will have the same effect after pulpotomy procedures remains to be seen. NaOCl lavage provides haemostasis without causing surface necrosis of the pulp and provides an antibacterial lavage to the wound. The disinfectant can be delivered through cotton pellets soaked in NaOCl and pressed gently over the pulp (Figure 6.16a). At present, there is no consensus on how long the pellet has to be in place with studies ranging evaluations from one to six minutes (48). Once the bleeding has completely stopped, the pulp capping procedure itself can be performed (Figure 6.16b,c). As an alternative to NaOCl, chlorhexidine can also be used, while the use of saline or water rinses should be avoided or limited to traumatic exposure (13, 61).

Placement of the Pulp Capping Material

Calcium hydroxide is no longer the material of choice for pulp capping procedures; however, its use is still recommended by some (83). HCSCs have replaced calcium hydroxide due to its poor mechanical characteristics, solubility and incomplete hard tissue bridge formation (56).

As suggested before (see section iv), in histological and clinical studies, hydraulic calcium silicate cement produced better results compared with calcium hydroxide materials (58, 60). Indeed, calcium hydroxide remains a product of the hydration reaction of HCSCs; however, these cements are far less aggressive on the pulp tissue and induce less inflammation (84).

Depending on the formulation of hydraulic calcium silicate cement used, the operative protocol may vary. Generally speaking, the material should be gently applied to the pulp once the bleeding has been arrested. A layer of at least 2–3 mm should be applied, and the surrounding sound dentine should be kept as clean as possible to increase the area for adhesion. Hand-mixed materials like MTA are the most difficult to handle (56). The hydraulic calcium silicate cement should be carefully mixed and carried to the exposure site using 'carriers' such as the MAP System (PD, Vevey, Switzerland) and compacted with a lightly moist paper point (Figure 6.5c). MTA has a long setting time that makes immediate restoration difficult; therefore, a slightly moist cotton pallet should be applied over the material before placing a temporary filling (85).

Biodentine is mixed in an amalgamator, which will result in a mix of thick creamy consistency that can be brought directly to the cavity with a hand instrument before compacting the material gently. The advantage of Biodentine is that it can be restored permanently after setting in one visit, or alternatively, the entire cavity can be filled and the Biodentine 'cut back' and permanently restored in a later appointment without the need for other temporary filling materials (Figure 6.17a,b).

Premixed materials are easy to manipulate and can be introduced in the cavity with a probe or a plugger. They can then be adapted over the exposure using a small brush. The initial setting time of these materials is generally fast, and many clinicians restore the tooth permanently after waiting for the initial setting rather than placing a temporary restoration (Figure 6.17c). Theracal is probably the easiest material to apply, having the consistency of a flowable composite and being delivered directly from a syringe. After its application, it can be light cured and the tooth restored permanently without delay. Unfortunately, the material cannot be recommended for direct pulp application as it has demonstrated the poorest pulpal responses (71–73).

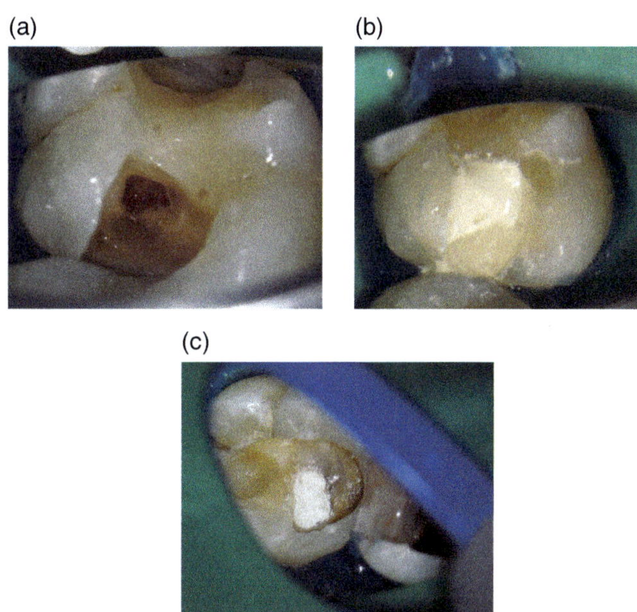

Figure 6.17 (a) After bleeding control, (b) the entire cavity is filled with Biodentine. Or (c) A putty HCSC has been placed over the pulpotomy, carefully limiting its presence to the capping area.

Placement of Final Restoration

Adequate coronal seal is a critical factor in determining the long-term success of VPT, as it prevents bacterial reinfection of the wound site. In VPT, not only the quality of restoration but also the timing appears to be important (13, 81). Although success has been reported with delayed permanent restoration, whenever possible, an immediate restoration should be preferred as the long-term outcome is more favourable (86–88). From a practical perspective, VPTs are often emergency procedures, and there could be a lack of time available for permanent restoration placement; however, the permanent coronal seal should still be applied as soon as possible, as the chance of failure increases if the temporary filling is left in place for more than two days (61). Currently, there is a paucity of literature regarding the bonding of RBCs to hydraulic calcium silicate cement, and further investigation is needed to understand which bonding protocol is the most appropriate. As a general rule, as much as possible, the peripheral dentine should be kept clean of cement in order to have a better surface for bonding (Figure 6.17c). In case of a delayed restoration, the entire cavity can be first sandblasted, the enamel can be selectively etched, and then primer and bonding applied (Figure 6.18a,b). After successful bonding, a first layer of flowable composite is applied to cover completely the hydraulic calcium silicate cement before restoring the tooth with bulk fill or incremental RBC (Figure 6.18c).

Outcomes of Pulpotomy

The objective of VPT is to maintain pulp vitality and prevent apical periodontitis. Evaluation of the outcome of the treatment should, therefore, assess if it achieved these objectives. This is often achieved as directly reported outcomes by patients or by clinicians during history and examination (clinical and radiographic).

Which Outcome to Assess?

Details of outcomes of VPT in general are discussed in Chapter 10. The most important patient-reported outcomes are pain and oral health-related quality of life (89). Pain is the main reason for patients to attend dental treatment; pain relief is the immediate outcome of pulpotomy. In this regard, pulpotomy is as effective as root canal treatment for postoperative pain relief (22). Other outcomes include response to pulp vitality/sensibility test, signs and symptoms suggestive of irreversible pulpitis or apical periodontitis, radiographic evidence of apical periodontitis, root resorption and canal calcifications, tooth survival and need for further intervention (16).

(a) (b) (c)

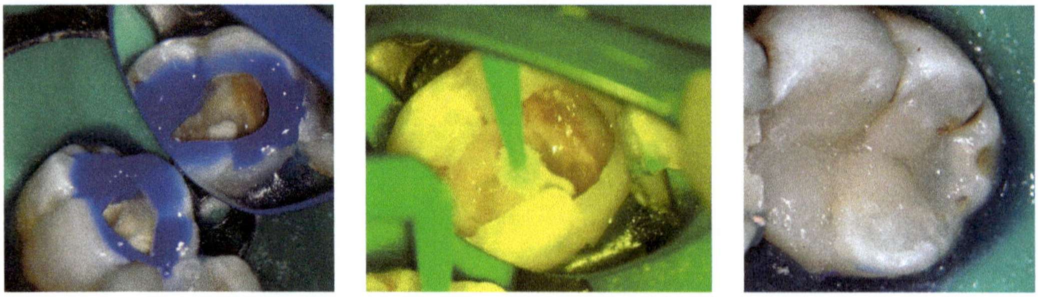

Figure 6.18 After setting the HCSC the tooth can be selectively etched and sandblasted (a). Prime and bond can be applied (b), and the tooth can be restored with an RBC (c).

When and How Outcomes Are Assessed?

Pulpotomy outcomes can be considered as short-term outcomes such as postoperative pain relief reported up to three months after treatment (90), or long-term outcomes that require longer follow-up to be evident including evidence clinical and radiographic evidence of pulpal and periapical disease and tooth survival. The ESE position statement (2019) recommended VPT procedures should be assessed 6 and 12 months postoperatively and at yearly intervals (if necessary) for four years thereafter. The assessment should be carried out clinically (signs and symptoms, including response to sensibility tests and clinical signs of infections) and radiographically. Success is often defined as the maintenance of pulp vitality with the absence of signs and symptoms of pulpal and periapical disease for at least one year (13).

Factors That May Influence the Outcomes of Pulpotomy

A number of tooth as well as patient-related factors have been suggested to influence the outcome of pulpotomy (90). Factors such as age, gender, tooth type and stage of root development were not shown to influence the outcome of pulpotomy (90). However, others outlined below could affect treatment outcomes, and many need to be discussed with patients in the treatment planning process as possible prognostic indicators.

- Caries depth and preoperative status of the pulp: Extremely deep caries are likely to be associated with bacterial infection of the pulp and, therefore, reduce the success of at least partial pulpotomy procedures (48). This same applies to cases with severe pulpitis (history of previous pain, spontaneous pain) that indicate an advanced level of inflammation that may not be treatable with partial pulpotomy. In this case, complete pulpotomy or even pulpectomy may be the treatment of choice.

In addition to these teeth-related factors, other operative factors including the use of the enhanced protocol with proper isolation with a dentaldam, disinfection, bleeding control, use of magnification, dressing with hydraulic calcium silicate cement and provision of high-quality coronal seals, are prerequisites for successful outcomes of both partial and complete pulpotomy (13, 90).

Conclusions

In summary, partial and full pulpotomy are minimally invasive pulp preservation therapies with many applications in modern endodontic practice. The procedure can be applied for the treatment of carious as well as traumatic pulp exposure using an enhanced protocol and appropriate case selection to ensure success. The current evidence suggests a high success rate for both procedures, even in teeth with a diagnosis suggestive of symptomatic irreversible pulpits; however, such evidence is derived from studies with a high risk of bias and should be interpreted with caution.

References

1 Bergenholtz G. Iatrogenic injury to the pulp in dental procedures: aspects of pathogenesis, management and preventive measures. *Int Dent J.* 1991;41(2):99–110.

2 Farges JC, Alliot-Licht B, Renard E, et al. Dental pulp defence and repair mechanisms in dental caries. *Mediat Inflamm.* 2015;2015:230251.

3 Galler KM, Weber M, Korkmaz Y, Widbiller M, Feuerer M. Inflammatory response mechanisms of the dentine-pulp complex and the periapical tissues. *Int J Mol Sci.* 2021;22(3):1480.
4 Cooper PR, Takahashi Y, Graham LW, Simon S, Imazato S, Smith AJ. Inflammation-regeneration interplay in the dentine-pulp complex. *J Dent.* 2010;38:687–97.
5 Bjørndal L, Simon S, Tomson PL, Duncan HF. Management of deep caries and the exposed pulp. *Int Endod J.* 2019;52:949–73.
6 El Karim IA, Cooper PR, About I, Tomson PL, Lundy FT, Duncan HF. Deciphering reparative processes in the inflamed dental pulp. *Front Dent Med.* 2021;2:1–10.
7 Dammaschke T. The history of direct pulp capping. *J Hist Dent.* 2008;56(1):9–23.
8 Careddu R, Plotino G, Cotti E, Duncan HF. The management of deep carious lesions and the exposed pulp amongst members of two European endodontic societies: a questionnaire-based study. *Int Endod J.* 2021;54:366–76.
9 European Society of Endodontology. Quality guidelines for endodontic treatment: consensus report of the European Society of Endodontology. *Int Endod J.* 2006;39:921–30.
10 Cushley S, Duncan HF, Lappin MJ, Tomson PL, Lundy FT, Cooper P, et al. Pulpotomy for mature carious teeth with symptoms of irreversible pulpitis: a systematic review. *J Dent.* 2019;88:103158.
11 Tomson PL, Grover LM, Lumley PJ, Sloan AJ, Smith AJ, Cooper PR. Dissolution of bio-active dentine matrix components by mineral trioxide aggregate. *J Dent.* 2007;35(8):636–42.
12 American Association of Endodontists Endodontic diagnosis. [Internet]. 2019. Available from: https://www.aae.org
13 Duncan HF, Galler KM, Tomson PL, Simon S, El-Karim I, Kundzina R, et al. European Society of Endodontology position statement: management of deep caries and the exposed pulp. *Int Endod J.* 2019;52(7):923–34.
14 Bjørndal L. The caries process and its effect on the pulp: the science is changing and so is our understanding. *J Endod.* 2008;34(7 Suppl):S2–5.
15 Bjørndal L, Fransson H, Bruun G, et al. Randomized clinical trials on deep carious lesions: 5-year follow-up. *J Dent Res.* 2017;96:747–53.
16 Cushley S, Duncan HF, Lundy FT, Nagendrababu V, Clarke M, El Karim I. Outcomes reporting in systematic reviews on vital pulp treatment: a scoping review for the development of a core outcome set. *Int Endod J.* 2022;55:891–909.
17 Alqaderi H, Lee CT, Borzangy S, Pagonis TC. Coronal pulpotomy for cariously exposed permanent posterior teeth with closed apices: a systematic review and meta-analysis. *J Dent.* 2016;44:1–7.
18 Galani M, Tewari S, Sangwan P, Mittal S, Kumar V, Duhan J. Comparative evaluation of postoperative pain and success rate after pulpotomy and root canal treatment in cariously exposed mature permanent molars: a randomized controlled trial. *J Endod.* 2017;43:1953–62.
19 Elmsmari F, Ruiz XF, Miró Q, Feijoo-Pato N, Durán-Sindreu F, Olivieri JG. Outcome of partial pulpotomy in cariously exposed posterior permanent teeth: a systematic review and meta-analysis. *J Endod.* 2019;45:1296–306.
20 American Association of Endodontists. *Glossary of Endodontic Terms*, 10th Ed., American Association of Endodontists, Chicago, 2020. Available from: https://www.aae.org/specialty/clinical-resources/glossary-endodontic-terms/.
21 Asgary S, Eghbal MJ, Bagheban AA. Long-term outcomes of pulpotomy in permanent teeth with irreversible pulpitis: a multi-center randomized controlled trial. *Am J Dent.* 2017;30:151–5.
22 Tomson PL, Vilela Bastos J, Jacimovic J, Jakovljevic A, Pulikkotil SJ, Nagendrababu V. Effectiveness of pulpotomy compared with root canal treatment in managing non-traumatic pulpitis associated with spontaneous pain: a systematic review and meta-analysis. *Int Endod J.* 2022. https://doi.org/10.1111/iej.13844.

23 Ather A, Patel B, Gelfond JAL, Ruparel NB. Outcome of pulpotomy in permanent teeth with irreversible pulpitis: a systematic review and meta-analysis. *Sci Rep.* 2022;12(1):19664.

24 Taha NA, Khazali MA. Partial pulpotomy in mature permanent teeth with clinical signs indicative of irreversible pulpitis: a randomized clinical trial. *J Endod.* 2017;43:1417–21.

25 Ramani A, Sangwan P, Tewari S, Duhan J, Mittal S, Kumar V. Comparative evaluation of complete and partial pulpotomy in mature permanent teeth with symptomatic irreversible pulpitis: a randomized clinical trial. *Int Endod J.* 2022;55:430–40.

26 Jassal A, Nawal RR, Yadav S, Talwar S, Yadav S, Duncan HF. Outcome of partial and full pulpotomy in cariously exposed mature molars with symptoms indicative of irreversible pulpitis: a randomized controlled trial. *Int Endod J.* 2023;56(3):331–44.

27 Altun C, Ozen B, Esenlik E, Guven G, Gürbüz T, Acikel C, et al. Traumatic injuries to permanent teeth in Turkish children, Ankara. *Dent Traumatol.* 2009;25:309–13.

28 Madhumita S, Chakravarthy D, Vijayaraja S, Ajith Kumar S, Kavimalar DS. The outcome of partial pulpotomy in traumatized permanent anterior teeth – a systematic review and meta-analysis. *Indian J Dent Res.* 2022;33(2):203–8.

29 Donnelly A, Foschi F, McCabe P, Duncan HF. Pulpotomy for treatment of complicated crown fractures in permanent teeth: a systematic review. *Int Endod J.* 2022;55:290–311.

30 Fuks A, Bielak S, Chosak A. Clinical and radiographic assessment of direct pulp capping and pulpotomy in young permanent teeth. *Pediatr Dent.* 1982;4(3):240–4.

31 Hecova H, Tzigkounakis V, Merglova V, Netolicky J. A retrospective study of 889 injured permanent teeth. *Dent. Traumatol.* 2010;26(6):466–75.

32 Wang G, Wang C, Qin M. Pulp prognosis following conservative pulp treatment in teeth with complicated crown fractures-a retrospective study. *Dent. Traumatol.* 2017;33(4):255–60.

33 Bo Bourguignon C, Cohenca N, Lauridsen E, Flores MT, O'Connell AC, Day PF, et al. International Association of Dental Traumatology guidelines for the management of traumatic dental injuries: 1. Fractures and luxations. *Dent. Traumatol.* 2020;36(4):314–30.

34 Krastl G, Weiger R, Filippi A, Van Waes H, Ebeleseder K, Ree M, et al. European Society of Endodontology position statement: endodontic management of traumatized permanent teeth. *Int Endod J.* 2021;54(9):1473–81.

35 Jepsen K, Dommisch E, Jepsen S, Dommisch H. Vital root resection in severely furcation-involved maxillary molars: outcomes after up to 7 years. *J Clin Periodontol.* 2020;47(8):970–9.

36 Pretzl B, Eickholz P, Saure D, Pfefferle T, Zeidler A, Dannewitz B. Endodontic status and retention of molars in periodontally treated patients: results after 10 or more years of supportive periodontal therapy. *J Clin Periodontol.* 2016;43(12):1116–23.

37 Eren B, Onay EO, Ungor M. Assessment of alternative emergency treatments for symptomatic irreversible pulpitis: a randomized clinical trial. *Int Endod J.* 2018;51(Suppl 3):e227–37.

38 Eghbal MJ, Haeri A, Shahravan A, Kazemi A, et al. Postendodontic pain after pulpotomy or root canal treatment in mature teeth with carious pulp exposure: a multicenter randomized controlled trial. *Pain Res Manag.* 2021;2020:5853412.

39 Koli B, Chawla A, Logani A, Kumar V, Sharma S. Combination of nonsurgical endodontic and vital pulp therapy for management of mature permanent mandibular molar teeth with symptomatic irreversible pulpitis and apical periodontitis. *J Endod.* 2021;47(3):374–81.

40 Bjørndal L, Reit C, Bruun G, et al. Treatment of deep caries lesions in adults: randomized clinical trials comparing stepwise vs. direct complete excavation, and direct pulp capping vs. partial pulpotomy. *Eur J Oral Sci.* 2010;118:290–7.

41 Bogen GC. Vital pulp therapy. In: Ingle JI, Bakland LK, Baumgartner JC (eds.) Ingle's Endodontics, BC Decker, Hamilton, ON, 2008, 1310–30.

42 Marques M, Wesselink P, Shemesh H. Outcome of direct pulp capping with mineral trioxide aggregate: a prospective study. *J Endod.* 2015;41(7):1026–31.

43 Bjørndal L. Caries pathology and management in deep stages of lesion formation. In: Bjørndal L, Kirkevang L-L, Whitworth J (eds.) Textbook of Endodontology, 3rd Ed., Wiley Blackwell, Oxford; UK, 2018, 61–78.

44 Patel S, Hamer S. A simple guide to using dental dam. *Br Dent J.* 2021;230(10):644–50.

45 Hörsted-Bindslev P, Vilkinis V, Sidlauskas A. Direct capping of human pulps with a dentin bonding system or with calcium hydroxide cement. *Oral Surg Oral Med Oral Pathol Oral Radiol Endod.* 2003;96(5):591–600.

46 Ng YL, Spratt D, Sriskantharajah S, Gulabivala K. Evaluation of protocols for field decontamination before bacterial sampling of root canals for contemporary microbiology techniques. *J Endod.* 2003;29(5):317–20.

47 Malyshev D, Dahlberg T, Wiklund K, Andersson PO, Henriksson S, Andersson M. Mode of action of disinfection chemicals on the bacterial spore structure and their Raman spectra. *Anal Chem.* 2021;93(6):3146–53.

48 Careddu R, Duncan HF. A prospective clinical study investigating the effectiveness of partial pulpotomy after relating preoperative symptoms to a new and established classification of pulpitis. *Int Endod J.* 2021;54:2156–72.

49 Stangvaltaite L, Schwendicke F, Holmgren C, Finet M, Maltz M, Elhennawy K, et al. Management of pulps exposed during carious tissue removal in adults: a multi-national questionnaire-based survey. *Clin Oral Investig.* 2017;21(7):2303–9.

50 Mutluay M, Arikan V, Sari S, Kisa V. Does achievement of hemostasis after pulp exposure provide an accurate assessment of pulp inflammation? *Pediatr Dent.* 2018;40(1):37–42.

51 Karabucak B, Li D, Lim J, Iqbal M. Vital pulp therapy with mineral trioxide aggregate. *Dent. Traumatol.* 2005;21(4):240–3.

52 Santini AH. Intraoral comparison of calcium hydroxide (Calnex) alone and in combination with Ledermixin first permanent mandibular molars using two direct inspection criteria. *J Dent.* 1985;13:52–9.

53 Munir A, Zehnder M, Rechenberg DK. Wound lavage in studies on vital pulp therapy of permanent teeth with carious exposures: a qualitative systematic review. *J Clin Med.* 2020;9:984.

54 Ballal NV, Duncan HF, Rai N, Jalan P, Zehnder M. Sodium hypochlorite reduces postoperative discomfort and painful early failure after carious exposure and direct pulp capping-initial findings of a randomized controlled trial. *J Clin Med.* 2020;9:2408.

55 Ballal NV, Duncan HF, Wiedemeier DB, Rai N, Jalan P, Bhat V, et al. MMP-9 levels and NaOCl lavage in randomized trial on direct pulp capping. *J Dent Res.* 2022;101:414–9.

56 Careddu R, Duncan HF. How does the pulpal response to biodentine and ProRoot mineral trioxide aggregate compare in the laboratory and clinic? *Br Dent J.* 2018;225:743–9.

57 Sangwan P, Sangwan A, Duhan J, Rohilla A. Tertiary dentinogenesis with calcium hydroxide: a review of proposed mechanisms. *Int Endod J.* 2013;46(1):3–19.

58 Nair PNR, Duncan HF, Pitt Ford TR, Luder HU. Histological, ultrastructural and quantitative investigations on the response of healthy human pulps to experimental capping with mineral trioxide aggregate: a randomized controlled trial. *Int Endod J.* 2008;41:128–50.

59 Kundzina R, Stangvaltaite L, Eriksen HM, Kerosuo E. Capping carious exposures in adults: a randomized controlled trial investigating mineral trioxide aggregate versus calcium hydroxide. *Int Endod J.* 2017;50:924–32.

60 Hilton TJ, Ferracane JL, Mancl L, Northwest Practice-based Research Collaborative in Evidence-based Dentistry (NWP). Comparison of CaOH with MTA for direct pulp capping: a PBRN randomized clinical trial. *J Dent Res.* 2013;92:16–22S.

61 Mente J, Leo M, Panagidis D, Sauni D, Pfefferle T. Treatment outcome of mineral trioxide aggregate: repair of root perforations – long-term results. *Int Endod J.* 2014;40(06):790–6.

62 Torabinejad M, Hong CU, McDonald F, Pitt Ford TR. Physical and chemical properties of a new root-end filling material. *J Endod.* 1995;21(7):349–53.

63 De-Deus G, Canabarro A, Alves GG, Marins JR, Linhares AB, Granjeiro JM. Cytocompatibility of the ready-to-usebioceramic putty repair cement iRoot BP Plus with primary humanosteoblasts. *Int Endod J.* 2012;45(6):508–18.

64 Mukhtar-Fayyad D. Cytocompatibility of new bioceramic-based materials on human fibroblast cells (MRC-5). *Oral Surg Oral Med Oral Pathol Oral Radiol.* 2011;112(6):137–42.

65 Willershausen I, Wolf T, Kasaj A, Weyer V, Willershausen B, Marroquin BB. Influence of a bioceramic root end material and mineral trioxide aggregates on fibroblasts and osteoblasts. *ArchOral Biol.* 2013;58(9):1232–7.

66 Chen I, Karabucak B, Wang C, Wang HG, Koyama E, Kohli MR, et al. Healing after root-end microsurgery by using mineral trioxide aggregate and a new calcium silicate-based bioceramic material as root-end filling materials in dogs. *J Endod.* 2015;41(3):389–99.

67 Nowicka A, Lipsky M, Parafinuk M, et al. Response of human dental pulp capped with biodentine and mineral trioxide aggregate. *J Endod.* 2013;39:743–7.

68 Taha NA, Abdulkhader SZ. Full pulpotomy with biodentine in symptomatic young permanent teeth with carious exposure. *J Endod.* 2018;44:932–7.

69 Awawdeh L, Al-Qudah A, Hamouri H, Chakra RJ. Outcomes of vital pulp therapy using mineral trioxide aggregate or Biodentine: a prospective randomized clinical trial. *J Endod.* 2018;44(11):1603–9.

70 Eskandari F, Razavian A, Hamidi R, Yousefi K, Borzou S. An updated review on properties and indications of calcium silicate-based cements in endodontic therapy. *Int J Dent.* 2022;2022:6858088.

71 Bakhtiar H, Nekoofar MH, Aminishakib P, et al. Human pulp responses to partial pulpotomy treatment with theracal as compared with. *J Endod.* 2017;43:1786–91.

72 Giraud T, Jeanneau C, Rombouts C, Bakhtiar H, Laurent P, About I. Pulp capping materials modulate the balance between inflammation and regeneration. *Dent Mater.* 2019;3:24–35.

73 Manaspon C, Jongwannasiri C, Chumprasert S, Sa-Ard-Iam N, Mahanonda R, Pavasant P, et al. Human dental pulp stem cell responses to different dental pulp capping materials. *BMC Oral Health.* 2021;26:21–209.

74 Kamburoglu K, Kolsuz E, Murat S, Yüksel S, Ozen T. Proximal caries detection accuracy using intraoral bitewing radiography, extraoral bitewing radiography and panoramic radiography. *Dentomaxillofac Radiol.* 2012;41(6):450–9.

75 Bjørndal L, Demant S, Dabelsteen S. Depth and activity of carious lesions as indicators for the regenerative potential of dental pulp after intervention. *J Endod.* 2014;40(4 Suppl):S76–81.

76 Demant S, Dabelsteen S, Bjørndal L. A macroscopic and histological analysis of radiographically well-defined deep and extremely deep carious lesions: carious lesion characteristics as indicators of the level of bacterial penetration and pulp response. *Int Endod J.* 2021;54(3):319–30.

77 Özyürek T, Demiryürek EÖ. Comparison of the antimicrobial activity of direct pulp-capping materials: mineral trioxide aggregate-Angelus and Biodentine. *J Conserv Dent.* 2016;19:569–72.

78 Uesrichai N, Nirunsittirat A, Chuveera P, Srisuwan T, Sastraruji T, Chompu-Inwai P. Partial pulpotomy with two bioactive cements in permanent teeth of 6- to 18-year-old patients with signs and symptoms indicative of irreversible pulpitis: a noninferiority randomized controlled trial. *Int Endod J.* 2019;52(6):749–59.

79 Wolters WJ, Duncan HF, Tomson PL, Karim IE, McKenna G, Dorri M, et al. Minimally invasive endodontics: a new diagnostic system for assessing pulpitis and subsequent treatment needs. *Int Endod J.* 2017;50(9):825–9.

80 Asgary S, Ehsani S. Permanent molar pulpotomy with a new endodontic cement: a case series. *J Conserv Dent.* 2009;12(1):31–6.

81 AAE position statement on vital pulp therapy. *J Endod.* 2021;47(9):1340–4.

82 Sadasiva K, Kumar KS, Rayar S, Shamini S, Unnikrishnan M, Kandaswamy D. Evaluation of the efficacy of visual, tactile method, caries detector dye, and laser fluorescence in removal of dental caries and confirmation by culture and polymerase chain reaction: an in vivo study. *J Pharm Bioallied Sci.* 2019;11(Suppl 2):S146–50.

83 Ricucci D, Loghin S, Siqueira JF Jr. Correlation between clinical and histologic pulp diagnoses. *J Endod.* 2014;40(12):1932–9.

84 Andrei M, Vacaru RP, Coricovac A, Ilinca R, Didilescu AC, Demetrescu I. The effect of calcium-silicate cements on reparative dentinogenesis following direct pulp capping on animal models. *Molecules (Basel, Switzerland).* 2021;26(9):2725.

85 Subay RK, Ilhan B, Ulukapi H. Mineral trioxide aggregate as a pulpotomy agent in immature teeth: long-term case report. *Eur J Dent.* 2013;7(1):133–8.

86 Barthel CR, Rosenkranz B, Leuenberg A, Roulet JF. Pulp capping of carious exposures: treatment outcome after 5 and 10 years: a retrospective study. *J Endod.* 2000;26(9):525–8.

87 Al-Hiyasat AS, Barrieshi-Nusair KM, Al-Omari MA. The radiographic outcomes of direct pulp-capping procedures performed by dental students: a retrospective study. *J Am Dent Assoc (1939).* 2006;137(12):1699–705.

88 Mente J, Geletneky B, Ohle M, Koch MJ, Friedrich Ding PG, Wolff D, et al. Mineral trioxide aggregate or calcium hydroxide direct pulp capping: an analysis of the clinical treatment outcome. *J Endod.* 2010;36(5):806–13.

89 Nagendrababu V, Vinothkumar TS, El-Karim I, Rossi-Fedele G, Doğramaci EJ, Dummer PMH, et al. Dental patient-reported outcomes in endodontics – a narrative review. *J Evid Based Dent Pract.* 2023;23(1):101805.

90 Duncan HF, El-Karim I, Dummer PMH, Whitworth J, Nagendrababu V. Factors that influence the outcome of pulpotomy in permanent teeth. *Int Endod J.* 2023;56(Suppl 2):62–81.

7

Vital Pulp Treatment – Material Selection

Renan Dal-Fabbro[1], *Isaac J. de Souza Araújo*[1,2], *and Marco C. Bottino*[1,3]

[1] *Department of Cariology, Restorative Sciences, and Endodontics, University of Michigan School of Dentistry, Ann Arbor, MI, USA*
[2] *Department of Bioscience Research, College of Dentistry, University of Tennessee Health Science Center, Memphis, TN, USA*
[3] *Department of Biomedical Engineering, College of Engineering, University of Michigan, Ann Arbor, MI, USA*

Introduction

Dental pulp tissue is a connective tissue found at the centre of the tooth, surrounded by dentine and enamel. When exposed through caries or tooth fractures, the dental pulp becomes highly susceptible to infections, which can lead to pain, necrosis, and severe infection of the alveolar bone and surrounding tissues (1). Currently, the most common treatment choice for pulp diseases in permanent teeth is orthograde root canal treatment (RCT), performed by a pulpectomy (complete removal of the damaged and healthy pulp inside the tooth), along with the possible use of dressing materials, filling with synthetic materials, and sealing to bring back masticatory function (2).

Vital pulp treatment (VPT) is a possible alternative to RCT, as it is a restorative dental procedure that aims to treat compromised dental pulp without completely removing the dental pulp tissue or excavating sound inner dentine walls (3). It can comprise indirect or direct pulp capping (applying a protective material that covers the pulp) and partial or complete/full pulpotomy (extirpation of part or all of the coronal pulp) (Figure 7.1A). It is more frequently performed in primary dentition (paediatric patients) due to incomplete root formation, ease of technique, and less trauma to young patients (7). Moreover, VPT is also indicated for secondary dentition (permanent), despite it not commonly being done for adults, precisely due to a lack of knowledge about the procedure and uncertainty regarding practitioners' success rates (8).

Both VPT and RCT achieve similar high and predictable success rates when properly performed (9). However, the less invasive technique may be advantageous to patients with secondary dentition, as it may help to extend the survival of the teeth, as orthograde endodontically treated teeth can be at risk for structural failure during mastication. In addition, these teeth are biologically inferior, since root canal filling materials have no biological immune defence (higher risk of reinfection) and have no innervation, thus causing loss of sensation of environmental changes (possibly leading to more or worse caries), reinfection, and development of apical periodontitis (10).

Critical factors are important for a successful VPT, such as the amount of infected tissue, bleeding control and maintenance of pulp free of bacteria during the procedure, the patient's age (since older patients have more fibrous pulp tissue and less blood supply), and healthy periodontium, in

Vital Pulp Treatment, First Edition. Edited by Henry F. Duncan and Ikhlas A. El-Karim.

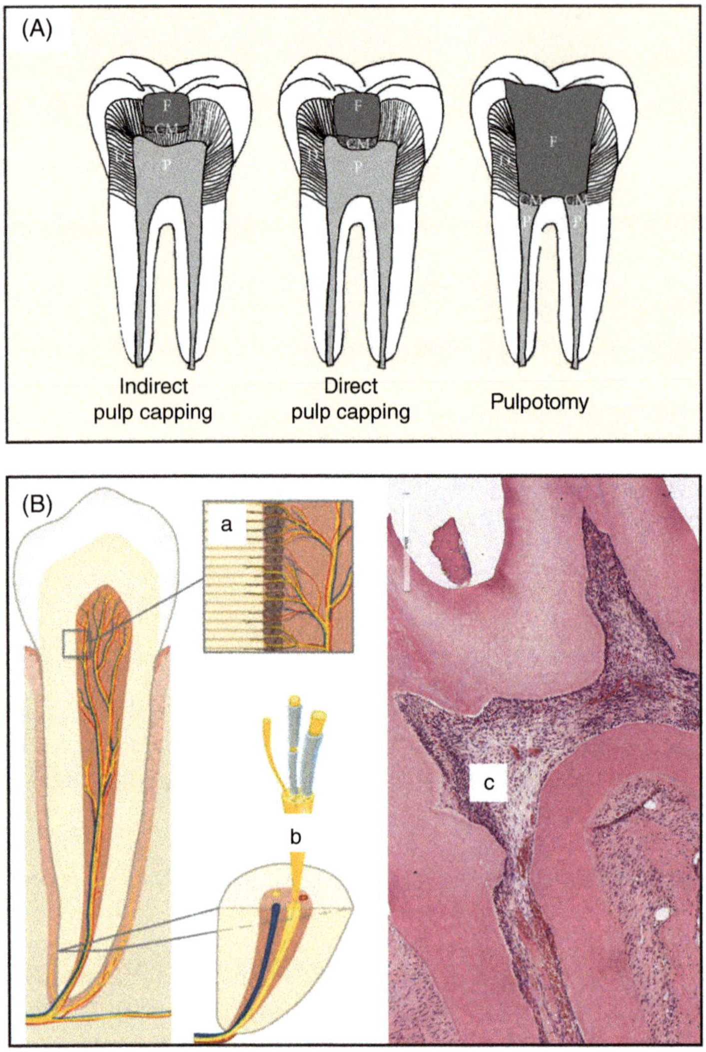

Figure 7.1 (A) Schematic representation of different VPT methods: Indirect pulp capping; Direct pulp capping; Pulpotomy. (D = Dentine; P = Pulp; CM = Capping material; F = Filling). (B) Pulp-dentinal complex vascularization and innervation: (a) Blood vessels (red and blue) and sensory nerves (yellow) from the pulp chamber to dentinal tubules forming the plexus of Raschkow; (b) Neurovascular bundle at tooth apex showing the nerve bundle; (c) Healthy pulp tissue showing the abundant presence of blood vessels. (C) Schematic representation showing the signalling pathways initiated following bacteria penetration due to tooth decay leading to inflammatory cytokines production. TLR: Toll-like receptor; Th: T helper; LPS: Lipopolysaccharides; LTA: Lipoteichoic acid; LT: Lipopeptide; MAPK: Mitogen-activated protein kinase; NFκB: nuclear factor-kappa light chain enhancer of activated B cells. (D) Histological aspects from pulp response to caries progression; p = pulp, d = dentine. Black arrows show bacteria and their components diffusing through the dentinal tubule until they reach the pulp. White arrows show reparative dentine deposited beneath the carious lesion with an apparent and localized inflammatory cell infiltrate (dotted line). Red arrows show cariogenic bacteria stained by Brown and Brenn in the same section. *Source:* Adapted with permission from Refs. (4–6).

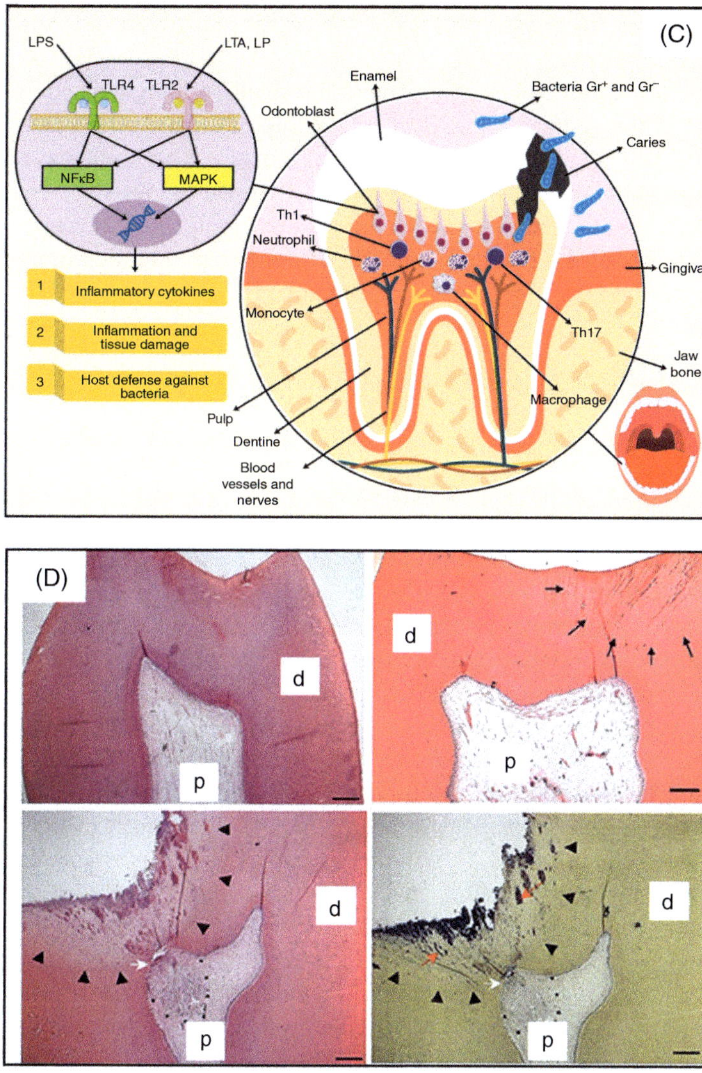

Figure 7.1 (Continued)

addition to the right selection of material for proper sealing and healing of the pulpal tissue and type of final restoration (3, 7, 11).

In this chapter, we will first describe native pulp conditions, its response to traumatic or carious injuries, and the decision-making process that determines the best treatment approach. The concepts, standard materials (properties, advantages, and drawbacks), tissue response biology and clinical evidence of successful treatment will be deeply addressed in the second section. The bulk of this chapter will give special attention to existing and next-generation regenerative-based biomaterials to be employed in VPT, aiming at the outcome of regenerative endodontics outcome.

Native Pulp Conditions

Pulp tissue originates from the proliferation and condensation of neural crest cells (ectomesenchyme) that are prime to the development of the dental papilla, later originating in mature pulp tissue residing in an inflexible chamber made by dentine, enamel, and cementum (12). This tissue has a layer of highly specialized cells and odontoblasts along its periphery that continuously secrete dentine after development is complete, both under normal and non-homeostatic conditions. In healthy pulp tissue, this dentine is called secondary and is slower-paced and deposited circumferentially (in tubular continuity with primary dentine) at a gradual speed during the life of a vital tooth (12, 13).

Pulp tissue is a highly vascularized tissue. Usually, pulp microcirculation is nourished through dental arteries that come from the maxillary artery, a branch of the external carotid artery. This blood supply enters the tooth via the apical foramen, feeding each tooth (1). Overall, the pulp vessels are organized in a hierarchical system with arterioles in the central capillaries, and their branches at the periphery of the pulp, all with the same objective as any other circulatory flow in the human body, supplying the odontoblasts and other constituent cells with oxygen, as well as a source of nutrients (14). The venules are likewise present in the central part and are responsible for draining waste products (1). The dental pulp also provides robust mechanical support and protection from the microbial-rich oral environment. Furthermore, this microcirculatory has an extraordinary incidence of innervation (mainly branches of the maxillary and mandibular divisions of the trigeminal nerve), which is involved in pulp pain perception and transduction, both of which are vital for warning of minimal changes from the healthy state (13) (Figure 7.1B).

Commonly, teeth with healthy pulp tissue have extra resistance to bacterial invasion into dentinal tubules compared to their endodontically treated counterparts, mainly due to the complex immune response and defence process evoked by resident cells. This cell complex combines to form a major robust immune cell population, namely, neutrophils, T lymphocytes, monocytes, dendritic cells, natural killer (NK) cells, B cells, and regulatory T cells (Tregs) (15). These immune cells are in homeostasis with adjacent odontoblasts, fibroblasts, and pulpal stem cells and are crucial for the immunological response when facing a microorganism attack (16).

These cells recognize potential threats via pattern-recognition receptors (PRRs) that acknowledge pathogen-associated molecular patterns (PAMPs) (17). The main PRRs are transmembrane receptors, referred to as toll-like receptors (TLRs) (18). While not their main function, odontoblasts are immunocompetent cells expressing PRRs and represent the first defence response once they are in the vicinity of the pulp, with their cell bodies residing in the pulp chamber and their cellular processes extending into the dentinal tubules, thus being able to elicit an inflammatory response (19). TLR-2 is activated by peptidoglycan, lipoteichoic acid (LTA), and lipoproteins, all of which are byproducts from gram-positive bacteria predominantly found in carious lesions (20). Typically, gram-positive bacteria dominate over gram-negative bacteria in pulp tissue. Therefore, the TLR-2 expression is initially more remarkable than TLR-4 in dental pulp exposed to the oral environment (21) (Figure 7.1C).

Pulp Response to Traumatic or Carious Injuries

According to the last World Health Organization report, carious lesions are the most frequent non-communicative disease, affecting almost half of the world's population, leading to direct–indirect financial costs reaching US$442 billion in 2010 (22). The response of pulp tissue to irritation (regardless of traumatic or carious origin) is inflammation. If unattended, the integrity of the structural pulp environment will be lost, leading to exacerbated inflammation and pulp necrosis (23) (Figure 7.1D).

Since pulp is relatively incompressible, the total blood volume within the pulp chamber cannot be significantly increased. In this way, minor alterations in pulp microcirculation are the first to occur with the onset of pulp inflammation, leading to increased tissue pressure (1). Subsequent compression of the blood vessels contributes to the origination of pulp inflammation and necrosis, which may spread to the adjacent alveolar bone at a later stage and evoke periapical pathosis (24). In severe cases, pulp necrosis can culminate in oral sepsis, which can be life-threatening if the infection spreads, causing purulent sinusitis, meningitis, and brain abscess from the maxillary teeth, or Ludwig's angina from the mandibular teeth (25).

In carious lesions, changes in the odontoblast cell layer occur even before the pulp tissue appears inflamed. As mentioned earlier, the odontoblasts and undifferentiated mesenchymal cells (which may differentiate into dentine-forming cells if stimulated) hold the capacity to form dentine throughout life, enabling pulp to compensate for the loss of enamel or dentine caused by caries, called tertiary dentine (1, 13). This tertiary dentine can be termed reactionary dentine (secreted by surviving post-mitotic odontoblasts) and reparative dentine (secreted by a new group of odontoblast-like cells derived from a progenitor cell population) in reaction to adverse stimuli, such as caries or operative procedures (detailed in Chapter 2). The rate seems to depend inversely on the rate of carious attack; that is, more dentine is formed in response to slowly progressing carious lesions (23).

During infections with gram-negative bacteria, PAMP lipopolysaccharide (LPS) represents the main byproduct released by bacteria and can produce inflammation (26). When bound to TLR-4, it evokes an activation of the inflammatory molecular cascade through the nuclear factor-kappa B pathway (NF-Kb), releasing several proinflammatory cytokines, such as interleukin IL-1 beta and tumour necrosis factor-alpha (TNF-a), which mediate innate immune responses by regulating phagocytosis and triggering antimicrobial activity (15). Chemokines recruit and activate tissue-resident and blood-borne immune/inflammatory cells at the site. As microorganisms keep invading the pulp, destruction of the odontoblast layer is observed, and the subjacent pulp fibroblasts are triggered to participate in the host response, similar to odontoblasts through TLRs (27). If not properly addressed, long-term irritation will cause chronic pulp inflammation, which further culminates in total pulp necrosis that will then be followed by infection of the periradicular space, since bacteria will have a pathway by which it can enter the area via foramen (24).

Similar to carious lesions, traumatic dental injuries (TDI) are another concern regarding dental pulp response, since they are also very frequent, with one in four individuals aged 6–50 years having evidence of TDI, according to a U.S. national survey (28). Mild injuries, such as enamel cracks or minor uncomplicated crown fractures, may cause mild localized inflammation in the pulp, which usually resolves by itself through continuous dentinal tubule deposition (29). On the other hand, in complicated crown fractures, the pulp is lacerated and exposed to the oral environment (30, 31). Unless the tooth is quickly restored, this will evoke localized haemorrhaging, bacteria and toxins penetrating the tissue, leading to liquefaction-type necrosis, similar to that seen following carious exposure (29).

Trauma causing the displacement of teeth from the alveolus will result in damage to the apical blood vessels. When affecting fully developed teeth, these blood vessels will not be able to heal and revascularize the pulp (29). Nevertheless, a young tooth with a wide root apical foramen probably will recover and re-establish blood flow (32). In aseptic necrotic pulp tissue, if the tooth remains intact, the necrotic pulp may remain sterile and poses no adverse effects on the surrounding periradicular tissues. However, due to the lack of blood supply and a competent immune system defending it, a secondary crack or fracture may provide a pathway for bacterial entry that will easily infect the root canal system and result in periapical and periodontal pathologies (24, 33).

Decision-making for Pulp Exposures

It is believed that several tooth extractions could be avoided if proper treatment was carried out at the first diagnostic appointment (34). However, due to the difficulty in identifying unclear symptoms and the inaccessibility of the pulp for clinical tests, the right diagnosis becomes difficult (35). Moreover, the presence of a referred toothache derived from tissues other than pulp hampers accurate identification. In this way, the professional should conduct an appropriate clinical examination and diagnostic tests.

As outlined in Chapter 3, pulpal diagnosis is based on the patient's pain history. Second, sensibility tests, such as applying cold, hot, and electric stimulus, provides the clinician with additional evidence to assist with diagnosis. In addition to such tests, percussion tests may infer a pulpal state from the presence of symptomatic apical periodontitis (36, 37). When there is a possibility of seeing pulp tissue, complete caries removal is indispensable to eliminating infected tissues and creating appropriate conditions to visualize the pulp tissue underneath, according to the American Association of Endodontists (AAE) (7, 38). However, a recent position statement by the European Society of Endodontology (ESE) recommended that selective carious-tissue removal is advocated (39). A lack of consensus among the experts regarding caries removal and how to manage deep caries is an evolving topic that forces new studies. Finally, intraoral radiographs evaluate the extent of root formation and apical foramen width (40).

Regarding signs and symptoms, spontaneous unprovoked pain, sinus tract, excessive mobility not associated with trauma, apical radiolucency, and radiographic evidence of internal or external resorption have a clinical diagnosis of irreversible pulpitis or necrosis, making them suitable candidates for RCT. On the other hand, induced or short-duration pain that ceases upon removal of the stimulus has a clinical diagnosis of reversible pulpitis and is eligible for VPT (7).

Since the primary goal of VPT is to create conditions for pulp tissue preservation and repair, the amount of remaining pulp tissue after disinfection must be based on operator evaluations, the overall treatment plan, and the patient's general oral and systemic health to allow for healing (41). The age of the patient is directly correlated with the pulp tissue's volume, since continuous deposition of secondary dentine throughout one's whole life leads to pulp recession and difficulty with execution of the VPT but does not affect outcomes when properly conducted (13, 42, 43). In addition to pulp volume, the patient's age also interferes with the level of root development and apical foramen diameter, where incompletely developed roots and open apex enhance the chances of a successful VPT (13, 29).

Also, the timeframe between pulp exposure to the oral environment and treatment is a determinant in deciding between RCT and VPT, as well as the location of the injury and how it happened (32). A delay in initiating endodontic treatment after a trauma incident in a contaminated environment increases the chances of the pulp becoming necrotic and unsuitable for VPT (32). Furthermore, the patient's ability to return for follow-up appointments should also be considered, since VPT requires numerous radiographs over the following year to assess the success of the technique (28).

Overall, many aspects should be considered quickly in order to apply the right pulp treatment. When the treatment plan is established, other considerations should be properly made, as in the case of materials selection for each case, which will be discussed in the following sections.

Historical Background on VPT Materials and Their Influence on Success

As discussed above, bacterial invasion caused by caries and dental trauma affects dental pulp and can lead to inflammation that, if left untreated, results in pulp necrosis (44–46). These damages imply the need for a variety of further treatments, depending on the injury's severity and timeframe. The materials used for vital pulp therapy in permanent teeth have evolved over time. The first materials used in VPT were likely basic materials, such as calcium hydroxide ($Ca(OH)_2$) and formocresol.

Formocresol, a mixture of formaldehyde, cresol and glycerin, was first introduced in the 1930s and was widely used for many years as a pulp therapy material. It has been shown to have strong antimicrobial properties, as well as the ability to fix tissue; however, due to concerns about its toxicity, formocresol has largely been replaced by other materials.

Calcium hydroxide has been used in dentistry as a pulp-capping material for over a century; it has been considered the gold standard for a long time and may still be effective in certain situations (41). Calcium hydroxide has been shown to have excellent antibacterial properties and, when applied to pulp tissue, stimulates the formation of a mineralized tissue barrier that helps to protect the pulp from further damage. Calcium hydroxide materials are commercially available as a powder or paste, according to their intended use. For indirect pulp capping, it is conventionally presented as a two-paste material that is mixed and applied as a liner on the internal walls of the cavity. In the meantime, direct pulp capping using $Ca(OH)_2$ is often applied as a pristine powder directly onto the exposed area. Due to its high alkalinity (pH ~12.5–12.8), $Ca(OH)_2$ creates a critical environment for bacteria, and the hydroxyl ions induce phospholipid membrane disruption that leads to bacterial death (47). In conjunction with this, due to the high pH of $Ca(OH)_2$, its direct contact with pulp or through micro exposures in indirect pulp capping induces an inflammatory response that acts as a signalling stimulus for dentine matrix secretion at the region of the injury (48). Furthermore, $Ca(OH)_2$ products also result in partial solubilization on the dentine matrix that releases bioactive molecules and consequent dental pulp stem cells (DPSCs) recruitment to the area of the damage (49). In the meantime, calcium and hydroxyl dissociate in contact with aqueous fluids and play pivotal roles in mineral deposition to form mineralized barriers (Figure 7.2C).

Despite its good properties, there are several disadvantages to using $Ca(OH)_2$, such as limited sealing ability – $Ca(OH)_2$ has a limited ability to seal the pulp and may allow bacteria to penetrate the pulp tissue, leading to further infection and inflammation; poor mechanical properties – $Ca(OH)_2$ is a weak material and can be easily displaced or washed out of the tooth during the procedure, thus reducing its effectiveness; long-term success rate – studies have shown that the long-term success rate of pulp capping and pulpotomy procedures using $Ca(OH)_2$ is lower than those using mineral trioxide aggregate (MTA) or other newer materials. Moreover, $Ca(OH)_2$ is not recommended for indirect pulp-capping procedures because it does not have enough antibacterial properties, and it can take several weeks to stimulate the formation of reparative dentin, which increases the risk of bacterial penetration.

Furthermore, the mineralized barriers formed by $Ca(OH)_2$ products are not homogeneous and present a poorly organized and non-tubular structure resembling the characteristics of osteodentine, instead of the native dentine organization (52). It can also present tunnel defects that result in improper sealing, which increases the risk of reinfection (52). Also, when $Ca(OH)_2$ is applied as a powder in direct pulp-capping procedures, the inflammatory response, due to its highly alkaline

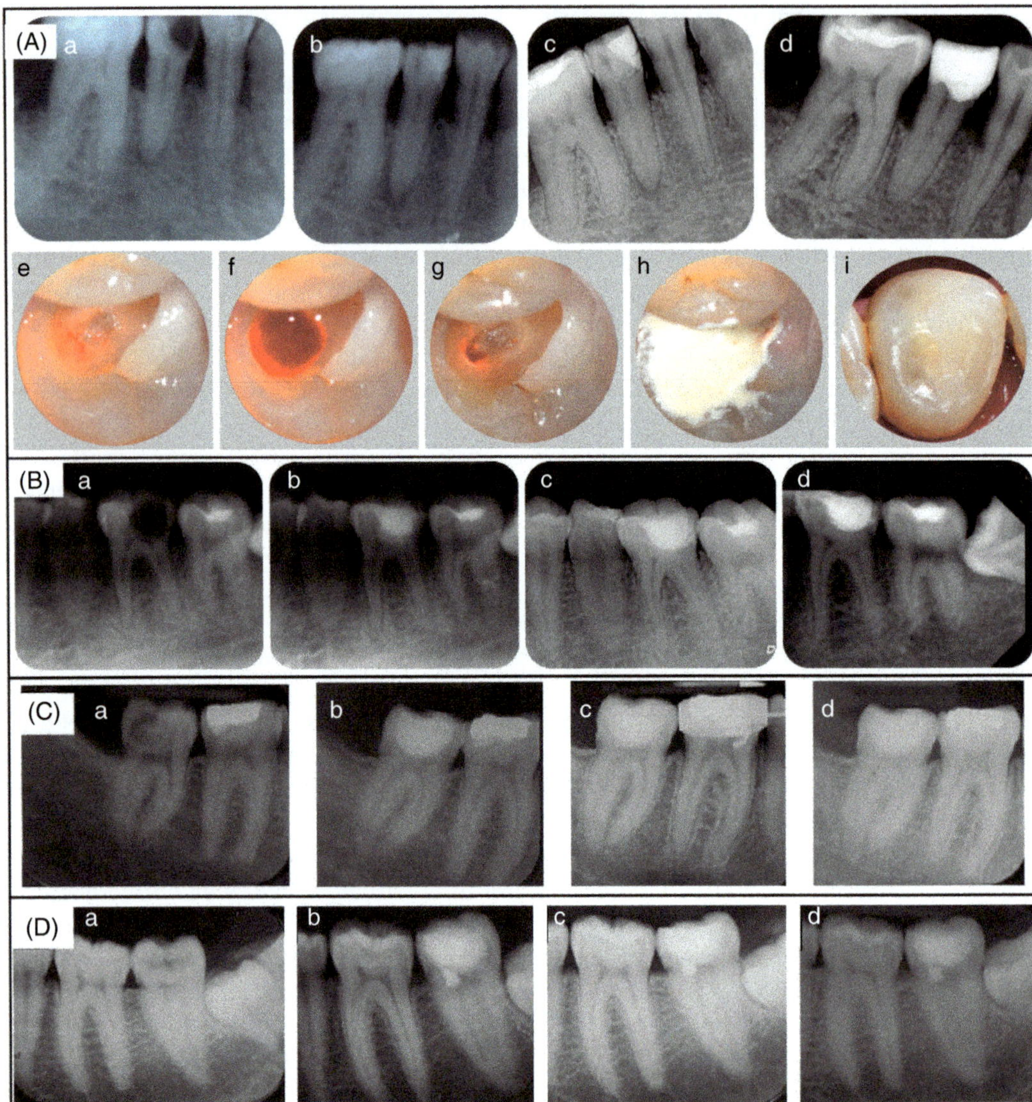

Figure 7.2 (A–B) Pulpotomy in Mature Permanent Teeth treated with Biodentine™. (A) Periapical radiographs: (a) preoperative; (b) after treatment; (c) six months postoperative; (d) 12 months postoperative. Intraoral photographs: (e–g) access opening for pulpotomy procedure; (h) placement of Biodentine™; (i) resin-based composite restoration. (B) Periapical radiographs: (a) preoperative; (b) after treatment; (c) six months postoperative; (d) 24 months postoperative. (C) A lower right second molar in a 22-year-old man with a clinical diagnosis of irreversible pulpitis: (a) the preoperative periapical radiograph; (b) the postoperative periapical radiograph after calcium hydroxide partial pulpotomy; (c) 12-month follow-up; (d) 26-month follow-up. (D) A lower left second molar in a 21-year-old female patient with a clinical diagnosis of irreversible pulpitis: (a) The preoperative periapical radiograph; (b) the postoperative periapical radiograph after MTA partial pulpotomy; (c) 12-month follow-up. (d) 28-month follow-up. *Source:* (a) Taha and Khazali (50)/From MDPI/CC BY 4.0. (b) Tran et al. (51)/Reproduced with permission from Elsevier.

pH and fast hydroxyl dissociation, creates superficial zones of necrosis (~1.5 mm deep) in the pulp. As hydroxyl diffuses through the pulp and dentinal tubules, the inflammatory reaction is usually controlled by the ability of the tissue to neutralize pH and the fast formation of the mineralized barrier in a competent tissue (47). On the other hand, in unfavourable conditions and infected tissues, the inflammation could be exacerbated by caustic conditions and can result in unsuccessful treatment.

Since the development of these early materials, many other materials have been introduced for VPT, including resin-based materials, tricalcium silicate-based materials, bioactive glasses, and various regenerative endodontic materials aiming to effectively promote pulp healing and tissue regeneration while minimizing the risk of adverse reactions or complications.

Current Gold Standard and Limitations of VPT Materials

From a materials perspective, ISO 23317:2014 (53) defines bioactivity as the specific biological interaction between material and substrate to form a layer of apatite-like tissue. Besides bioactivity, some of the prerequisites for a successful material in VPT include antimicrobial potential; adherence to dentine and restorative materials; mechanical stability to support masticatory forces; tight seal of the exposed area; low solubility; and radiopacity (41). However, one should notice that there is no material that presents all the characteristics mentioned above for consideration as the only choice for pulp-capping strategies.

Calcium hydroxide in improved formulations (Dycal®, Sealapex®, UltraCal®, etc.) and calcium silicate-based materials (BioRoot® MTA, Biodentine®, Theracal®, etc.) are the standard choices for VPT, mostly due to their ability to stimulate competent odontoblast or differentiated odontoblast-like cells to form mineralized barriers (or dentine bridges) which are, by definition, characterized as a bioactive mechanism.

For indirect pulp capping, the two-paste system is the most common mechanism of $Ca(OH)_2$ delivery for pulp protection. These agents are a mixture of $Ca(OH)_2$, resins, initiators, and radiopaque components presented in separate containers (base and catalyst) with easy handling, mixing and application. They undergo a chemical reaction and present a fast-setting time after the mixture. Its use on the pulpal walls of deep cavities has demonstrated effectiveness in promoting sclerotic dentine formation and partial remineralization of affected dentin, which contributes to preserving pulp vitality (47). Major clinical concerns about these materials include their high solubility and poor mechanical properties. Therefore, no excess cement should be left on the external walls or the margins of the cavity for the restorative procedure, and the $Ca(OH)_2$ layer should be covered by a base agent, such as glass ionomer cement, before insertion of the restorative material. To circumvent the issues related to solubility and poor mechanical stability, some manufacturers also incorporated methacrylate monomers and photo-initiators in single-paste $Ca(OH)_2$ preparations. However, the entrapment of $Ca(OH)_2$ on the polymeric chain of these formulations limits its ability to induce mineralized tissue formation.

Calcium silicate-based materials, first named MTA, are tri- and di-calcium silicates derived from Portland cement. The original formulation, currently still predominant, contains tricalcium silicate, tricalcium aluminate, tricalcium oxide, silicate oxide and bismuth oxide. The main differences from Portland cement are the presence of bismuth oxide (radiopacity), the particles' size, and their distribution (54). It is possible to label several commercial names of MTA available in the market, including ProRoot MTA (Dentsply Sirona Inc., York, PA, USA) – the first commercially available, Angelus MTA (Angelus, Londrina-PR-Brazil), MTA BioAggregate

(Innovative BioCeramix, Inc, BC, Canada), MTA Vitalcem (Avalon Biomed, Houston, TX, USA), MTA Plus (Prevest DenPro Limited, Jammu, India), MTA Repair HP (Avalon Biomed), Endocem MTA (Maruchi USA, Anheim, CA, USA), NeoMTA Plus (Avalon Biomed), BioMTA (Septodont, Saint-Maur-des-Fossés, France), MTA Flow (Ultradent Products, Inc., South Jordan, UT, USA), and EndoSequence Root Repair Material (Brasseler USA Dental Instrumentation, Savannah, GA, USA). It is important for the clinician to carefully evaluate the specific properties of each product to select the most appropriate material for a given case, in addition to looking for recent scientific publications evaluating their success rates.

Most of these materials are set in contact with water by forming a hydrated matrix with an elevated pH similar to calcium hydroxide. Moreover, their ability to form mineralized barriers is related to the formation of calcium hydroxide as part of the setting reaction. MTA has demonstrated superior chemical stability and mechanical properties, compared to calcium hydroxide, with less inflammatory reaction induction and better outcomes concerning dentine bridge formation (52) (Figure 7.2D). However, MTA still has drawbacks regarding its manipulation, where many powder/liquid ratio disproportions could occur and affect the material's properties. MTA also presents a long setting time, and bismuth oxide leads to tooth discoloration (55–57).

A further development in the calcium silicate cement-based material area is Biodentine (Septodont Ltd., Saint Maur des Fausse's, France). It is a tri- and di-calcium silicate powder that also contains calcium carbonate and calcium oxide with zirconium oxide as its opacifier. Different from MTA, the mixing liquid in Biodentine presents calcium chloride to accelerate the reaction and reduce the issue with setting time and a hydrosoluble polymer to act as a water-reducing agent to prevent the formation of cracks in the matrix (58). The material is presented in a capsule to be triturated using an amalgamator after adding the liquid, and according to the manufacturer, the setting time is about 12 minutes. The trituration process reduces the formation of bubbles and manipulation mistakes in terms of the powder/liquid ratio. Biodentine hydrated matrix is mostly like all the conventional tricalcium silicate-based materials that release calcium ions and induce mineralized barrier formation. In a recent meta-analysis, Biodentine had comparable clinical and radiographic success to that of MTA when used as a direct pulp-capping material in mature permanent teeth (59). Although both MTA and Biodentine are constituted of tricalcium silicate cores, Biodentine overcomes the disadvantages of MTA in terms of discoloration and brittleness but still has a long setting time, high cost, handling difficulties, limited working time, and sensitivity reaction as disadvantages (60) (Figure 7.2A,B).

In an attempt to overcome the setting time limitation, TheraCal LC® was developed as a light-curable calcium silicate-based cement. TheraCal LC is commercialized as a paste that contains Portland cement type III, silica, metallic oxides for radiopacity, and methacrylate monomers for polymerization using dental light curing units (61). Although the complete set is only achieved after the chemical reaction of the calcium-rich hydraulic matrix, the presence of the resin matrix allows control over the initial setting time. According to the manufacturer, this material is recommended for pulp capping and as a liner associated with other restorative materials. It has been reported that TheraCal LC hydration does not form calcium hydroxide as part of the chemical reaction. Moreover, the calcium release from TheraCal LC is limited by the resin matrix, possibly reducing its bioactivity, compared to other calcium silicate-based materials (62). Therefore, the clinician should be aware that differences in the current composition of calcium silicate-based materials impact calcium ions' release and result in various outcomes regarding bioactivity (63).

Continuous comparisons among calcium hydroxide and various calcium silicate-based materials have been performed to establish the best alternative material for VPT. Overall, $Ca(OH)_2$ induces the highest inflammatory reaction and consequent zone of necrosis in direct pulp capping. This fact is mainly associated with the fast dissociation and release of calcium and hydroxyl from calcium hydroxide compared to tricalcium silicate materials. Regarding hard tissue bridge formation, MTA and Biodentine provide better organization of the mineralized tissue when compared to calcium hydroxide *in vivo* (64). In the meantime, there are also differences among the calcium silicate-based materials, where the conventional hydraulic types of cement (MTA, Biodentine) present better outcomes than TheraCal regarding time, thickness, and continuity of the mineralized barrier (9, 65).

From a clinical standpoint, calcium hydroxide and calcium silicate-based materials have been compared in clinical studies with various outcomes (50, 66, 67). MTA induces a lower inflammatory reaction than calcium hydroxide, and a meta-analysis reported that the formation of dentine bridges with MTA is also more predictable (52). However, the authors also highlighted limitations regarding the small sample size and unclear description of randomization methods for the randomized clinical trials, which implies the need for further prospective clinical studies with appropriate designs.

Biology of the Tissue Response and Mechanisms of Repair – Matrix Proteins, Signalling Molecules and Pathways

The success rate of VPT is dependent on the clinical conditions of the pulp, the choice of treatment (indirect pulp capping, direct pulp capping, or pulpotomy), and materials selection. As we previously discussed the aspects related to the decision-making and characteristics of the materials, we also present the biological mechanisms involved with healing of the tissue in response to VPT. Biologically, the chemotactic dynamics and stem-cell differentiation that results in complete tissue repair rely on the need for optimal conditions, which is hard to find in a clinical situation. Thus, the most successful scenario is still limited to the formation of osteodentine and pulp-like tissue partially resembling the native dentine-pulp complex (68–70).

Nonetheless, it is well understood that bioactive molecules, such as growth factors and non-collagenous proteins, guide specific cascades of events that result in cell proliferation or differentiation and mineral deposition (71, 72). Therefore, biomolecules like the Transforming growth factor beta (TGF-β) family and small integrin-binding ligand N-linked glycoprotein (SIBLING proteins, e.g. dentine matrix acidic phosphoprotein 1 – DMP1 and dentine sialophosphoprotein – DSPP) are involved in the odontoblastic differentiation, synthesis of the dentine matrix, and regulation of calcium and phosphate deposition to mineralize the newly deposited matrix (73–75). For instance, TGF-β1 is the predominant isoform of TGF-β in dentin, and it appears to participate in the formation of tertiary dentine while regulating deposition of the dentine matrix via odontoblasts' stimulation (76). It is also reported that bone morphogenetic protein (BMP), a member of the TGF-β family, participates in the mechanisms that regulate stem-cell differentiation into the odontoblastic lineage and dentine sialophosphoprotein (DSPP) expression (77).

On the other hand, non-collagenous proteins are more involved in the process of calcium and phosphate deposition and the hierarchical organization of hydroxyapatite crystals (73). The negatively charged domains of phosphorylated DMP1 and DSPP are responsible for attracting calcium ions and stabilizing mineral sites on the collagen templates during biomineralization (75). DSPP is the predominant non-collagenous protein in the dentine structure, and it presents high expression levels in active, fully differentiated odontoblasts (78). DSPP also binds to collagen fibrils and forms spatially organized structures that favour calcium ions to aggregation during hydroxyapatite nucleation and growth (75). Meanwhile, DMP1 is directly involved in hydroxyapatite crystals' nucleation, where its C-terminal appears to organize the crystallographic plans, while the N-terminal stabilizes the amorphous phase during mineralization (79). DMP1 is also highly expressed during odontoblast differentiation and in recently polarized cells in their secretory stage, but it is downregulated after dentine mineralization (80).

Besides the TGF-β family and SIBLING proteins, other biomolecules and signalling mechanisms have been reported to be involved in the mechanisms of pulp-dentine complex formation and repair. Complement activation via pulp-capping materials apparently regulates the tissue response towards inflammation or DPSC recruitment for regeneration (81). Moreover, the Wnt/β-catenin pathway seems to be activated and accumulates in pulp cells located in the region beneath cavity preparations, which indicates involvement of the Wnt signalling pathway in the dentine repair (82).

It is important to note that all those biomolecules work in balance during the stages of development and natural repair, while conditions during injuries could lead to a critical environment for regulation of the cascade of events occurring after VPT. Therefore, comprehension of the cellular and molecular mechanisms requested for complete pulp-dentine complex repair is essential for developing specific strategies that provide the most favourable conditions for prolonging tooth lifespan. However, such strategies demand targeting bioengineering and regenerative approaches, as further discussed in this chapter.

Opportunities and Next-generation VPT Materials

The gold standard techniques applied for VPT still rely on the use of $Ca(OH)_2$ and calcium silicate-based materials even though pulp-capping agents are not effective chemotactic mediators and do not form homogeneous native-like dentine tissues. However, the advent of dental tissue engineering has provided some relevant insights and contributions toward complete regeneration of the dentine-pulp complex.

One of the issues to be addressed regarding conventional materials for VPT is to reduce the inflammatory reaction induced by bacteria, caries removal and caustic pH from the materials. For instance, the exposed pulp is an LPS-rich environment as a sign of the inflammatory reaction. In that regard, nanofibrous scaffolds containing simvastatin demonstrated the ability to reduce important proinflammatory markers' activity and provided favourable conditions for the pulp-dentine complex regeneration (83).

Besides the ability to control inflammation, the materials' capacity to form an organized tubular dentine-like structure is critical for the process of repair in VPT. Thus, functionalized scaffolds have been used to mimic the extracellular matrix, optimize dentine bridges' formation and guide the transition from hard to soft tissue. Another future perspective of materials for VPT is the use of nanotechnology to enhance the properties and performance of dental materials, since it can also facilitate the delivery of bioactive molecules.

Nanofibrous scaffolds containing drugs such as dexamethasone, well-known for their ability to stimulate differentiation into osteo- and dental-like lineages, were synthesized as possible alternatives for pulp-capping strategies (84). Similarly, self-assembling peptide-containing electrospun scaffolds also demonstrated their potential to regulate dental stem-cell differentiation and mineralized tissue formation (85) (Figure 7.3). Combining the ability of nanofibrous scaffolds to mimic ECM with the non-collagenous proteins-like mechanism of self-assembling peptide provided an auspicious environment to guide differentiation and could indicate an interesting approach for future application in dentine regeneration.

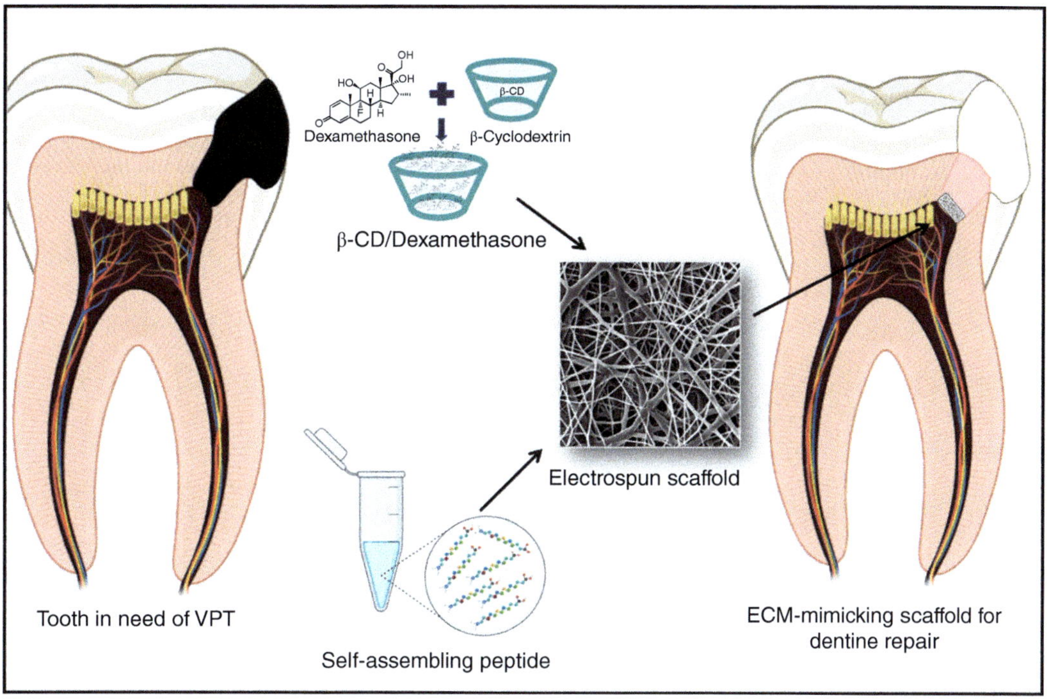

Figure 7.3 Schematic representation of the proposed application of functionalized electrospun scaffolds for dentine regeneration. Biomolecules incorporated on the nanofibers work as agents that induce mineralization and target specific pathways, while the nanofibrous scaffolds recapitulate the collagenous structure and ECM-like environment. β-Cyclodextrin/Dexamethasone inclusion complexes (84) or self-assembling peptides (85) are current examples of compounds added to the nanofibers to induce mineralized tissue regeneration. *Source:* de Souza Araújo et.al. (85)/Reproduced with permission from Elsevier.

Moreover, chitosan scaffolds containing either collagen or calcium-based materials have indicated their potential to recapitulate the extracellular matrix conditions and provide optimal conditions for DPSC differentiation toward an odontoblast lineage with the upregulation of important markers for dentine formation, such as DMP1, DSPP, and Collagen I (86, 87) (Figure 7.4A). Apart from that, sponges and hydrogels containing GSK3-inhibitors have stimulated odontogenic differentiation through Wnt-signalling pathway activation (89, 90). Although the complex phenomena involved in Wnt activation and its role in dentine regeneration are not completely elucidated, its activation resulted in tubular structures replicating the native organization of dentine *in vivo* as early as four weeks after treatment with better outcomes than the application of MTA.

Regarding the use of biomolecules to target specific phenomena in dentine repair, oligo peptides derived from DMP1 have also promoted mineralization in contact with proper amounts of calcium and phosphate and could be applied in future strategies for dentine remineralization (91). Another study investigated the encapsulation of growth factors involved in dentine-pulp complex healing (TGF-β and FGF-2) into polymeric matrices as a possible mechanism for the controlled release of these biomolecules for regenerative strategies (92). Besides, alginate and dentine matrix-derived bioink demonstrated the ability to induce dental stem-cell differentiation and expression of osteo/odontogenic markers, which could be promising for customized 3D printed constructs containing specific molecules for dentine regeneration in the future (93).

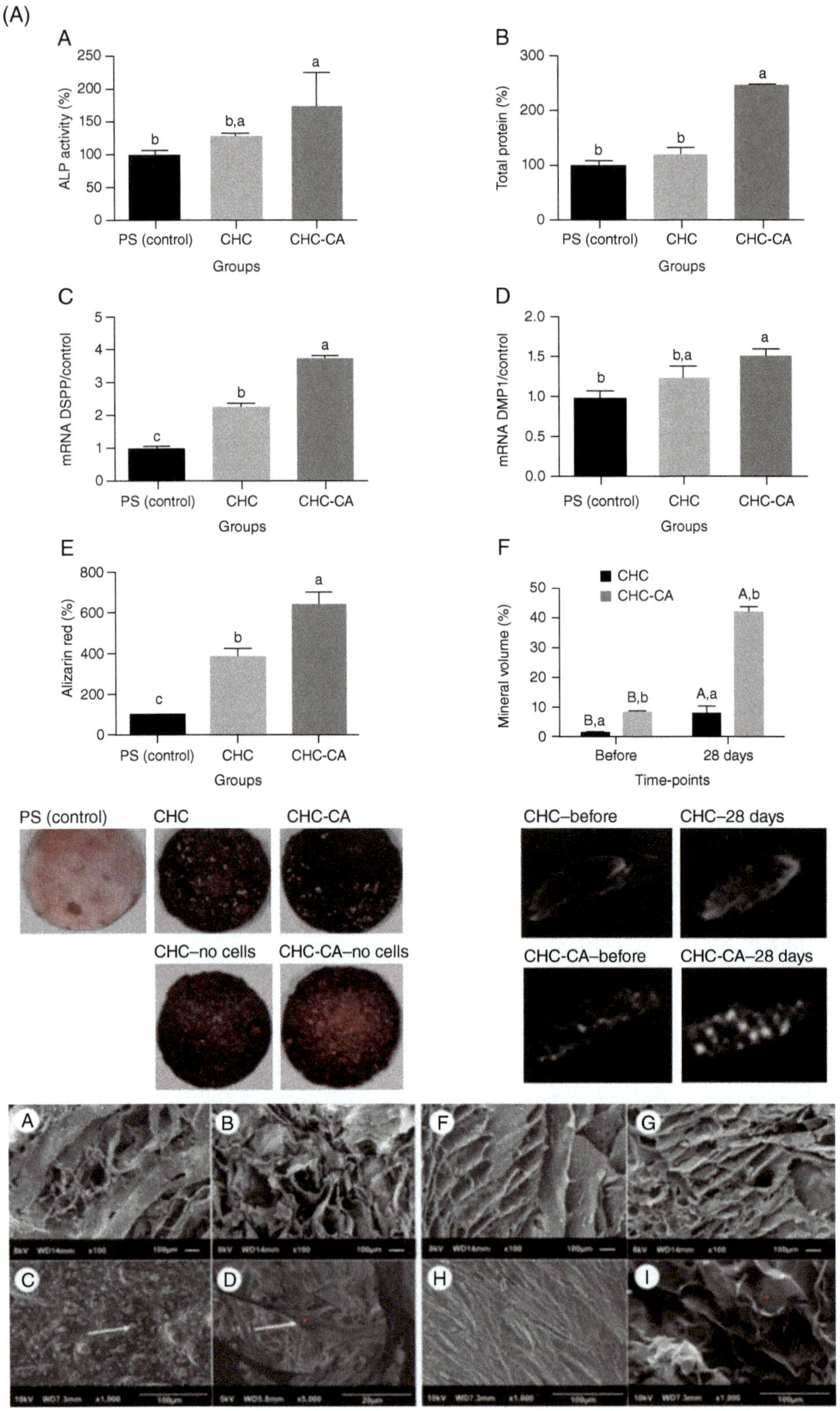

Figure 7.4 Regenerative strategies for dentine-pulp complex regeneration. (A) Chitosan/calcium-rich scaffolds upregulate osteogenic and odontogenic markers expression and provide favourable microenvironment conditions for stem-cell differentiation. *Source:* Soares et al. (87)/Springer Nature.
(B) Laser-ablation technology creates micro islands on gelatin-based fibrous scaffolds to recapitulate the dentine matrix, and guide cell commitment and single-cell polarization toward an odontoblast morphology. *Source:* Ma et al. (88)/John Wiley & Sons/CCBY 4.0.

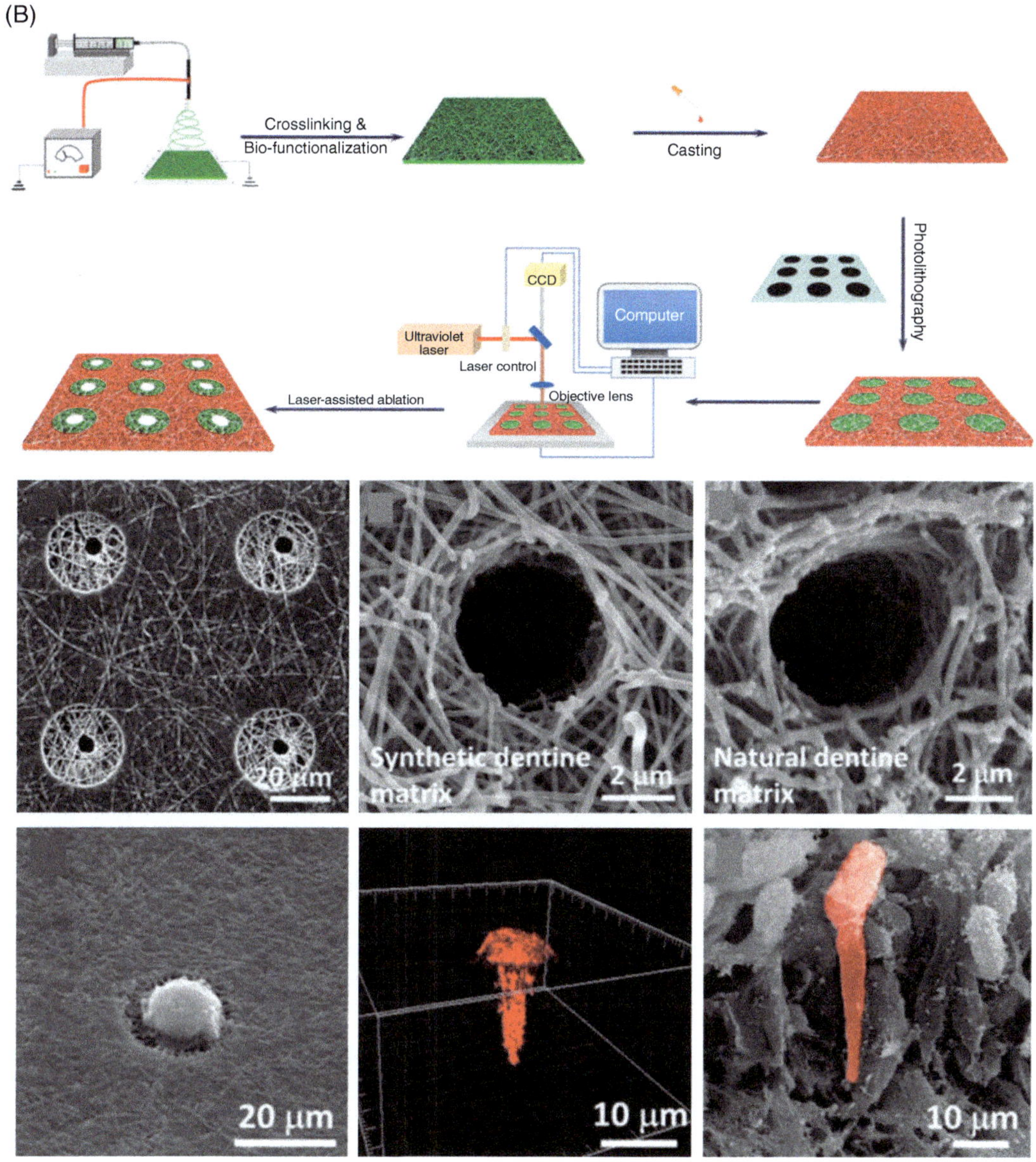

Figure 7.4 (Continued)

Complementary to that, guiding cell commitment and orientation for either preserving or inducing odontoblast layer activity after regeneration is also of interest for tissue engineering strategies in VPT. One should note that, due to the accelerated process occurring to repair the dentin-pulp complex injury, stem-cell differentiation in VPT usually results in a layer of matrix-secreting odontoblast-like cells, instead of fully differentiated odontoblasts. Odontoblasts are very specialized cells, and their differentiation occurs only in the early stages of differentiation during tooth development (94). In addition, the odontoblast processes extend into the dentinal tubules and are responsible for the secretion of dentine matrix throughout the whole life of a healthy tooth (94). Since pulp exposures compromise or lead to the death of a portion of the odontoblast layer, guiding the cell fate to obtain morpho-functional characteristics in the regenerated tissue is preferred. Laser-ablated micropatterned constructs were developed to create islands for single-cell housing and to guide DPSC polarization to address that aspect. The ECM-like structure contains ablated micro-islands oriented DPSC polarization and cytoplasmic extension, such as odontoblast processes into the dentinal tubules (88, 95) (Figure 7.4B).

The principles and techniques for regeneration of the dentine-pulp complex still require further exploration and clinical validation. Nevertheless, constant improvements in materials and technologies and the above-mentioned findings could open horizons for regenerative strategies that pave the path toward DPSC differentiation into odontoblast lineages and the homogeneous reestablishment of morphological and functional characteristics of the dentin-pulp complex after exposures for successful and predictable VPT.

Overall, while regenerative-based strategies for VPT are still relatively new, they offer exciting possibilities for the regeneration of damaged pulp tissue and the preservation of natural teeth. However, more research is needed to determine the optimal techniques and materials for these procedures and to assess their long-term outcomes.

Acknowledgements

M.C.B. acknowledges the National Institutes of Health (NIH – National Institute of Dental and Craniofacial Research/NIDCR, R01DE026578). The content is solely the responsibility of the authors and does not necessarily represent the official views of the NIH.

References

1 Yu C, Abbott PV. An overview of the dental pulp: its functions and responses to injury. *Aust Dent J.* 2007;52(1 Suppl):S4–16.

2 León-López M, Cabanillas-Balsera D, Martín-González J, Montero-Miralles P, Saúco-Márquez JJ, Segura-Egea JJ. Prevalence of root canal treatment worldwide: a systematic review and meta-analysis. *Int Endod J.* 2022;55(11):1105–27.

3 Edwards D, Stone S, Bailey O, Tomson P. Preserving pulp vitality: part two - vital pulp therapies. *Br Dent J.* 2021;230(3):148–55.

4 Zhang W, Yelick PC. Vital pulp therapy-current progress of dental pulp regeneration and revascularization. *Int J Dent.* 2010;2010:856087.

5 El Karim IA, Cooper PR, About I, Tomson PL, Lundy FT, Duncan HF. Deciphering reparative processes in the inflamed dental pulp. *Front Dent Med.* 2021;2.

6 Khorasani MMY, Hassanshahi G, Brodzikowska A, Khorramdelazad H. Role(s) of cytokines in pulpitis: latest evidence and therapeutic approaches. *Cytokine.* 2020;126:154896.

7 AAE position statement on vital pulp therapy. *J Endod.* 2021;47(9):1340–4.

8 Scalzilli PA, Jara CM, Flores D, Heinzmann D, Figueiredo JAP, Scarparo RK. Decision-making for dental pulp exposure: a survey in graduate programs at Brazilian universities. *Braz Oral Res.* 2022;36:e087.

9 Leong DJX, Yap AU. Vital pulp therapy in carious pulp–exposed permanent teeth: an umbrella review. *Clin Oral Investig.* 2021;25(12):6743–56.

10 Lin LM, Ricucci D, Saoud TM, Sigurdsson A, Kahler B. Vital pulp therapy of mature permanent teeth with irreversible pulpitis from the perspective of pulp biology. *Aust Endod J.* 2020;46(1):154–66.

11 Duncan HF. Present status and future directions-vital pulp treatment and pulp preservation strategies. *Int Endod J.* 2022;55 Suppl 3(Suppl 3):497–511.

12 Ghannam MG, Alameddine H, Bordoni B. *Anatomy, Head and Neck, Pulp (Tooth)*, StatPearls Publishing LLC, Treasure Island (FL), 2022.

13 Hargreaves KM, Berman LH. *Cohen's Pathways of the Pulp*, 12th Ed., Elsevier, St. Louis (Mo.), 2021. xii, 979 pages : illustrations (chiefly color), portraits p.

14 Rombouts C, Giraud T, Jeanneau C, About I. Pulp vascularization during tooth development, regeneration, and therapy. *J Dent Res.* 2017;96(2):137–44.

15 Galler KM, Weber M, Korkmaz Y, Widbiller M, Feuerer M. Inflammatory response mechanisms of the dentine-pulp complex and the periapical tissues. *Int J Mol Sci.* 2021;22(3):1480.

16 Jontell M, Gunraj MN, Bergenholtz G. Immunocompetent cells in the normal dental pulp. *J Dent Res.* 1987;66(6):1149–53.

17 Amarante-Mendes GP, Adjemian S, Branco LM, Zanetti LC, Weinlich R, Bortoluci KR. Pattern recognition receptors and the host cell death molecular machinery. *Front Immunol.* 2018;9:2379.

18 Kawasaki T, Kawai T. Toll-like receptor signaling pathways. *Front Immunol.* 2014;5:461.

19 Yumoto H, Hirao K, Hosokawa Y, Kuramoto H, Takegawa D, Nakanishi T, et al. The roles of odontoblasts in dental pulp innate immunity. *Jpn Dent Sci Rev.* 2018;54(3):105–17.

20 Farges JC, Carrouel F, Keller JF, Baudouin C, Msika P, Bleicher F, et al. Cytokine production by human odontoblast-like cells upon Toll-like receptor-2 engagement. *Immunobiology.* 2011;216(4):513–7.

21 Mutoh N, Tani-Ishii N, Tsukinoki K, Chieda K, Watanabe K. Expression of toll-like receptor 2 and 4 in dental pulp. *J Endod.* 2007;33(10):1183–6.

22 World Health Organization. *Sugars and Dental Caries*, World Health Organization, Geneva, 2017. 2017. Contract No.: WHO/NMH/NHD/17.12.

23 Bjørndal L, Simon S, Tomson PL, Duncan HF. Management of deep caries and the exposed pulp. *Int Endod J.* 2019;52(7):949–73.

24 Nair PN. Pathogenesis of apical periodontitis and the causes of endodontic failures. *Crit Rev Oral Biol Med.* 2004;15(6):348–81.

25 Candamourty R, Venkatachalam S, Babu MR, Kumar G. Ludwig's angina-an emergency: a case report with literature review. *J Nat Sci Biol Med.* 2012;3(2):206–8.

26 Liu Y, Gao Y, Zhan X, Cui L, Xu S, Ma D, et al. TLR4 activation by lipopolysaccharide and Streptococcus mutans induces differential regulation of proliferation and migration in human dental pulp stem cells. *J Endod.* 2014;40(9):1375–81.

27 Nakanishi T, Takegawa D, Hirao K, Takahashi K, Yumoto H, Matsuo T. Roles of dental pulp fibroblasts in the recognition of bacterium-related factors and subsequent development of pulpitis. *Jpn Dent Sci Rev.* 2011;47(2):161–6.

28 Petti S, Glendor U, Andersson L. World traumatic dental injury prevalence and incidence, a meta-analysis—one billion living people have had traumatic dental injuries. *Dent Traumatol.* 2018;34(2):71–86.

29 Yu CY, Abbott PV. Responses of the pulp, periradicular and soft tissues following trauma to the permanent teeth. *Aust Dent J.* 2016;61(Suppl 1):39–58.

30 Feliciano KMPC, Caldas AF Jr. A systematic review of the diagnostic classifications of traumatic dental injuries. *Dent Traumatol.* 2006;22(2):71–6.

31 Petersson E, Andersson L, Sörensen S. Traumatic oral vs non-oral injuries. *Swed Dent J.* 1997;21(1-2):55–68.

32 Krastl G, Weiger R, Filippi A, Van Waes H, Ebeleseder K, Ree M, et al. Endodontic management of traumatized permanent teeth: a comprehensive review. *Int Endod J.* 2021;54(8):1221–45.

33 Nair PN. Apical periodontitis: a dynamic encounter between root canal infection and host response. *Periodontol.* 2000;1997(13):121–48.
34 Glickman GN. AAE consensus conference on diagnostic terminology: background and perspectives. *J Endod.* 2009;35(12):1619–20.
35 Schweitzer JL. The endodontic diagnostic puzzle. *Gen Dent.* 2009;57(6):560–7. quiz 8-9, 95, 679.
36 Jafarzadeh H, Abbott PV. Review of pulp sensibility tests. Part II: electric pulp tests and test cavities. *Int Endod J.* 2010;43(11):945–58.
37 Jafarzadeh H, Abbott PV. Review of pulp sensibility tests. Part I: general information and thermal tests. *Int Endod J.* 2010;43(9):738–62.
38 Asgary S, Hassanizadeh R, Torabzadeh H, Eghbal MJ. Treatment outcomes of 4 vital pulp therapies in mature molars. *J Endod.* 2018;44(4):529–35.
39 Duncan HF, Galler KM, Tomson PL, Simon S, El-Karim I, Kundzina R, et al. European Society of Endodontology position statement: management of deep caries and the exposed pulp. *Int Endod J.* 2019;52(7):923–34.
40 Setzer FC, Lee SM. Radiology in endodontics. *Dent Clin North Am.* 2021;65(3):475–86.
41 Ibrahim S, Perez Alfayate R, Prichard J. Vital pulp therapy an insight over the available literature and future expectations. *Eur Endod J.* 2020;5(1):46–53.
42 Asgary S, Eghbal MJ, Fazlyab M, Baghban AA, Ghoddusi J. Five-year results of vital pulp therapy in permanent molars with irreversible pulpitis: a non-inferiority multicenter randomized clinical trial. *Clin Oral Investig.* 2015;19(2):335–41.
43 Kang CM, Sun Y, Song JS, Pang NS, Roh BD, Lee CY, et al. A randomized controlled trial of various MTA materials for partial pulpotomy in permanent teeth. *J Dent.* 2017;60:8–13.
44 Albuquerque MT, Valera MC, Nakashima M, Nor JE, Bottino MC. Tissue-engineering-based strategies for regenerative endodontics. *J Dent Res.* 2014;93(12):1222–31.
45 Galler KM. Clinical procedures for revitalization: current knowledge and considerations. *Int Endod J.* 2016;49(10):926–36.
46 Münchow EA, Bottino MC. Current and future views on biomaterial use in regenerative endodontics. In: Duncan HF, Cooper PR (eds.) Clinical Approaches in Endodontic Regeneration: Current and Emerging Therapeutic Perspectives, Springer International Publishing, Cham, 2019, 77–98.
47 Farhad A, Mohammadi Z. Calcium hydroxide: a review. *Int Dent J.* 2005;55(5):293–301.
48 Accorinte MLR, Loguercio AD, Reis A, Carneiro E, Grande RHM, Murata SS, et al. Response of human dental pulp capped with MTA and calcium hydroxide powder. *Oper Dent.* 2008;33(5):488–95.
49 Graham L, Cooper PR, Cassidy N, Nor JE, Sloan AJ, Smith AJ. The effect of calcium hydroxide on solubilisation of bio-active dentine matrix components. *Biomaterials.* 2006;27(14):2865–73.
50 Taha NA, Khazali MA. Partial pulpotomy in mature permanent teeth with clinical signs indicative of irreversible pulpitis: a randomized clinical trial. *J Endod.* 2017;43(9):1417–21.
51 Tran XV, Ngo LTQ, Boukpessi T. BiodentineTM full pulpotomy in mature permanent teeth with irreversible pulpitis and apical periodontitis. *Healthcare.* 2021;9(6):720.
52 Li Z, Cao L, Fan M, Xu Q. Direct pulp capping with calcium hydroxide or mineral trioxide aggregate: a meta-analysis. *J Endod.* 2015;41(9):1412–7.
53 International-Organization-for-Standardization. ISO 23317:2014 Implants for surgery—In vitro evaluation for apatite-forming ability of implant materials. 2014.
54 Rao A, Rao A, Shenoy R. Mineral trioxide aggregate—a review. *J Clin Pediatr Dent.* 2009;34(1):1–8.

55 Parirokh M, Torabinejad M. Mineral trioxide aggregate: a comprehensive literature review—part III: clinical applications, drawbacks, and mechanism of action. *J Endod.* 2010;36(3):400–13.
56 Vallés M, Mercadé M, Duran-Sindreu F, Bourdelande JL, Roig M. Color stability of white mineral trioxide aggregate. *Clin Oral Investig.* 2013;17(4):1155–9.
57 Vallés M, Mercadé M, Duran-Sindreu F, Bourdelande JL, Roig M. Influence of light and oxygen on the color stability of five calcium silicate–based materials. *J Endod.* 2013;39(4):525–8.
58 About I. Biodentine: from biochemical and bioactive properties to clinical applications. *G Ital Endod.* 2016;30(2):81–8.
59 Alsubait S, Aljarbou F. Biodentine or mineral trioxide aggregate as direct pulp capping material in mature permanent teeth with carious exposure? a systematic review and meta-analysis. *Oper Dent.* 2021;46(6):631–40.
60 Torabinejad M, Parirokh M, Dummer PMH. Mineral trioxide aggregate and other bioactive endodontic cements: an updated overview - part II: other clinical applications and complications. *Int Endod J.* 2018;51(3):284–317.
61 Arandi NZ, Rabi T. TheraCal LC: from biochemical and bioactive properties to clinical applications. *Int J Dent.* 2018;2018:3484653.
62 Camilleri J. Hydration characteristics of Biodentine and Theracal used as pulp capping materials. *Dent Mater.* 2014;30(7):709–15.
63 Gandolfi MG, Siboni F, Botero T, Bossù M, Riccitiello F, Prati C. Calcium silicate and calcium hydroxide materials for pulp capping: biointeractivity, porosity, solubility and bioactivity of current formulations. *J Appl Biomater Funct Mater.* 2015;13(1):43–60.
64 Chicarelli LPG, Webber MBF, Amorim JPA, Rangel ALCA, Camilotti V, Sinhoreti MAC, et al. Effect of tricalcium silicate on direct pulp capping: experimental study in rats. *Eur J Dent.* 2020;15(01):101–8.
65 Kayad M, Koura A, El-Nozahy A. A comparative histological study of the effect of TheraCal LC and biodentine on direct pulp capping in rabbits: an experimental study. *Clin Oral Investig.* 2022;27:1013–22.
66 Nowicka A, Lipski M, Parafiniuk M, Sporniak-Tutak K, Lichota D, Kosierkiewicz A, et al. Response of human dental pulp capped with biodentine and mineral trioxide aggregate. *J Endod.* 2013;39(6):743–7.
67 Taha NA, Al-Rawash MH, Imran ZA. Outcome of full pulpotomy in mature permanent molars using 3 calcium silicate-based materials: a parallel, double blind, randomized controlled trial. *Int Endod J.* 2022;55(5):416–29.
68 Ward J. Vital pulp therapy in cariously exposed permanent teeth and its limitations. *Aust Endod J.* 2002;28(1):29–37.
69 Orti V, Collart-Dutilleul P-Y, Piglionico S, Pall O, Cuisinier F, Panayotov I. Pulp regeneration concepts for nonvital teeth: from tissue engineering to clinical approaches. *Tissue Eng Part B: Rev.* 2018;24(6):419–42.
70 Shang W, Zhang Z, Zhao X, Dong Q, Schmalz G, Hu S. The understanding of vital pulp therapy in permanent teeth: a new perspective. *Biomed Res Int.* 2022;2022:8788358.
71 Kim SG. Biological molecules for the regeneration of the pulp-dentin complex. *Dent Clin North Am.* 2017;61(1):127–41.
72 Murray PE, Garcia-Godoy F, Hargreaves KM. Regenerative endodontics: a review of current status and a call for action. *J Endod.* 2007;33(4):377–90.
73 Moradian-Oldak J, George A. Biomineralization of enamel and dentin mediated by matrix proteins. *J Dent Res.* 2021;100(10):1020–9.

74 Jung C, Kim S, Sun T, Cho Y-B, Song M. Pulp-dentin regeneration: current approaches and challenges. *Journal of tissue engineering.* 2019;10:2041731418819263.

75 George A, Veis A. Phosphorylated proteins and control over apatite nucleation, crystal growth, and inhibition. *Chem Rev.* 2008;108(11):4670–93.

76 Cassidy N, Fahey M, Prime SS, Smith AJ. Comparative analysis of transforming growth factor-beta isoforms 1-3 in human and rabbit dentine matrices. *Arch Oral Biol.* 1997;42(3):219–23.

77 Aksel H, Huang GTJ. Combined effects of vascular endothelial growth factor and bone morphogenetic protein 2 on odonto/osteogenic differentiation of human dental pulp stem cells in vitro. *J Endod.* 2017;43(6):930–5.

78 D'souza RN, Cavender A, Sunavala G, Alvarez J, Ohshima T, Kulkarni AB, et al. Gene expression patterns of murine dentin matrix protein 1 (Dmp1) and dentin sialophosphoprotein (DSPP) suggest distinct developmental functions in vivo. *J Bone Miner Res.* 1997;12(12):2040–9.

79 Gajjeraman S, Narayanan K, Hao J, Qin C, George A. Matrix macromolecules in hard tissues control the nucleation and hierarchical assembly of hydroxyapatite*. *J Biol Chem.* 2007;282(2):1193–204.

80 Hao J, Zou B, Narayanan K, George A. Differential expression patterns of the dentin matrix proteins during mineralized tissue formation. *Bone.* 2004;34(6):921–32.

81 Giraud T, Rufas P, Chmilewsky F, Rombouts C, Dejou J, Jeanneau C, et al. Complement activation by pulp capping materials plays a significant role in both inflammatory and pulp stem cells' recruitment. *J Endod.* 2017;43(7):1104–10.

82 Yoshioka S, Takahashi Y, Abe M, Michikami I, Imazato S, Wakisaka S, et al. Activation of the Wnt/β-catenin pathway and tissue inhibitor of metalloprotease 1 during tertiary dentinogenesis. *J Biochem.* 2012;153(1):43–50.

83 Soares DG, Zhang Z, Mohamed F, Eyster TW, de Souza Costa CA, Ma PX. Simvastatin and nanofibrous poly(l-lactic acid) scaffolds to promote the odontogenic potential of dental pulp cells in an inflammatory environment. *Acta Biomaterialia.* 2018;68:190–203.

84 Daghrery A, Aytac Z, Dubey N, Mei L, Schwendeman A, Bottino MC. Electrospinning of dexamethasone/cyclodextrin inclusion complex polymer fibers for dental pulp therapy. *Colloids Surf B Biointerfaces.* 2020;191:111011.

85 de Souza Araujo IJ, Ferreira JA, Daghrery A, Ribeiro JS, Castilho M, Puppin-Rontani RM, et al. Self-assembling peptide-laden electrospun scaffolds for guided mineralized tissue regeneration. *Dent Mater.* 2022;38(11):1749–62.

86 Soares DG, Bordini EAF, Cassiano FB, Bronze-Uhle ES, Pacheco LE, Zabeo G, et al. Characterization of novel calcium hydroxide-mediated highly porous chitosan-calcium scaffolds for potential application in dentin tissue engineering. *J Biomed Mater Res B Appl Biomater.* 2020;108(6):2546–59.

87 Soares DG, Rosseto HL, Scheffel DS, Basso FG, Huck C, Hebling J, et al. Odontogenic differentiation potential of human dental pulp cells cultured on a calcium-aluminate enriched chitosan-collagen scaffold. *Clin Oral Investig.* 2017;21(9):2827–39.

88 Ma C, Chang B, Jing Y, Kim H, Liu X. Bio-inspired micropatterned platforms recapitulate 3D physiological morphologies of bone and dentinal cells. *Adv Sci.* 2018;5(12):1801037.

89 Alaohali A, Salzlechner C, Zaugg LK, Suzano F, Martinez A, Gentleman E, et al. GSK3 inhibitor-induced dentinogenesis using a hydrogel. *J Dent Res.* 2021;101(1):46–53.

90 Neves VCM, Babb R, Chandrasekaran D, Sharpe PT. Promotion of natural tooth repair by small molecule GSK3 antagonists. *Sci Rep.* 2017;7(1):39654.

91 Padovano JD, Ravindran S, Snee PT, Ramachandran A, Bedran-Russo AK, George A. DMP1-derived peptides promote remineralization of human dentin. *J Dent Res.* 2015;94(4):608–14.

92 Mathieu S, Jeanneau C, Sheibat-Othman N, Kalaji N, Fessi H, About I. Usefulness of controlled release of growth factors in investigating the early events of dentin-pulp regeneration. *J Endod.* 2013;39(2):228–35.

93 Athirasala A, Tahayeri A, Thrivikraman G, França CM, Monteiro N, Tran V, et al. A dentin-derived hydrogel bioink for 3D bioprinting of cell laden scaffolds for regenerative dentistry. *Biofabrication.* 2018;10(2):024101.

94 Kawashima N, Okiji T. Odontoblasts: specialized hard-tissue-forming cells in the dentin-pulp complex. *Congenital Anomalies.* 2016;56(4):144–53.

95 Chang B, Ma C, Liu X. Nanofibrous tubular three-dimensional platform for single dental pulp stem cell polarization. *ACS Appl Mater Interfaces.* 2020;12(49):54481–8.

8

Vital Pulp Treatment for Traumatic Dental Injuries

Bill Kahler[1] *and Giampiero Rossi-Fedele*[2]

[1] *Faculty of Medicine and Health, Department of Restorative and Reconstructive Dentistry, Sydney Dental School, The University of Sydney, Surry Hills, NSW, Australia*
[2] *Adelaide Dental School, The University of Adelaide, Adelaide, SA, Australia*

Introduction

The treatment of teeth that have sustained a traumatic dental injury (TDI) with vital pulp treatment (VPT) is not new, as it was pioneered by Cvek in 1978 (1). Maintaining pulp vitality to allow further root maturation is the principal goal of VPT, as pulp necrosis or injudicious removal of a healthy pulp has unfortunate consequences, particularly for immature teeth (2). Purported advantages of maintaining pulp vitality for mature and immature teeth include an improved likelihood of survival (3) plus the maintenance of dentine deposition and further repair mechanisms, immunological response and proprioceptive functions, among others (4). Interest in VPT in mature teeth has been reinvigorated recently due to an increased understanding of the reparative processes of the pulp, multiple improvements in the management of dental tissues, the availability of bioactive hydraulic calcium silicate cement (HCSCs), its less-invasive nature and its reported successful outcomes (4).

It is the purpose of this chapter to outline the developments and outcomes when mature and immature teeth with complicated crown fractures (CCFs) with luxation or root fractures are treated with VPT and showcase the current techniques with contemporary materials.

Traumatic Dental Injuries

TDI have the fifth highest incidence in diseases and conditions are commonly unreported (5). TDIs are mostly associated with children and young adults; therefore, subjects potentially present with mature and immature permanent teeth (6). Of TDIs in the permanent dentition, crown fractures are the most prevalent and are classified as either complicated or uncomplicated, depending on whether the pulp is exposed (7).

CCFs and root fractures involve the enamel, dentine and dental pulp (8, 9). Similarly, the dental pulp is commonly involved in crown-root fractures when the tooth in question has fully erupted. The cement and surrounding periodontal tissues are involved in root fractures and may be involved in crown-root fractures (8, 9). Crown-root fractures often have a limited displacement of the

Vital Pulp Treatment, First Edition. Edited by Henry F. Duncan and Ikhlas A. El-Karim.

coronal segment and a transverse direction, with a more coronal position in the buccal aspect of the tooth when compared with the palatal/lingual surface. In addition, luxation includes further damage to the periodontium and a subsequent displacement of the coronal segment in question with further injury to the dental pulp (10).

Teeth with CCFs are the most likely to undergo pulp necrosis without appropriate management and the most likely to benefit from VPT, though it has been shown that inflammation is limited in the earlier stages of exposure (11). Clinically, there are various presentations ranging from a slight haemorrhage to the formation of a pulp polyp, depending on the degree of contamination and the ability of the pulp to respond to the injury, with immature teeth expected to have more favourable outcomes compared with mature ones. Other TDIs, such as avulsion and luxation, are less likely to be treatable with VPT as the vasculature is compromised (12). Concomitant crown fractures and luxation injuries in permanent mature teeth are significantly associated with pulp necrosis (13, 14). In general, for most root fractures, the apical part of the pulp will remain vital, with no treatment required other than repositioning and fragment stabilization (15). Significant clinical factors that influence the healing of intra-alveolar fractures include mobility and dislocation of the coronal fragment, plus the diastasis between fragments which have been associated with rupture and/or stretching of the tissues (15).

Outcome measures considered in the literature have varied with time. In the classic literature, for CCFs in particular the absence of clinical symptoms, absence of radiographic radiolucency suggestive of pathosis, continuous root development and the presence of a hard-tissue bridge as well as a response to pulp sensibility testing were considered important (1, 16). Whereas loss of the injured tooth is a possible complication of root fractures (17). More recently, a core outcome set for TDIs in children and adults has been developed by the International Association of Dental Traumatology (IADT) (18). These include generic outcomes, such as injury activity (periodontal and pulpal healing), physical consequences of disease (pain and discolouration), functional status (tooth loss), social outcomes and quality of life (quality of life and aesthetics), side effects of therapy (dental anxiety) and health resource utilization (number of clinical visits) (18). In addition, injury-specific outcomes have been proposed, those relevant to this chapter being quality and loss of restoration for both types of injuries and mobility for crown-root fractures (18).

Therefore, the focus of this chapter relates to VPT for the management of CCFs associated with luxation and crown-root fractures and will also aim to discuss, when available, the core outcome measures of relevance.

Diagnosing the Pulp Condition

An accurate diagnosis is essential for any management and therefore is critical for predictable outcomes. The trauma is sudden, emotional, the impact is visually notable and often associated with soft tissue lacerations and swelling. Therefore, achieving an accurate diagnosis is challenging in traumatic injuries, especially in children. In fact, TDIs present most often in children aged between 6 and 12 years (19, 20) and it is understandable that obtaining an accurate diagnosis in this cohort will be difficult.

TDIs most commonly involve the maxillary central and lateral incisors (21), and CCFs may encompass a third of TDIs (19, 20) involving the maxillary central incisor in particular (22).

In the presence of CCFs, sensitivity to thermal changes is a common symptom. Pulp sensibility testing may be unreliable in children for emotional reasons such as anxiety and distress, difficulty in interpretation and inadequate neural development as the plexus of Rashkow does not fully develop for up to five years after a tooth erupts (23), in addition to the issues caused by laceration of the pulp tissues. Furthermore, pulpal oedema from the traumatic injury can lead to a temporary loss of sensibility (24). Thus, a non-response to pulp sensibility testing is not conclusive for pulp necrosis in TDIs (25–28). The concerns in a reliable assessment of the status of the traumatized pulp are outlined in the European Society of Endodontology (ESE) position statement: Endodontic Management of Traumatized Permanent Teeth (ESE 2021) (29).

A series of radiographic examinations at varying vertical angulations is required to diagnose concomitant TDIs such as luxations and root fractures. Cone beam computed tomography (CBCT) can particularly assist in assessing the extent and position of crown-root fractures (30). This is important as luxation injuries may synergistically affect the viability of VPT for the treatment of CCFs due to disturbance to the neuro-vascular bundle at the apical foramina. Diagnostic issues, nonetheless, are common even when three-dimensional imaging is used during the management of TDIs.

Direct Pulp Capping and Pulpotomies for Managing Traumatised Teeth

The IADT (2020) (31), the ESE position statement on Endodontic Management of Traumatised Permanent Teeth (ESE, 2021) (29) and The American Association of Endodontics "Treatment of Traumatic Injuries" (AAE 2013) (32) all advocate the use of VPT by either pulp capping or pulpotomy for CCFs and crown-root fractures (29, 31, 32). However, there are some inconsistencies in the recommendations/guidelines regarding the management of the exposed pulp. The IADT (2020) and AAE (2013) guidelines recommend either a pulp cap or a partial pulpotomy (ESE 2021). The IADT (2020) guidelines list partial pulpotomy followed by direct pulp capping, whereas AAE (2013) lists pulp capping first, followed by partial pulpotomy. Neither the IADT (2020) nor the AAE (2013) makes specific indication as to when either pulp capping or pulpotomy would be indicated as the first treatment choice. However, the ESE (2021) is more specific and recommends a partial pulpotomy for large exposures or when there is a treatment delay, and advocates pulp capping for minor exposures that have occurred within a few hours of the trauma, as it is considered that there has been less microbial challenge to the pulp, therefore a reduced risk of demise. The ESE (2021) further clarifies that root canal treatment is only indicated if there is a concomitant luxation injury or the restorative requirements indicate that a post is needed to restore the tooth. Both the IADT (2020) and AAE (2013) have specific guidelines for complicated crown-root fractures in which pulpotomy is recommended for immature teeth with incomplete root development and a pulpectomy is advised for a mature tooth if the tooth can be retained. Pulpectomy is also indicated if restoration with a post is required and may also involve either orthodontic extrusion with or without periodontal re-contouring of the gingiva or surgical extrusion. Autotransplantation is another option.

What is the Evidence for the Preferred Treatment Choice?

Several studies have shown a higher incidence of pulp necrosis for teeth treated with pulp capping rather than pulpotomy (16, 17, 33). A study of 76 teeth with CCFs reported a success rate of 92% for teeth treated with calcium hydroxide pulpotomy and 81.5% for teeth treated with direct pulp capping (16). However, there were also differences in the pre-operative status of the groups, as 38 of the teeth were mature and presented with pinpoint exposures treated by direct pulp capping, whereas the remaining 38 teeth were immature and treated with a pulpotomy. In another study of 76 teeth with CCFs followed for five years, pulp survival was only 32%. Unfortunately, the reason for the poor outcome was that most mature teeth had the pulp extirpated in primary care prior to referral. In teeth treated with VPT, pulp vitality rose to 75.8%. However, the incidence of pulp necrosis was higher for pulp capping (45.5%) when compared to partial pulpotomy (13.6%) over five years of review (17). In a more recent study of 375 teeth, the incidence of pulp necrosis for pulp capping was 57.1%, whereas teeth treated with partial pulpotomy was 10.1% and 9.8% for coronal pulpotomy and just 6.1% required retreatment with either a partial or coronal pulpotomy after the tooth had been initially treated by direct pulp capping (33). In this study, the retreatment of the pulp capping by pulpotomy offered a much better outcome than direct pulp capping and comparable outcomes to an initial treatment with pulpotomy. Twenty-eight teeth were retreated with pulpotomy and 75% (21/28 teeth) were retreated in less than 24 hours, 14.8% (4/28 teeth) in 24–72 hours and 11.2% (3/28 teeth) in more than 72 hours (33).

A recent systematic review has suggested that partial pulpotomy as opposed to pulp capping, should be the preferred treatment option for both mature and immature teeth that have sustained CCFs (34). However, the severity of the traumatic injury, the size of the pulp exposure, the presence of a concomitant luxation injury and any delay in treatment being initiated may influence pulp healing and the potential for pulp necrosis (1, 16, 35).

A recent study in a major hospital setting reported a success rate of only 61% for 56 teeth that had sustained either CCFs or complicated crown-root fractures (CCRF) that were treated with the Cvek protocol (36). Pulp survival was reported as 54.1% and 73.7% for teeth treated with partial and full coronal pulpotomies, respectively. Pulp survival for four teeth with CCRF was 50%. A concomitant luxation injury was noted in 30% of treated teeth. The experience and training of the clinician impacted the outcome. Pulp survival was reported in 70.4% and 71.4% of the teeth treated by post-graduate registrars and paediatric specialists, respectively. In contrast, pulp survival for teeth treated by general dental practitioners was 33%. This suggests that VPT is a clinically sensitive technique, and clinical experience can account for differences in outcome. The important factor of a concomitant luxation injury emphasises the need for a complete diagnosis prior to treatment.

Overall experience of the clinician in treating trauma is another barrier to treating CCFs with VPT. As stated above, Hecova et al. (17) reported poor outcomes for teeth with CCFs in most mature teeth when the pulp was extirpated in the primary care setting. Another study reported that the initial treatment for CCFs was pulp extirpation (44% overall; 61% of mature teeth and 35% of immature teeth), which was generally provided outside the hospital setting (37). These authors advocated the use of a pulp 'bandage' using a glass-ionomer cement restoration in the primary care setting prior to referral for the appropriate treatment. This is indeed suitable, as teeth treated with pulpotomies as either primary care or secondary to the emergency placement of a pulp cap were reported to be successful treatment approaches. Importantly, several studies show similar outcomes for either mature or immature teeth treated with pulpotomies (36, 38, 39), so a mature tooth should be treated with VPT rather than pulp extirpation except when it is considered that a post would be required for successful restoration of the tooth.

Several recent reviews have been published on VPT in CCFs (34, 40, 41). The relevant studies assessing pulp survival are included in Table 8.1. If pulp necrosis develops, it is generally within the first six months (16, 54), although other studies have reported one year (49) and others report two years (13).

Table 8.1 VPT studies related to CCFs.

Author	Number of teeth	Tooth Mature/ Immature	Intervention	Material	Restoration	Pulp survival %	Follow-up (years)
Cvek (1)	60	28/32	Cvek P	CH	ZOE and CR later	96	1–5
Fuks et al. (16)	76	38/38	Cvek P	CH	CR	P: 92 DPC: 81.5	7.5–11
Klein et al. (42)	34	NR	Partial P	CH	CR or SSBC	94.1	1–3
Gelbier and Winter (43)	175	NR	Full P	CH	NR	79.4	2
Cvek (38)	178	90/88	Cvek P	CH	ZOE and CR later	Immature 95.3 Mature 93.75	3–15
Fuks et al. (44)	40	NR	Partial P	CH	CR	94	1–5
De Blanco (45)	30	10/20	Cvek P	CH	ZOE/GIC/SSBC	100	1–8
Koyuncuoglu et al. (46)	13	13/0	Partial P	WMTA	GIC + CR	10	2
Caprioglio et al. (47)	27	27/0	Partial P	MTA	Temporary cement and CR	85.1	1–3
Xu (48)	70	NR	Partial P	CH	NR	75	1
Wang et al. (33)	375	333/42	DPC: 28 Partial P: 109 Full P: 205	DPC: Dycal P: CH or MTA	NR	DPC: 42.9 P: 90.1 DPC RTx P 93.9	11
Albuelniel et al. (49)	50	50/0	Full P	BioD: 25 WMTA: 25	GIC + CR	BioD 76 WMTA 84	1.5
Haikal et al. (50)	51	29/22	Partial P	BioD	NR	91	2
Rao et al. (39)	205	77/128	Partial P	Iroot BP Plus and CH	Ketac cement and CR or Reattachment	Mature 97.4 Immature 95.3	1–2

Yang et al. (51)	110	110/0	Partial P	Iroot BP Plus and CH	CR	CH	2
Bissinger et al. (52)	127	NR	DPC or Partial P	CH MTA	CR Reattachment	MTA: 80.5 CH: 71	1.5
Wu et al. (53)	69	69/0	DPC: 21 P: 48	DPC: CH P: MTA	DPC: CR P: GIC + CR	P: 100	0.5–3
Yu et al. (36)	56	56/0	Partial P & Coronal P	CH	GIC/CR/ Reattachment	61	1–5

Legend: BioD: Biodentine; CH: calcium hydroxide; CR: crown; DPC: direct pulp capping; GIC: Glass-Ionomer Cement; MTA: mineral trioxide aggregate; NR: not reported; P: pulpotomy; reattachment (of the fractured fragment); RTx: retreatment; SSBC: stainless steel basket crowns; WMTA: White Mineral Trioxide Aggregate; ZOE: zinc oxide eugenol.

Factors that Affect Outcomes of VPT in TDI

Restorations

Restorations are of relevance in the event of CCF, as these have a significant functional role in mastication, aesthetics and to address potential sensitivity to various stimuli such as air, cold and sweets and protect the pulp from further contamination long-term (31). In fact, quality and loss of restoration are injury-specific core outcomes relevant to CCFs and root fractures (18), with loss and breakdown of the restoration being considered unfavourable outcomes. Rebonding of the fractured fragment after rehydration is the preferred first option as it reconstitutes the original tooth form and over time is likely to have the most aesthetic appearance. However, Bücher et al. (55) reported that bonded fragments were three times more likely to fail than direct restorations. A recent systematic review of pulpotomies for the management of CCFs found that no studies assessed the quality of the restoration and its impact on pulp necrosis and/or apical periodontitis (34). However, one study excluded from analysis cases where there had been either partial or complete loss of the restoration, so loss of the restoration was not assessed (39). In a different component study, lost restorations were reported for 24 of 54 (46.7%) teeth, with 13 (54.2%) of the teeth with a lost restoration demonstrating pulp healing and 11 (45.8%) of the teeth developing pulp necrosis (36). In this study, rebonding of the fragment was preferred, with 11 rebonded fragments; of these, 5 rebonded fragments failed over a 2- to 51-month period. The teeth were then retreated with full-coverage composite resin strip crowns. When the tooth fragment was rebonded in the 11 cases, 8 (72.7%) demonstrated pulp healing, whereas 3 teeth (27.2%) developed pulp necrosis. Of the 27 teeth restored with strip crowns, 15 (55.6%) teeth demonstrated pulp healing, while 12 (44.4%) teeth developed pulp necrosis (36).

A retrospective study of 98 teeth that sustained CCFs reported that 67% of the pulp-capped teeth and 47% of the pulpotomies relied on an emergency bandage, as the teeth were restored with glass-ionomer cement rather than a definitive composite/compomer restoration. The mean survival time for pulp vitality was improved with the use of a bonded restoration as the definitive restoration. Using a definitive bonded restoration at the initial presentation significantly reduced the risk of developing pulp necrosis (22).

Overall, the research supports that a definitive restoration should be placed without delay and preferably immediately after VPT, to minimize the risk of coronal leakage and subsequent pulp infection in CCFs (24). A restoration will be necessary in root fractures if the coronal fragment becomes necrotic and infected or in case of discolouration.

Figures 8.1–8.5 illustrate cases of teeth with CCF treated with either reattachment of the bonded fragment, immediate restoration with composite and cases where the bonded fragment failed and was then replaced with a composite restoration. Figure 8.5 shows a tooth with a CCRF restored with composite.

Mobility

Tooth mobility is an injury-specific core outcome for root fractures (18). At the same time, pre-operative mobility of the coronal fragment has a negative influence on the survival of the coronal pulp and on fracture healing with hard tissue, the latter being considered a positive outcome for this type of injury (15). For crown-root fractures, there is often mobility of the retained fractured segment, which has some attachment to the PDL apparatus. Different healing patterns in intra-alveolar root fractures are possible. These include the interposition of soft tissue exclusively or the

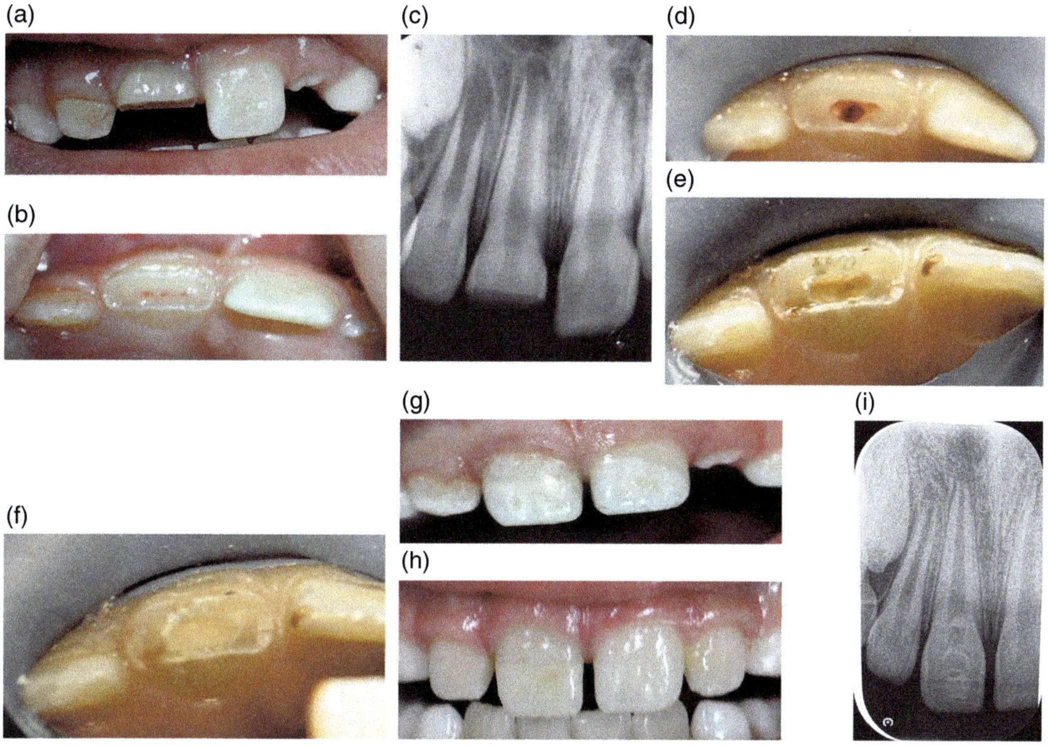

Figure 8.1 (a) A clinical photograph of a complicated crown fracture in an eight-year-old boy. (b) A clinical photograph of the incisal fractured surface. (c) A pre-treatment periapical radiograph revealing an open apex. (d) The pulp was accessed to a depth of 2 mm, and haemostasis was obtained by placing a microbrush soaked in 1% NaOCl. (e) UltraCal and Life (calcium hydroxide cavity liner) were inserted onto the pulp. (f) Glass-ionomer cement was placed on the Life to fill the pulp access cavity. (g) The fractured fragment was rebonded. The tooth and the fragment were etched with phosphoric acid and cemented with RelyX. (h) A clinical photograph was taken at a two-year review. (i) A periapical radiograph taken at the two-year review showing complete root maturation.

presence of chronic inflammatory tissue – that should be described as "non-healing", which may be associated with increased mobility compared with healing that includes hard tissue, at least partially (15). Regarding CCFs, mobility is likely to be associated with a concomitant luxation injury, and the crown should be promptly restored as described above.

Delay in Treatment

TDIs are among the most urgent dental presentations in clinical practice. Nonetheless, although the importance of early diagnosis needs to be reiterated, the necessity for prompt treatment will differ based on the injury type, and treatment delay may not negatively affect treatment outcomes in specific clinical presentations. For CCFs, according to a recent review (34), four studies assessed the time delay for treatment with a pulpotomy following injury and found no impact on pulp survival and the absence of apical periodontitis (16, 38, 42, 44). However, one of these studies did find a significant difference in successful outcomes for teeth treated within 72 hours following trauma compared to longer delays before treatment (38). Another study of 175 teeth treated with a pulpotomy reported that 12% of teeth treated within 24 hours of the injury lost pulp vitality, compared

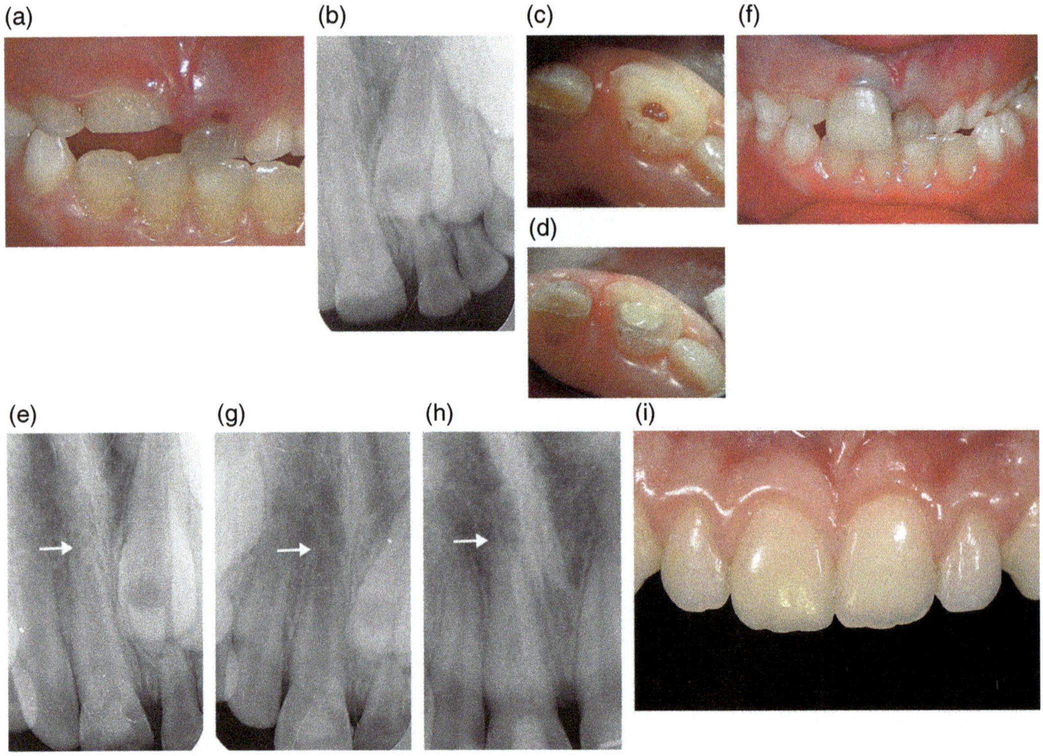

Figure 8.2 A seven-year-old male patient referred after trauma displaying a horizontal coronal fracture of the maxillary right central incisor (11) with a pulp exposure covered with a glass-ionomer cement by the general dentist and a retained deciduous left central incisor (56). (a) Clinical photograph showing a horizontally fractured right maxillary incisor and retained deciduous left central incisor. (b) Periapical radiograph reveals open apex for tooth 11 and unerupted maxillary left permanent incisor 21. In addition, a mesiodens is visible at the location of 21. (c) Photograph after shallow Cvek coronal pulpotomy. (d) View of access cavity after haemostasis using NaOCl and placement of 3–4 mm Biodentine (Septodont, Saint-Maur-des-Fossés, France) plug. (e) Radiograph after pulpotomy and temporary restoration placement with an open apex (white arrow). (f) Clinical photograph three days after verified Calcium Silicate Cement setting and reattachment of the fractured coronal segment after bonding. (g) Radiograph Tooth 11 with bonded crown segment reattachment showing immature open apex (white arrow). (h) Five-year radiographic review Tooth 11 demonstrating complete radicular maturation (white arrow). The incisor responded positive to cold testing. (i) Clinical photograph at five years after finishing of a resin composite veneer created with a layering technique on Tooth 11. *Source:* Courtesy of Dr Marga H. Ree. Reprinted with permission. Courtesy of George Bogen. From Bogen G et al. Cohens Pathways of the Pulp, 12th ed. (57).

with 32% for teeth treated after 24 hours (43). In a primate study of mechanically exposed pulps that were pulp capped with either setting calcium hydroxide Dycal (Batch Catalyst 070929, Base 070979, L. D. Caulk, Milford, DE 19963, USA). or Life (Batch Base 9-1207, Cat. 9-1226, Sybron/Kerr Dental Products Division. Romulus, MI 48174, USA), favourable outcomes were reduced from 93% to 56% when treatment was delayed from one hour to seven days (59). This would suggest that where there is a significant delay in treatment for CCF, a pulpotomy may be the preferred option for treatment. It would be prudent to treat all CCFs as early as possible after the trauma, especially when the patient is in pain. However, where treatment is delayed, VPT can maintain pulp vitality and should be the preferred treatment option. Regarding root fractures, no significant relationship

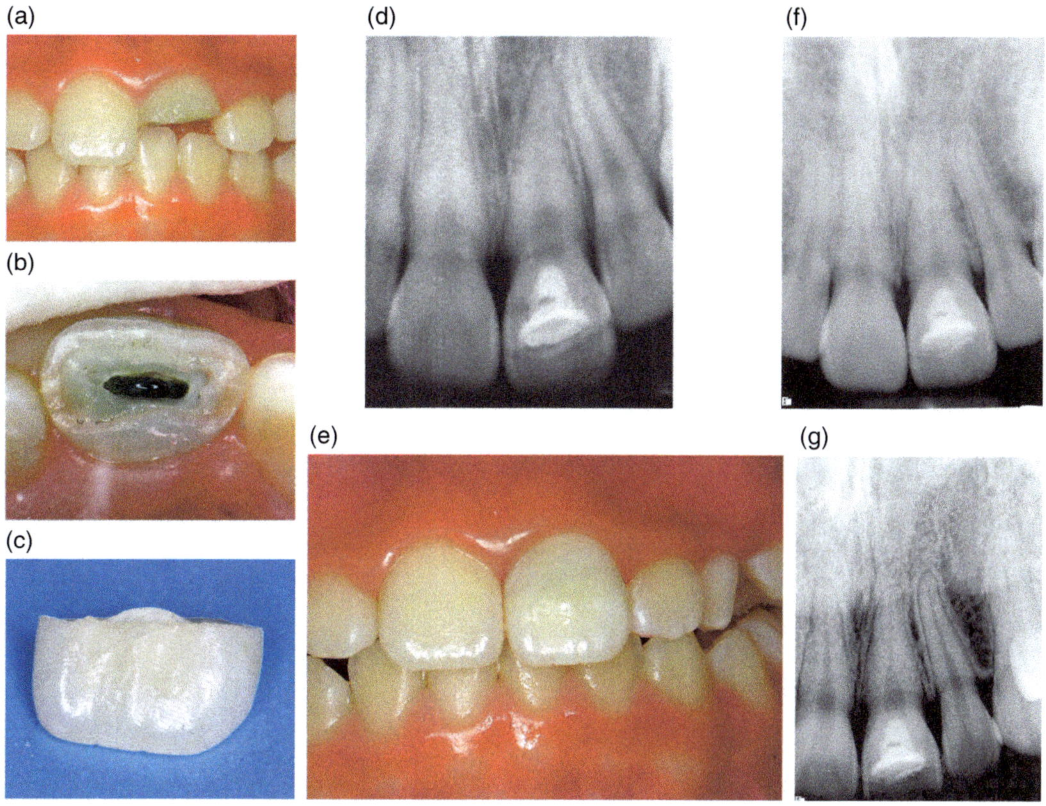

Figure 8.3 An 11-year-old female presented three hours after trauma with a horizontal coronal fracture of the maxillary left central incisor. (a) Clinical photograph showing mid-coronal horizontal fracture. The pulp was exposed and exhibited normal vitality. (b) Photograph of access cavity after Cvek pulpotomy and placement of GMTA (ProRoot MTA, Tulsa/Dentsply, Tulsa, OK, USA). (c) Photograph of the fractured incisal segment before bonding and reattachment. (d) Six-month radiograph with a bonded fractured segment showing initial reparative bridge formation with the absence of apical pathosis. The incisor was asymptomatic and normally responded to cold sensibility testing. (e) Clinical photograph of the restored tooth. (f) Eight-year radiographic review. (g) Eleven-year radiographic recall. The tooth was asymptomatic with normal mobility, probings and a positive response to cold test. *Source:* Courtesy of Dr. Winston Chee and Dr. Stefan Zweig. From Bogen G et al. Cohens Pathways of the Pulp, 12th ed. (57). Reprinted with permission). Courtesy of George Bogen.

was found in a seminal study between treatment delay and type of healing, even if the time length was more than three days after the TDI occurred (60).

Size of Pulp Exposure

The dental pulp has a remarkable ability to withstand exposure to the oral cavity. Cvek (1), in a study of 60 teeth where the pulp exposure associated with CCF varied from 0.5 to 4.0 mm, demonstrated that the pulp chamber size was not a critical factor for pulp healing, with most cases being treated 30 or fewer hours after the accident. Few studies have assessed the effect of pulp exposure size on outcomes. However, the determining factor is the vitality of the treated pulp rather than the size of the pulp exposure (44, 56). Therefore, the ability to achieve haemostasis following amputation of the superficial layer of the pulp as per the Cvek protocol is the more important determining

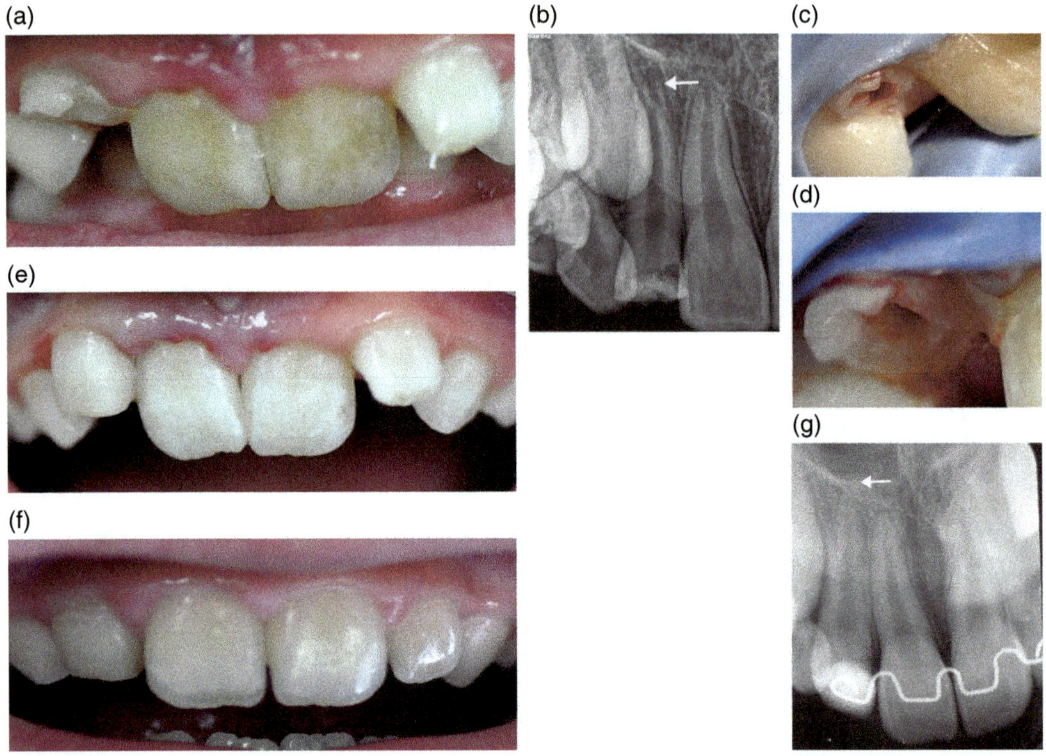

Figure 8.4 (a) A clinical photograph of a complicated crown fracture on which a GIC emergency bandage had been placed for an eight-year-old girl on the right lateral incisor following a blow with a hockey stick. Note the Class II Division II malocclusion. (b) A pre-treatment periapical radiograph revealing an open apex (white arrow). (c) The GIC emergency bandage has been removed to reveal a bleeding pulp. (d) The pulp was accessed to a depth of 2 mm and haemostasis was obtained by placing a microbrush soaked in 1% NaOCl. (e) The tooth was restored with an acid-etched composite resin. (f) Anterior teeth post-orthodontic treatment. (g) A periapical radiograph taken at the post-orthodontic treatment with an orthodontic retention splint in place to prevent relapse. Note that completed root maturation is evident (white arrow).

variable on outcomes. The ESE (2021) guidelines advise a partial pulpotomy for large exposures as the preferred treatment but do not define what is a large exposure (29). The IADT (2020) and AAE (2013) guidelines make no recommendation on the size of the pulp exposure (31, 32).

The size of pulp exposure is difficult to assess for root fractures. Interestingly, cervical location with more likelihood of exposure of the pulp to the oral cavity is slightly associated with a more favourable type of healing (no pulp necrosis and a fracture repair by hard and/or soft tissue), when compared with fractures located in the middle and apical thirds of the root (15). These authors suggested this might be explained by the shorter distance required for revascularization in the cervical region, or the fact that a certain number of severely displaced teeth with cervical fractures were extracted, skewing the data (15).

Stage of Root Development

VPT is particularly desirable in immature teeth; however, it should be considered a valid alternative to root canal treatment in mature teeth. In fact, the stage of root development is not a likely determining variable on the outcome, even in cariously exposed pulps treated with VPT, though

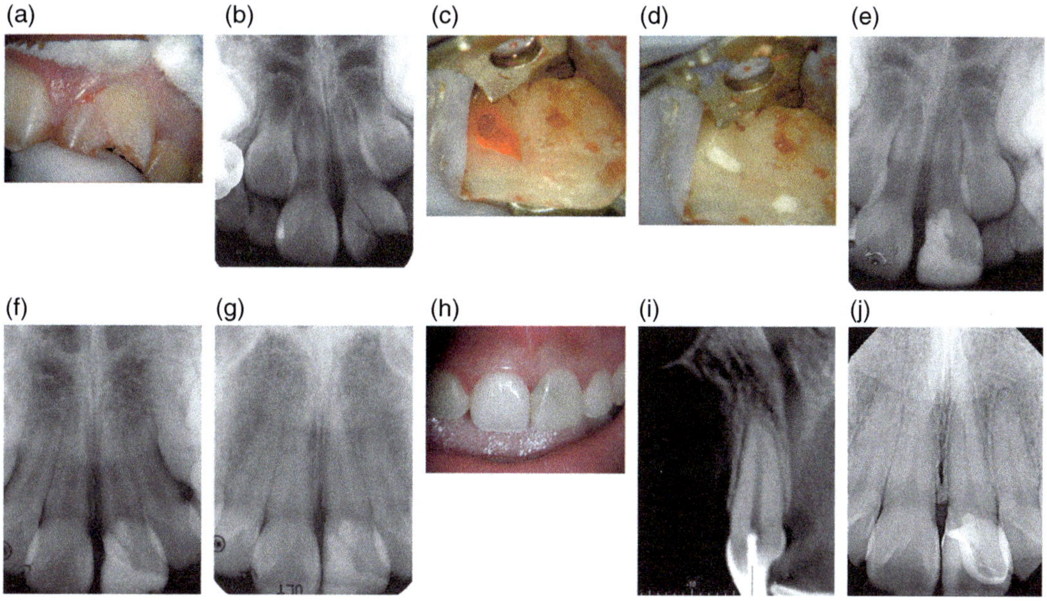

Figure 8.5 (a) Clinical photograph of a traumatized maxillary left central incisor in an eight-year-old male patient. (b) Periapical radiograph showing two oblique coronal fractures and open apex. (c) Clinical photograph of pulp exposure. (d) Cvek pulpotomy using white MTA after NaOCl haemostasis. (e) Radiograph of completed pulpotomy and bonded composite restoration. (f) Two-year radiographic follow-up. (g) Five-year radiographic follow-up. (h) Clinical photograph at a seven-year recall. (i) CBCT sagittal image at 9.5-year follow-up. (j) A Periapical radiograph taken at an 11-year review. *Source:* Courtesy Dr Paul Anstey. From: Kang ML, Bogen G. Endodontic Prognosis (58).

contrasting evidence is available in the literature for the latter. For example, Cvek's seminal study (1) reported similar outcomes for immature and mature roots, whereas a more recent study reported a significant impact of tooth maturity on pulp survival (33).

The treatment modality (pulp capping vs. pulpotomy) has similar pulp survival rates following stratification according to tooth maturity (17). The critical factor is the complete removal of the inflamed pulp rather than the stage of root development (61), as previously highlighted. There is a paucity of evidence assessing the role of root maturity in the healing of root fractures; therefore, no conclusion can currently be made on this issue.

Material Choice for CCFs

Different bioactive endodontic materials aiming to stimulate a biological seal have been used throughout the history of endodontics. Calcium hydroxide was used in the original Cvek study (1) with Calasept placed on the pulp, which was then covered with zinc oxide eugenol. The 58 out of 60 teeth that had a successful outcome were reviewed from 14 to 60 months (average 31 months) until a continuous hard-tissue barrier was observed radiographically. The interim restoration and calcium hydroxide were then removed, and the tooth was definitively restored with a hard-setting calcium hydroxide (Dycal) and with an acid-etched resin composite (1). Calcium hydroxide was used due to its anti-microbial properties and action as a hard-tissue stimulating material. The disadvantages of calcium hydroxide are its solubility, lack of adhesion (62) and tunnel defects in the hard-tissue barrier formed (63).

HCSCs have attracted the interest of researchers and have been used clinically more commonly in the last decades. Mineral trioxide aggregate (MTA) has been utilized due to its superior physical properties, where a more homogenous hard-tissue barrier is formed. MTA is primarily composed of calcium and silicates and has minimal or no solubility, with well-documented sealing and biocompatibility properties (64). The disadvantages of using MTA include the risk of discolouration (49) and a prolonged setting time (65). Other comparable materials used are Biodentine, iRoot PB Plus and Acemannan. Biodentine™ (Septodont Ltd., Saint Maur des Fausse's, France) is an HCSC with similar properties to MTA regarding biocompatibility and formation of a hard-tissue barrier. However, there is less coronal discolouration as well as an improved mixing encapsulated delivery system with a shorter setting time to facilitate the handling of the material (66). iRoot BP Plus (Innovative Bioceramix Inc, Vancouver, Canada) is also a calcium silicate-based bioactive ceramic with purportedly improved mixing and handling properties (39, 67). Finally, Acemannan (Spectrum System 2000; PerkinElmer, Waltham, MA, USA) is a natural polysaccharide extracted from aloe vera (68). It is worth highlighting that the scientific evidence to support the usage of more recently proposed HCSCs is limited when compared with the use of established materials, such as calcium hydroxide, MTA and Biodentine.

Time Taken to Achieve Haemostasis

Bleeding is a cardinal sign of inflammation; therefore, the haemostasis of inflamed pulp should be considered less predictable than that of healthy pulp. Teeth with traumatic exposures should not have an underlying pulp inflammation if treatment is timely, and the level of pulpotomy should take into consideration this factor. Therefore, arresting of bleeding should be easily achieved when pressure is applied with either saline, local anaesthetic or sodium hypochlorite-soaked cotton pellets after five minutes (24). One study assessing pulpotomies on teeth that have suffered CCFs measured bleeding time and found haemostasis was achieved in five minutes (39). Interestingly, the time taken for haemostasis to occur after pulp amputation impacts the prognosis for VPT in teeth with carious exposures (69). Failure to achieve haemostasis or to initiate bleeding for teeth that sustained CCFs is likely to indicate a concomitant luxation injury contributing towards pulp demise.

Time or Patient Limited Options

Patients do not always seek treatment immediately following an injury and operators often have limited time allocated to the management of dental emergencies, including TDIs. Two studies reported that only 43–54% of patients sought treatment on the day of the injury (22, 37). Several other studies have assessed the impact of delay in seeking treatment with a pulpotomy on pulp survival and demonstrated that a certain time delay was not a significant variable (16, 33, 38, 42). This is likely due to the inflammatory infiltrate being superficial following a pulp exposure, even over a seven-day period. These clinical findings are supported by a histological study in monkeys, which reported that in pulps exposed after 48 hours, the inflammatory infiltrate extended 1.5–2 mm (mean 1.8 mm), while after seven days, the depth was only 0.8–2.2 mm (mean 1.6 mm) (70). From a biological perspective, it is expected that a non-inflamed pulp will respond to VPT; therefore, this treatment modality should not be excluded *a priori* if a delay in treatment occurs, providing the inflamed tissue is managed adequately.

Initial Pulp Cap Followed by a Later Partial Pulpotomy

Wang et al. (33) reported that direct pulp capping with Dycal was five times more likely to result in pulp necrosis than treatment with a pulpotomy. Consistent with other studies (22, 71), these authors noted that emergency treatment undertaken was often a pulp capping followed by restoration. The outstanding finding of the study from Wang et al. (33) was that in teeth referred for specialist paediatric care retreated with a pulpotomy, success rates were similar to teeth initially treated with a pulpotomy.

The IADT guidelines are not clear on whether treatment with pulp capping or pulpotomy is indicated in the presence of CCFs. Considering the difference in success rates for pulp capping when compared to either partial or coronal pulpotomy, further treatment may well be warranted if the clinician is skilled in the provision of VPT. Figure 8.6 illustrates a case where retreatment with a VPT was undertaken on a tooth associated with persistent symptoms following the restoration of a crown fracture. It is possible that an undiagnosed CCF was present, as pulp exposures can be difficult to identify, as seen in Figure 8.7. An example of a partial or a Cvek pulpotomy is illustrated in Figures 8.4, 8.5 and 8.8. An example of a full pulpotomy is shown in Figures 8.2 and 8.9.

Complications from VPT in Traumatised Teeth

Pulp Canal Calcification

Pulp canal calcification leading towards partial or total radiographic obliteration (PCO) can be a sequela of a crown fracture (73) or root fracture (74). Some studies considered the presence of PCO following VPT as a successful outcome (39), while other studies considered PCO as a

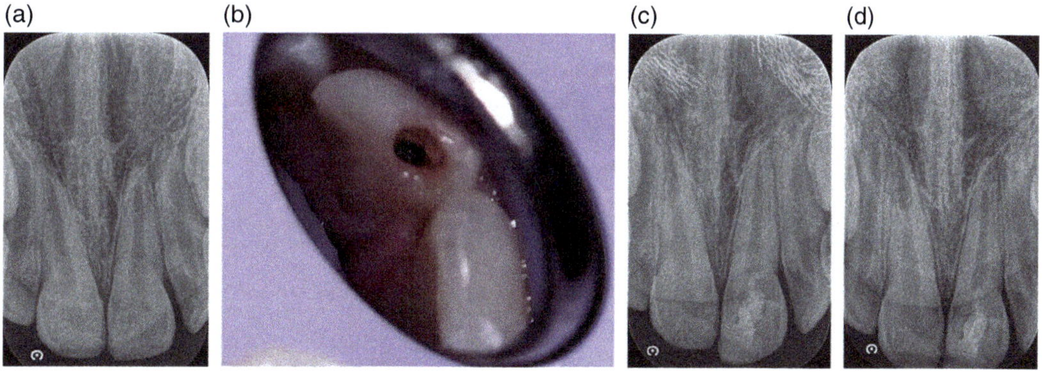

Figure 8.6 (a) A periapical radiograph taken 11 days post-injury when two uncomplicated crown fractures were restored with composite resin on the day of the injury. (b) Note the proximity of the restoration to the pulp horns, especially in the left maxillary central incisor. Both teeth were responsive to cold pulp sensibility testing, with the left central incisor acutely responsive. The patient was unable to tolerate cold liquids. While it was not possible to determine the extent of the pulpitis, the parent wanted any treatment that could potentially avoid the tooth requiring a root filling. The possibility that the symptoms were related to a micro-exposure that would have benefited from a VPT could not be excluded. A photograph of the pulp which was accessed to a depth of 2 mm, and haemostasis was obtained by placing a microbrush soaked in 1% NaOCl. (c) A post-treatment periapical radiograph showing radiopaque material in the pulp space consisting of UltraCal, Life and glass-ionomer cement. The access cavity was finally restored with acid-etched composite resin. (d) A periapical radiograph taken at a six-month review. Both the central incisors were asymptomatic and responsive to cold pulp sensibility testing in a comparable range.

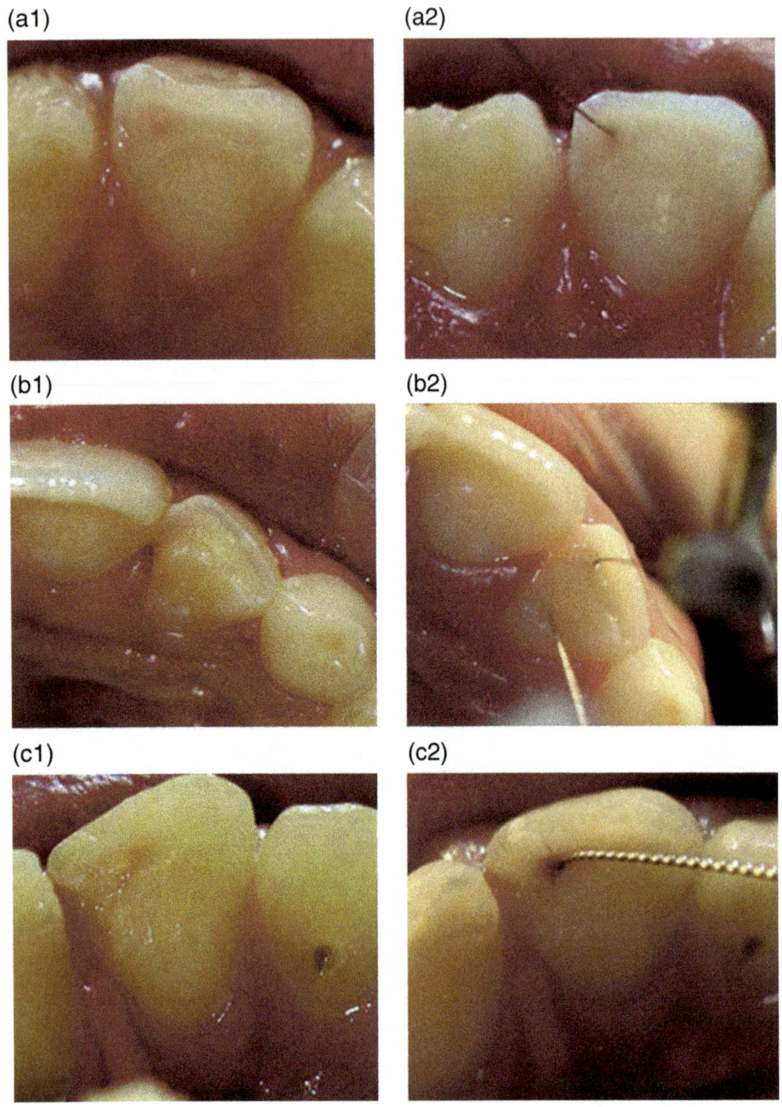

Figure 8.7 An example of three study cases with crown fractures presenting with micro-exposures. Despite (a1, b1, c1) no evident exposure point, (a2, b2, c2) gentle and meticulous exploration of the fracture site using a sterile K-file #8 can lead to the identification of pulp exposure. These cases require vital pulp therapy for proper management. *Source:* Shahmohammadi et.al. (72)/Reproduced with permission from Elsevier.

failure (16, 38), with a further one correlating rapid calcification with the development of a periapical radiolucency after several years in one-fifth of cases with total obliteration (74). Therefore, the presence of PCO *per se* indicates ongoing vitality as new mineralized tissue has developed that requires long-term recall as late complications may follow (69). Cases needing treatment will likely require referral as this complication should be considered as a high-difficulty case.

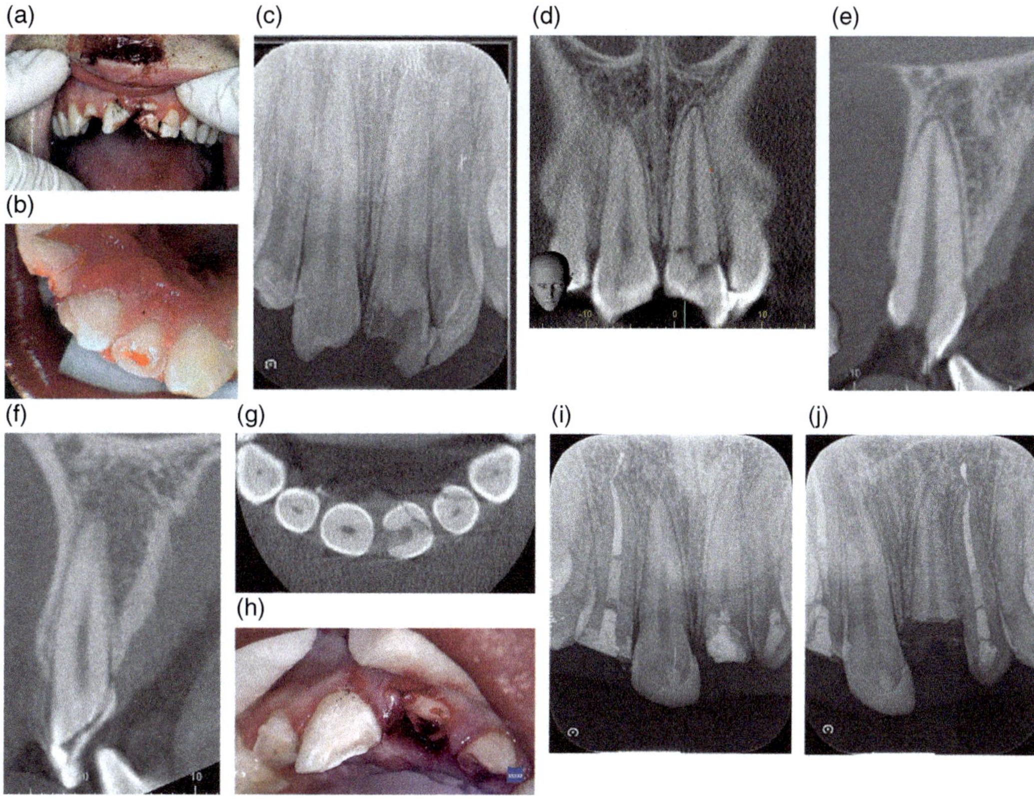

Figure 8.8 This case features two complicated crown fractures and two complicated crown-root fractures with different fracture patterns and differing treatment options due to the extent of the fracture(s). (a) A clinical photograph taken on presentation to the general dentist immediately following the injury from the hospital. Bitumen staining is evident on the buccal aspect of the maxillary right central incisor following a fall from a bicycle in a 15-year-old boy. (b) A clinical photograph taken by the general dentist revealing a complicated crown fracture for the right lateral incisor, a possible micro-exposure of the right central incisor and a crown-root fracture of the left central incisor. (c) A pre-treatment periapical radiograph showing a glass-ionomer emergency bandage has been placed on the exposed pulp of the right lateral incisor. Extensive crown fractures are evident in the left central and lateral incisors. (d) A coronal CBCT view showing the extent of the fractures in the left central incisor. (e) A sagittal CBCT view of the left central incisor showing one of the fractures extends below the level of the alveolar crest. (f) A sagittal CBCT view revealing the extent of the crown-root fracture of the left lateral incisor. (g) An axial CBCT review revealing the fractures in the left central and lateral incisors. (h) A clinical image revealing the glass-ionomer emergency bandage on the right lateral incisor, the micro-pulp exposure is evident in the right lateral incisor, and the fractured fragments were removed from the left central and lateral incisors. (i) The right lateral incisor was root-filled, and a slurry of UltraCal was placed in the post space. The access cavity was closed with Cavit and glass-ionomer cement. The right central incisor was treated with a Cvek pulpotomy with Biodentine. A radiopacity at the pulp horn for the VPT is evident. The tooth was restored with an acid-etched composite restoration. The left central incisor has been provisionally restored with an emergency glass-ionomer cement bandage where calcium hydroxide (UltraCal) was placed on the pulp. This tooth was deemed to be unrestorable, and treatment planned for decoronation and submergence of the root to maintain alveolar bone for eventual replacement with an implant-retained crown. (j) The post-endodontic treatment radiograph of the left central incisor where the crown was decoronated and a blood clot was induced in the pulp canal space after the root was submerged. The left lateral incisor was root-filled and a post space was filled with a slurry of UltraCal. The access cavity was closed with Cavit and glass-ionomer cement. The Biodentine placed in the pulp horn of the right central incisor is also evident.

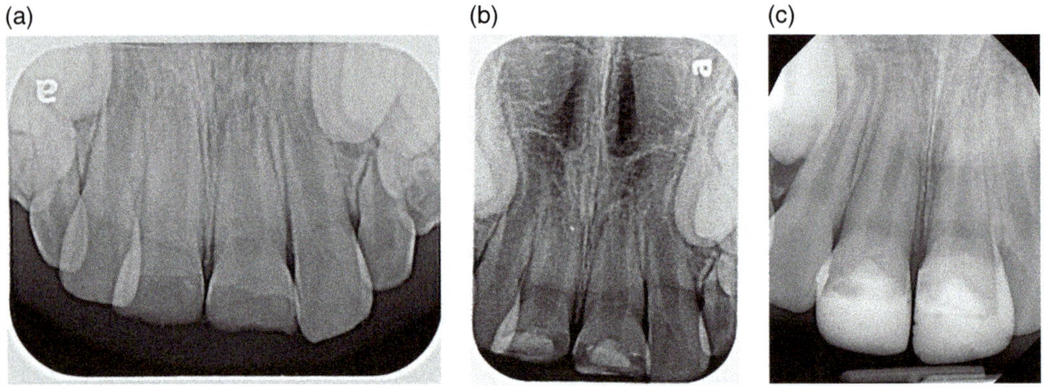

Figure 8.9 (a) The maxillary central incisors sustained complicated crown fractures in a seven-year-old boy. A periapical radiograph shows wide open apices and thin dentinal root walls. (b) The teeth were treated with calcium hydroxide pulpotomies. The teeth were restored with acid-etched composite resins. (c) A periapical radiograph taken at an 18-month review shows complete root maturation. The teeth were responsive to cold pulp sensibility testing. *Source:* Courtesy of Dr Zameera Fida.

Discolouration

Tooth discolouration is a crucial patient-reported outcome measure and is considered by the IADT a consequence of disease but also of relevance for social outcomes due to the contribution of aesthetic factors. CCFs would be associated with discolouration due to the use of materials having this adverse effect. Conversely, teeth with root fractures may suffer from discolouration in those cases where the coronal segment becomes necrotic.

A recent systematic review of pulpotomies for the management of CCFs showed that no studies reported discolouration of teeth as a complication from treatment (34). A more recent study reported 13 of 56 teeth (27.1%) discoloured post-treatment when calcium hydroxide was the medicament selected, which included six teeth that had healing of the pulp and seven teeth that were diagnosed with pulp necrosis (36). Another recent study using Biodentine as the repair material reported that 17% of teeth showed only slight discolouration (50). A recent randomized trial comparing MTA and Biodentine in a study of 50 traumatized immature permanent teeth with CCFs reported no significant differences in radiographic outcomes shown by further root maturation, but there was a greater incidence of discolouration for the MTA cohort (49). The difference in the discolouration rate may be due to the differences in material used but may also be due to the higher success rate of 91% of the 55 teeth treated with Biodentine pulpotomies, where only four teeth developed pulp necrosis. Rao et al. (39) compared iRoot BP Plus and calcium hydroxide as pulpotomy materials and selected iRoot BP Plus as it was considered to not cause discolouration of the crown. However, discolouration was not a reported variable in this study, so no inference can be drawn. Discolouration is a patient-reported treatment outcome; thus, the patient, parents or caretakers should be advised of this potential complication at the informed consent stage. Nonetheless, in the shared decision-making process, the selection of material should take into consideration the relevant clinical outcome measures, such as pulp survival for VPT. It has been shown that discolouration caused by MTA can be successfully reversed with internal bleaching, with the tooth remaining vital (75). Figures 8.10–8.12 illustrate a tooth that was discoloured and successfully bleached.

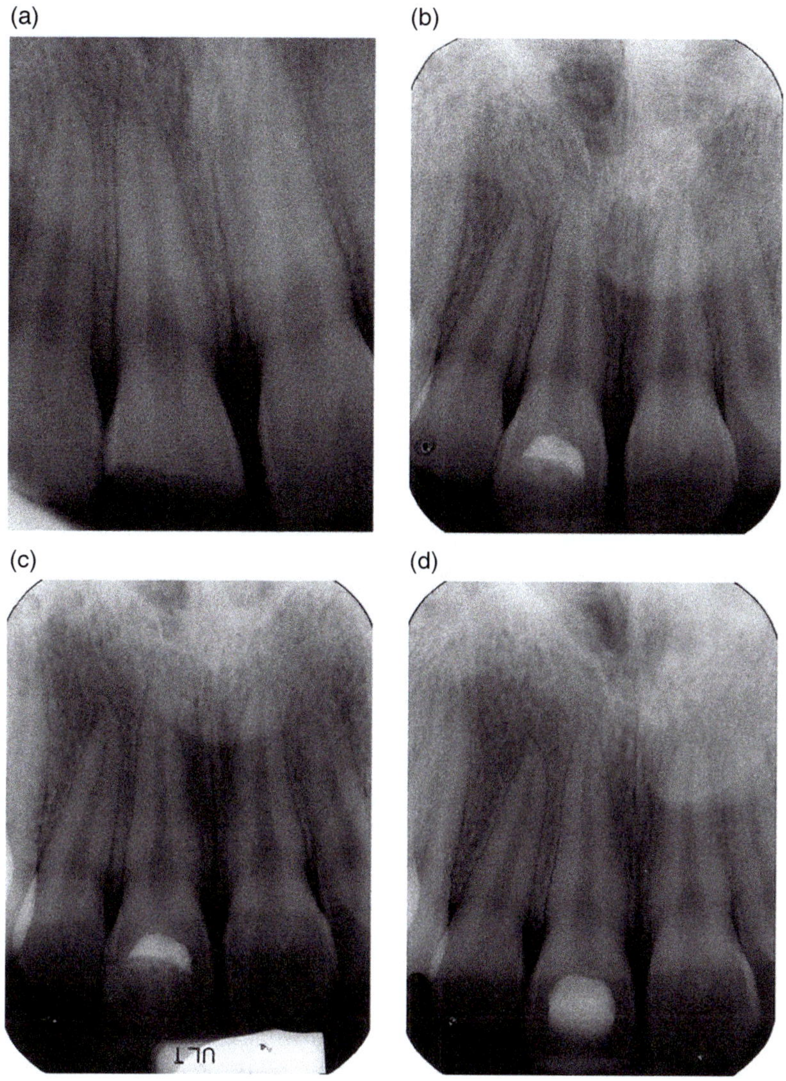

Figure 8.10 (a) A periapical radiograph of maxillary right central incisor upon presentation. (b). The immediate postoperative radiograph showing the placement of WMTA and the reattachment of the coronal fragment. (c) A radiograph at 17 months showing the formation of a hard-tissue bridge and root maturation. (d) A radiograph post-bleaching and restoration of the access cavity. *Source:* Belobrov and Parashos (75) Reproduced with permission from Elsevier. Courtesy of Prof. Peter Parashos.

Resorption

Various types of tooth resorption are possible complications of TDIs in general (31). The incidence of resorption for teeth with CCFs is low and when present is associated with teeth that also sustained a concomitant luxation injury (55). If treatment is unsuccessful and infection occurs, inflammatory resorption related to apical periodontitis is relatively common (76). Similarly, a possible unfavourable outcome in the management of root fractures is the presence of inflammation in the fracture line (31). The role of long-term recall following TDIs should be reiterated, as late resorption is a possible sequela of TDIs (31).

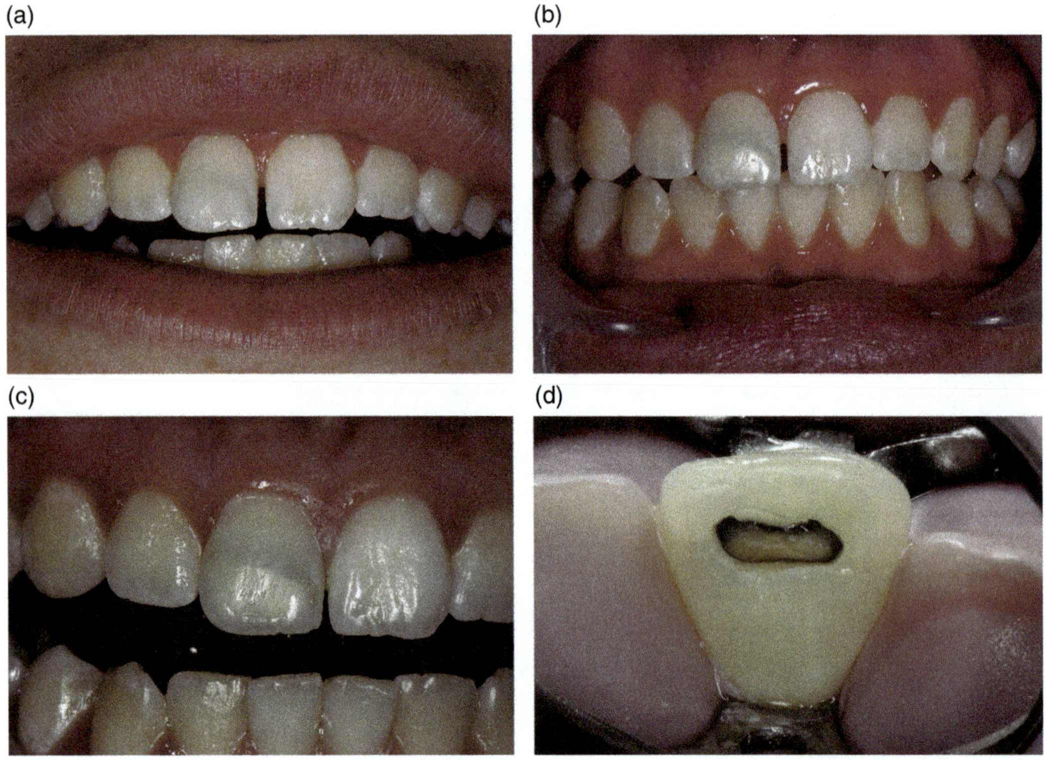

Figure 8.11 (a) An intraoral photograph at the one-month follow-up. Note the slight grey discolouration apical to the fracture line. (b) Further crown discolouration at the five-month recall. (c) Distinctly noticeable crown discolouration 17 months after partial pulpotomy with WMTA. (d) The removal of discoloured WMTA.
Source: Belobrov and Parashos (75) Reproduced with permission from Elsevier. Courtesy of Prof. Peter Parashos.

Oral Health-Related Quality of Life

Social outcomes and oral health-related quality of life (OHRQoL) are part of the core outcome set listed by the IADT in 2018 (18). Unfortunately, there is a paucity of evidence assessing OHRQoL regarding VTP in the management of CCFs and root fractures. Regarding CCFs, fractures involving dentine and/or pulp have been associated with a negative impact compared with subjects without TDIs; however, their management was not described in detail (77). Other studies have failed to detect significant differences since CCFs are relatively uncommon compared with other injury types; therefore, analyses assessing the impact of CCFs on OHRQoL have low statistical power (78–80). Finally, for root fractures, as population studies rarely include radiographic examination, this type of injury remains unaccounted for in most studies assessing OHRQoL (81).

Differences Between Trauma and Caries Management

Several studies over the last five decades reported successful outcomes for VPT in mature permanent teeth with carious exposure (Table 8.2). These studies have been summarized in several systematic reviews (60, 89, 100–102). VPT for cariously exposed pulp requires removal of the inflamed pulp and haemostasis, as well as covering the pulp with calcium hydroxide, MTA, Biodentine or

(a) (b) (c) (d)

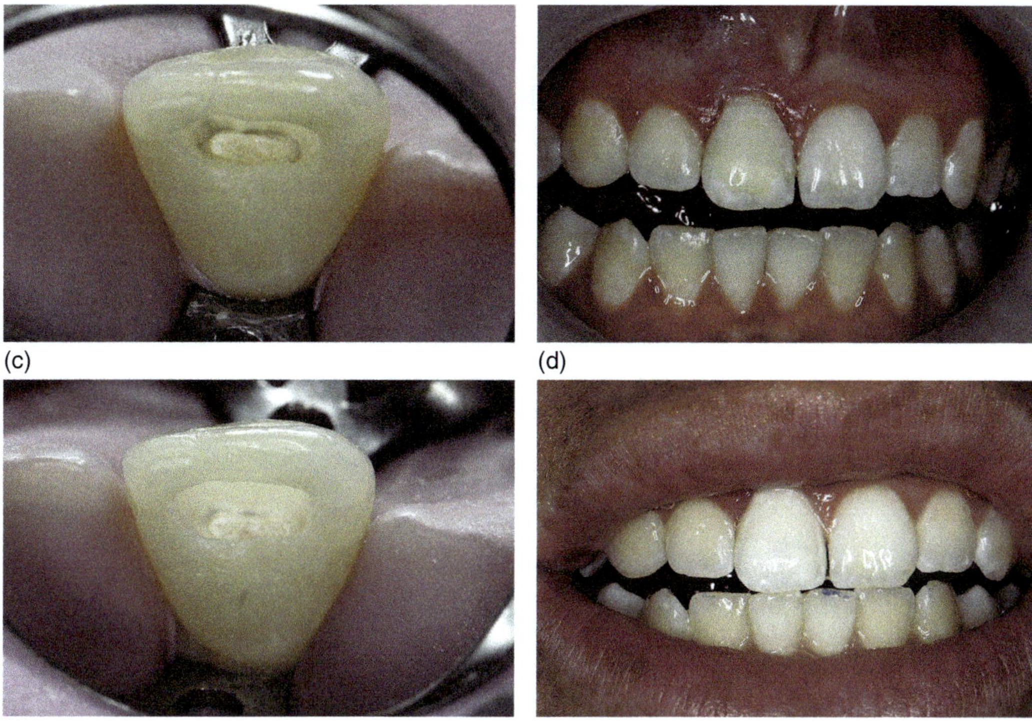

Figure 8.12 (a) All discoloured WMTA was removed until a hard-tissue bridge was reached. (b) A noticeable improvement in the colour of the crown could be seen immediately after the removal of discoloured WMTA. (c) The dentine colour after one week of internal bleaching. (d) The excellent aesthetic result after the removal of discoloured WMTA and internal bleaching. *Source:* Belobrov and Parashos (75) Reproduced with permission from Elsevier. Courtesy of Prof. Peter Parashos.

Table 8.2 Studies undertaking a pulpotomy on mature teeth.

Authors	Age of participants (years)	Number of teeth	Aetiology	Material	Follow-up	Pulp survival (%)
Santini (82)	9–62	20	CE	CH (Calnex)	5 years	65
Caliskan (83)	10–22	21	IP	CH	1–4 years	91.6
Çalışkan (84)	10–24	26	IP	CH	16–72 months	92.3
Da Rosa (85)	14–70	26	CE	CH	14–88 months	65
Asgary and Ehsani (86)	14–62	12	CE & IP	NEC	15.8 months	100
Asgary et al. (87)	9–65	205	CE & IP	CEM	1 year	97.6
Barngkgei et al. (88)	27–54	11	CE & RP	MTA	24–42 months	100
Alqaderi et al. (89)	10–15	29	CE	MTA	25 ± 14 months	90
Asgary et al. (90)	9–65	205	CE & IP	CEM	5 years	78.1
Asgary et al. (91)	9–40	34	CE & IP	CEM & MTA	2–5 years	>98
Taha et al. (92)	11–51	44	CE & IP	MTA	3 years	92.7

(Continued)

Table 8.2 (Continued)

Authors	Age of participants (years)	Number of teeth	Aetiology	Material	Follow-up	Pulp survival (%)
Galani et al. (93)	15–36	18	CE	MTA	1.5 years	84.6
Taha and Abdulkhader (94)	9–17	20	CE & IP	Biodentine	1 year	95
Taha and Abdulkhader (95)	19–69	63	CE & IP	Biodentine	1 year	100 Clinical 98.4 Radio
Asgary et al. (96)		69	71% RP 29% IP	CEM	1 year	93.5
Awadeh et al. (97)	16–59	68	CE	Biodentine MTA	3 years	Biodentine 91.7% MTA 96%
Ricucci et al. (98)	Mean age 22.7 years ± 10.3	225	CE	$Ca(OH)_2$ Powder + Dycal	35 years	100%, 95%, 95%, 86% and 89% at 1, 5, 10, 20 and 35 years

Legend: IP – irreversible pulpitis; RP – reversible pulpitis; CE – carious exposure; NEC – new endodontic cement; CH – Dycal (Dentsply Caulk, Milford, DE, USA); CEM – calcium enriched material; MTA – mineral trioxide aggregate.
Source: Adapted from Lin et al. (99).

other bioactive materials, as presented in Table 8.2. Clinical protocols are comparable to those for VPT following CCFs; nonetheless, dental caries is a slow process compared with TDIs. A recent study that reviewed teeth over 35 years reported the main variable influencing pulp survival after VPT in carious teeth was the quality of the coronal restoration (98). Histologically, healing of exposed pulps has been reported in immature and mature teeth (103–105), generally by reparative dentinogenesis (106, 107). This is also supported by histological studies in pulps with CCFs subsequently removed for prosthodontic reasons that demonstrated healing (108). This is due to the inflammatory infiltrate following exposure of the pulp being limited to the superficial layers of the pulp tissue, where histological studies show that only 2 mm of the pulp should be removed, even for a treatment delay of up to seven days after the injury (70). Animal studies have also shown that experimentally exposed pulps in monkeys to a depth of 2 mm will develop a hard-tissue barrier over the original wound surface with dentine-like tissue and a non-inflamed pulp (109).

The outcomes reported for permanent mature teeth are comparable to outcomes for the treatment of CCFs with VPT. Success and outcomes should be considered from the perspective of pulp biology, where wound healing generally occurs by repair, not regeneration, which would depend on the resident postnatal stem cells and micro-environmental cues (99).

Complicated Crown Fracture with Luxation and Complex Injuries

Complex TDIs may encompass multiple teeth, their periodontium and the hard plus soft tissues in the oral cavity. The most common injury associated with CCFs is a luxation. Any trauma to the teeth can cause significant damage, and a concomitant luxation injury has been suggested as a

Table 8.3 Studies that reported concomitant luxation injuries.

Author	Number of teeth	Intervention	Concomitant trauma	Pulp survival %	Follow-up (years)
Klein et al. (42)	34	Partial pulpotomy	8 concussion 3 luxation	94.1	1–3
Robertson et al. (110)	103	DPC or Partial	69	No luxation 100 Luxation 75	1–11
Lauridson et al. (13)	70	DPC	30 concussion	100	1–5
Lauridson et al. (14)	21	DPC	7 subluxation	85.7	1–2.25
Haikal et al. (50)	51	Biodentine pulpotomy	28 luxations 8 concussion 17 subluxation 2 lateral luxation 1 extrusion	91	1.25
Yu et al. (36)	56	Pulpotomy	13 luxations	61 Overall 53.8 with luxation	1–5

Legend: DPC, direct pulp cap.

significant reason for developing pulpal necrosis due to damage to the pulpal circulation where there is a displacement of the root, and the neurovascular bundle is either stretched or ruptured.

Several clinical studies have assessed the association between CCFs and luxation injuries (Table 8.3). In a study of 98 teeth with CCFs, 30% of teeth with open apices and 28% of mature teeth sustained a concomitant luxation injury (22). Caprioglio et al. (47) reported 22 of the 27 teeth were tender to percussion and all had increased mobility except for one, indicating an underlying luxation injury in the majority of the teeth. A study of 103 teeth with CCFs reported that 69 of the teeth also had damage to the periodontal attachment apparatus, which increased the risk of pulp necrosis from 0% to 14%. Incidentally, the risk of pulp necrosis was up to 28% for teeth with uncomplicated crown fractures, further emphasizing the risks associated with a concomitant luxation injury where the pulp circulation is compromised (110). Other studies have also shown that teeth with crown fractures and only mild luxation injuries of concussion and subluxation have an increased risk of pulp necrosis, especially when the tooth did not respond to electric pulp testing at the initial assessment (13, 14). A further study reported that all failed teeth with CCFs had a concomitant luxation but still reported an overall success rate of 91% following pulpotomy (50). Bissinger et al. (52) also reported on teeth with crown fractures and found a greater risk of pulp necrosis when there was a concomitant luxation injury. In addition, the highest reported success rates for VPT and CCFs were studies that excluded luxation injuries, with Cvek (38) reporting 95% and Rao et al. (39) reporting 96%. Root fractures may be a concomitant injury with CCFs (31). However, this presentation should be considered less common.

The different vascular response that may occur in pulp tissue is illustrated in Figure 8.13. Figure 8.10 illustrates a case where three CCFs and CCF with an associated root fracture (CCRF) were treated according to the clinical scenario. Figure 8.14 illustrates a case with an underlying alveolar fracture with displacement of the maxilla.

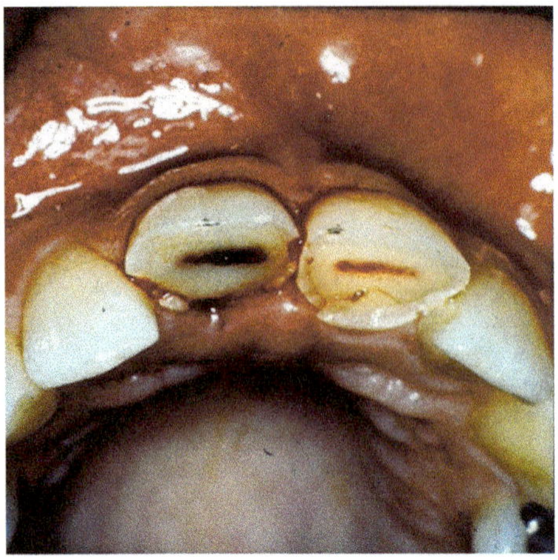

Figure 8.13 A clinical photograph of two complicated crown-root fractured maxillary central incisors. Both teeth have mobile fractured fragments extending sub-gingivally. The pulp in the right central incisor has a cyanotic appearance, suggesting a concomitant luxation injury and a disturbance to the pulp vascularity. The clinical appearance of the left central incisor suggests the pulp circulation has not been disturbed by a luxation injury. *Source:* Picture reprinted with permission. Andreasen FM et al. In Andreasen JO. et al. (Eds) Textbook and Color Atlas of Traumatic Injuries to the Teeth. 5th ed. (11) (Courtesy of Dr Frances Andreasen, Copenhagen, Denmark).

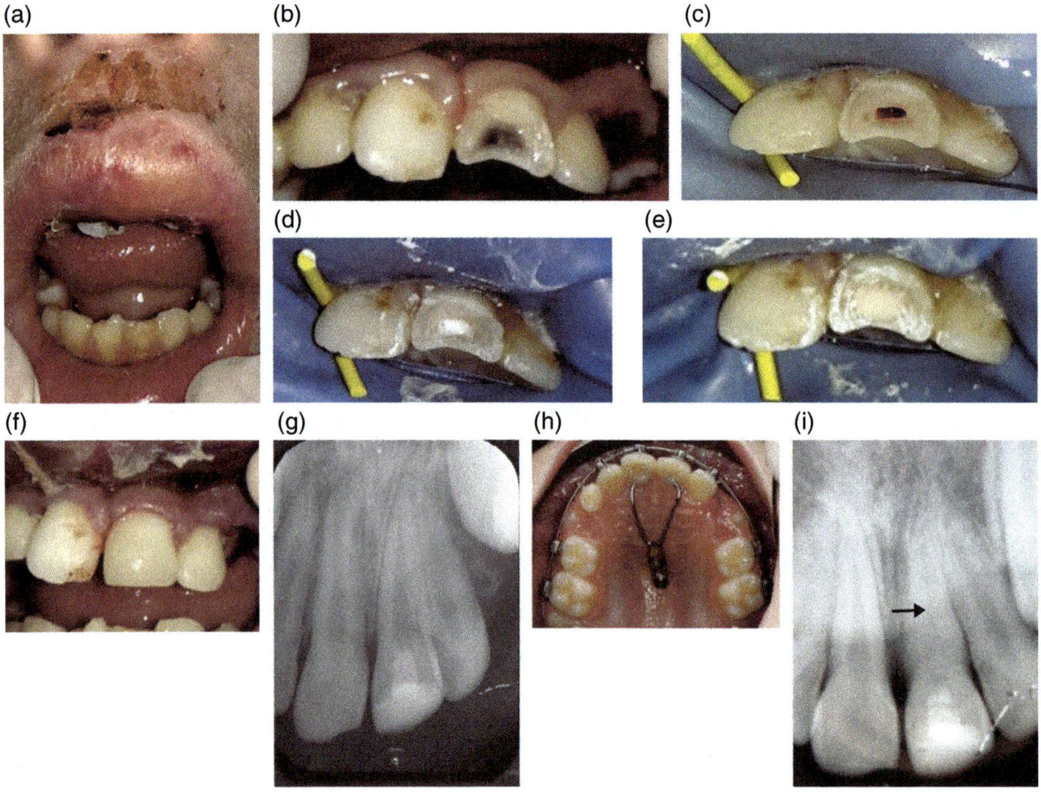

Figure 8.14 (a) Trauma to the teeth, lips, soft tissues and a fracture to the premaxilla from fielding a cricket ball five days earlier. The damage to the mandibular incisors was uncomplicated crown fractures. (b) A clinical photograph of a complicated crown fracture on the maxillary left central incisor where the exposed pulp has a cyanotic appearance, and there is a slough on the surface of the pulp. Cvek reported that the prognosis for pulpotomy was not diminished even when treatment was delayed for up to seven days, so the preferred treatment option was a pulpotomy if bleeding and haemostasis could be achieved. (c) The pulp was accessed with a diamond bur to a depth where bleeding commenced. Haemostasis was obtained by placing a microbrush soaked in 1% NaOCl. (d) Ultracal was placed on the exposed pulp. (e) The pulp access cavity was restored with Life and glass-ionomer cement. (f) The tooth was restored with composite resin. (g) A post-treatment radiograph. (h) There was a concomitant fracture of the premaxilla and an oral surgeon suggested orthodontic management as the displacement was slight. The referring orthodontist (Dr Ashley Smith, Toowoomba, Australia) devised a precision attachment anchored into the palate with temporary anchorage devices and fixed orthodontic appliances that reduced the fracture. (i) A periapical radiograph taken at the 18-month review revealing a calcific bridge adjacent to the calcium hydroxide pulpotomy (white arrow) as well as intracanal calcification of the pulp space, which is considerably reduced when compared to the right central incisor (black arrow).

The findings of recently published systematic reviews agree with those from the above clinical studies. A recent review reported that the only variable that affected pulp vitality for CCFs was a concomitant luxation injury (41). Another review summarized that the studies that did not control for luxation injuries also had good outcomes, which suggested that a concomitant luxation injury and CCFs did not preclude management with VPT (34), though the literature available in the field overall suggests better outcomes in the absence of luxation injuries overall.

Clinical Protocols for Direct Pulp Capping and Pulpotomy

Pulpotomy

Local anaesthesia should be administered, and the affected tooth/teeth should be isolated with a dental dam. The pulp is accessed with a sharp high-speed diamond bur to a level of 2 mm, as recommended by Cvek (1, 38). Haemostasis is generally achieved within five minutes (24). Haemostatic agents such as sodium hypochlorite (NaOCl), local anaesthetic with a vasoconstrictor or saline to assist in controlling bleeding are recommended as these agents have been shown not to adversely affect the pulp (111). Considering that the ability to achieve haemostasis is critical for achieving a successful outcome, if bleeding is not controlled the pulp should be resected to a deeper level. Finally, if bleeding is not controlled, a pulpectomy is indicated.

The choice of material for a pulpotomy is either calcium hydroxide or HCSCs. Figures 8.1–8.4 illustrate cases with these three materials. The advantages and disadvantages of these materials were discussed above, and all these materials have been utilized with successful outcomes.

If the fractured tooth fragment is available, it should be hydrated before reattachment. There may be some initial colour difference between the tooth and the reattached fragment, which generally disappears over 12 months (112). There are a variety of different adhesive systems including total-etch and self-etch applications. Intermediate materials used for reattachment can be resin cement, glass-ionomer cement, composite and self-adhesive cement. Systematic reviews revealed no ideal technique or material for tooth fragment reattachment (113, 114). Some techniques advocate for further retention with dentine grooves and bevelling of enamel. However, a recent systematic review recommends reattachment without modification (113). The tooth/teeth should be checked for occlusal disturbances including lateral and protrusive guidance. Appropriate finishing and polishing should be undertaken to achieve a pleasing aesthetic result.

When the fragment is not available, a restoration with a resin-based composite is recommended. Strip crowns have the advantage of allowing a more predictable shape for the restoration. Studies show strip crowns have been used successfully (36). However, the survival rate of strip crowns for permanent teeth was 95.2% over 2 years, which reduced to 88.9% after 10 years (115).

Direct Pulp Capping

Direct pulp capping, isadvocated by the ESE 2021 position statement for minor exposures treated within the first few hours after injury. The treatment follows a similar protocol as for a pulpotomy described above but without mechanical penetration of the pulp space (29).

Follow-up Protocol

For CCFs, the IADT guidelines advocate clinical and radiographic evaluations at 6–8 weeks, after three months, after six months and then one year (31). However, if there is an associated luxation or root fracture, follow-ups to five years and longer are recommended (31). Possible adverse sequelae following trauma generally involve pulp necrosis, pulp canal obliteration and/or resorption of the root, plus lack of further development in immature teeth. Restorative outcomes include quality and loss of restoration in the form of fragment debonding, marginal caries and discolouration of the tooth and/or the restoration.

The treatment of root fractures has been described in the relevant Trauma Guidelines (31) and is not included in the present chapter as they are not necessarily considered a modality of VPT.

Future Directions

VPT for the management of CCFs and root fractures has been used for more than five decades with outstandingly favourable clinical outcomes. Further understanding of the role of bioactive materials, in particular the more recently commercialized HCSCs, as well as the clinical translation of molecular biomarkers for the diagnosis of the status of the pulp, are required.

The evidence available in the field consists mostly of retrospective studies, case reports and case series, as these were study designs commonly used before the introduction of evidence-based dentistry. Recently, some randomized controlled trials in the field have been published, which represent a higher level of evidence.

Further high-quality studies that encompass the core outcome set for VPT in CCFs and root fractures are recommended, as most of the literature currently available focuses on clinician-reported outcome measures.

References

1 Cvek M. A clinical report on partial pulpotomy and capping with calcium hydroxide in permanent incisors with complicated crown fracture. *J Endod.* 1978;4:232–7.
2 Cvek M. Prognosis of luxated non-vital maxillary incisors treated with calcium hydroxide and filled with gutta-percha. A retrospective clinical study. *Endod Dent Traumatol.* 1992;8:45–55.
3 Eckerbom M, Magnusson T, Martinsson T. Reasons for and incidence of tooth mortality in a Swedish population. *Endod Dent Traumatol.* 1992;8:230–4.
4 Duncan HF. Present status and future directions-vital pulp treatment and pulp preservation strategies. *Int Endod J.* 2022;55(Suppl 3):497–511.
5 Petti S, Andreasen JO, Glendor U, Andersson L. NA0D – the new traumatic dental injury classification of the World Health Organization. *Dent Traumatol.* 2022;38:170–4.
6 Andersson L. Epidemiology of traumatic dental injuries. *Pediatr Dent.* 2013;35:102–5.
7 DiAngelis AJ, Andreasen JO, Ebeleseder KA, Kenny DJ, Trope M, Sigurdsson A, et al. Guidelines for the management of traumatic dental injuries: 1. Fractures and luxations of permanent teeth. *Pediatr Dent.* 2016;38:358–68.
8 Andreasen JO, Andreasen FM, Tsukoboshi M, Eichelsbachere. Crown-root fractures. In: Andreasen JO et al. (eds.) Textbook and Color Atlas of Traumatic Injuries to the Teeth, 5th Ed., John Wiley & Sons Ltd, Hoboken, NJ, USA, 2019, 355–76.
9 Andreasen FM, Andreasen JO, Tsilingaridis G. Root fractures. In: Andreasen JO et al. (eds.) Textbook and Color Atlas of Traumatic Injuries to the Teeth, 5th Ed., John Wiley & Sons Ltd, Hoboken, NJ, USA, 2019, 377–412.

10 Andreasen FM, Lauridsen E, Andreasen JO. Extrusive luxation and lateral luxation. In: Andreasen JO et al. (eds.) Textbook and Color Atlas of Traumatic Injuries to the Teeth, 5th Ed., John Wiley & Sons Ltd, Hoboken, NJ, USA, 2019, 450–68.

11 Andreasen FM, Lauridsen E, Andreasen JO. Crown fractures. In: Andreasen JO et al. (eds.) Textbook and Color Atlas of Traumatic Injuries to the Teeth, 5th Ed., John Wiley & Sons Ltd, Hoboken, NJ, USA, 2019, 327–54.

12 Andreasen FM, Kahler B. Pulpal response after acute dental injury in the permanent dentition: clinical implications – a review. *J Endod.* 2015;41:299–308.

13 Lauridsen E, Hermann NV, Gerds TA, Ahrensburg SS, Kreiborg S, Andreasen JO. Combination injuries 1. The risk of pulp necrosis in permanent teeth with concussion injuries and concomitant crown fractures. *Dent Traumatol.* 2012;28:364–70.

14 Lauridsen E, Hermann NV, Gerds TA, Ahrensburg SS, Kreiborg S, Andreasen JO. Combination injuries 2. The risk of pulp necrosis in permanent teeth with subluxation injuries and concomitant crown fractures. *Dent Traumatol.* 2012;28:371–8.

15 Andreasen JO, Andreasen FM, Mejàre I, Cvek M. Healing of 400 intra-alveolar root fractures. 1. Effect of pre-injury and injury factors such as sex, age, stage of root development, fracture type, location of fracture and severity of dislocation. *Dent Traumatol.* 2004;20:192–202.

16 Fuks AB, Bielak S, Chosak A. Clinical and radiographic assessment of direct pulp capping and pulpotomy in young permanent teeth. *Pediatr Dent.* 1982;4:240–4.

17 Hecova H, Tzigkounakis V, Merglova V, Netolicky J. A retrospective study of 889 injured permanent teeth. *Dent Traumatol.* 2010;26:466–75.

18 Kenny KP, Day PF, Sharif MO, et al. What are the important outcomes in traumatic dental injuries? An international approach to the development of a core outcome set. *Dent Traumatol.* 2018;34:4–11.

19 Altun C, Ozen B, Esenlik E, Guven G, Gürbüz T, Acikel C, et al. Traumatic injuries to permanent teeth in Turkish children, Ankara. *Dent Traumatol.* 2009;25:309–13.

20 Diaz JA, Bustos L, Brandt AC, Fernandez BE. Dental injuries among children and adolescents aged 1–15 years attending to public hospital in Temuco, Chile. *Dent Traumatol.* 2010;26:254–61.

21 Glendor U. Epidemiology of traumatic dental injuries – a 12 year review of the literature. *Dent Traumatol.* 2008;24:603–11.

22 Maguire A, Murray JJ, Al-Majed I. A retrospective study of treatment provided in the primary and secondary care services for children attending a dental hospital following complicated crown fracture in the permanent dentition. *Int J Paediatr Dent.* 2000;10:182–90.

23 Johnsen DC. Innervation of teeth: qualitative, quantitative, and developmental assessment. *J Dent Res.* 1985;64:555–63.

24 Krastl G, Weiger R, Filippi A, Van Waes H, Ebeleseder K, Ree M, et al. Endodontic management of traumatized permanent teeth: a comprehensive review. *Int Endod J.* 2021;54:1221–45.

25 Dummer PM, Hicks R, Huws D. Clinical signs and symptoms in pulp disease. *Int Endod J.* 1980;13:27–35.

26 Kaletsky T, Furedi A. Reliability of various types of pulp testers as a diagnostic aid. *J Am Dent Assoc.* 1935;22:1559–74.

27 Teitler D, Tzadik D, Eidelman E, Chosack A. A clinical evaluation of vitality tests in anterior teeth following fracture of enamel and dentin. *Oral Surg Oral Med Oral Pathol.* 1972;34:649–52.

28 Zadik D, Chosack A, Eidelman E. The prognosis of traumatized permanent anterior teeth with fracture of the enamel and dentin. *Oral Surg Oral Med Oral Pathol.* 1979;47:173–5.

29 European Society of Endodontology (ESE) developed by, Krastl G, Weiger R, Filippi A, et al. European Society of Endodontology position statement: endodontic management of traumatized permanent teeth. *Int Endod J.* 2021;54:1473–81.

30 Andreasen FM, Kahler B. Diagnosis of acute dental trauma: the importance of standardized documentation: a review. *Dent Traumatol.* 2015;31:340–9.

31 Bourguignon C, Cohenca N, Lauridsen E, et al. International Association of Dental Traumatology guidelines for the management of traumatic dental injuries. 1. Fractures and luxations. *Dent Traumatol.* 2020;36:314–30.

32 The Recommended Guidelines of the American Association of Endodontists for the Treatment of Traumatic Dental Injuries. Available at: https://www.aae.org/specialty/wp-content/uploads/sites/2/2019/02/19_TraumaGuidelines.pdf.

33 Wang G, Wang C, Qin M. Pulp prognosis following conservative pulp treatment in teeth with complicated crown fractures – a retrospective study. *Dent Traumatol.* 2017;33:255–60.

34 Donnelly A, Foschi F, McCabe P, Duncan HF. Pulpotomy for treatment of complicated crown fractures in permanent teeth: a systematic review. *Int Endod J.* 2022;55:290–311.

35 Andreasen JO, Andreasen FM, Skeie A, Hjorting-Hansen E, Schwartz O. Effect of treatment delay upon pulp and periodontal healing of traumatic dental injuries – a review article. *Dent Traumatol.* 2002;18:116–28.

36 Yu L, Kahler B, Nanayakkara S, Prabhu N. Retrospective analysis of the outcomes of pulpotomies in traumatised permanent anterior teeth. *Dent Traumatol.* 2022;38:505–11.

37 Jackson NG, Waterhouse PJ, Maguire A. Factors affecting treatment outcomes following complicated crown fractures managed in primary and secondary care. *Dent Traumatol.* 2006;22:179–85.

38 Cvek M. Partial pulpotomy in crown-fractured incisors-results 3 to 15 years after treatment. *Acta Stomatologica Croatica.* 1993;27:168–73.

39 Rao Q, Kuang J, Mao C, Dai J, Hu L, Lei Z, et al. Comparison of iRoot BP Plus and calcium hydroxide as pulpotomy materials in permanent incisors with complicated crown fractures: a retrospective study. *J Endod.* 2020;46:352–7.

40 Matoug-Elwerfelli M, ElSheshtawy AS, Duggal M, Tong HJ, Nazzal H. Vital pulp treatment for traumatized permanent teeth: a systematic review. *Int Endod J.* 2022;55:613–29.

41 Tzanetakis GN, Tsiouma O, Mougiou E, Koletsi D. Factors related to pulp survival after complicated crown fracture following vital pulp therapy: a systematic review and meta-analysis. *J Endod.* 2022;48:457–78.

42 Klein H, Fuks A, Eidelman E, Chosack A. Partial pulpotomy following complicated crown fracture in permanent incisors: a clinical and radiographical study. *J Pedod.* 1985;9:142–7.

43 Gelbier MJ, Winter GB. Traumatised incisors treated by vital pulpotomy: a retrospective study. *Br Dent J.* 1988;21(164):319–23.

44 Fuks AB, Gavra S, Chosack A. Long-term follow-up of traumatized incisors treated by partial pulpotomy. *Pediatr Dent.* 1993;15:334–46.

45 Blanco LP. Treatment of crown fractures with pulp exposure. *Oral Surg Oral Med Oral Pathol Oral Radiol Endod.* 1996;82:564–8.

46 Koyuncuoglu G, Gorken FN, Ikikarakayali G, Zorlu S, Erdem AP, Sepet E, et al. Management of open apices in thirteen traumatized permanent incisors using mineral trioxide aggregate: case series. *Ped Dent J.* 2013;23:51–6.

47 Caprioglio A, Conti V, Caprioglio C, Caprioglio D. A long-term retrospective clinical study on MTA pulpotomies in immature permanent incisors with complicated crown fractures. *Eur J Paediatr Dent.* 2014;15:29–34.

48 Xu H. *Success rate of Cvek pulpotomies in permanent teeth with complicated crown fractures* (Master's Thesis), The Ohio State University, Ohio, USA.

49 Abuelniel GM, Duggal MS, Kabel N. A comparison of MTA and Biodentine as medicaments for pulpotomy in traumatized anterior immature permanent teeth: a randomized clinical trial. *Dent Traumatol.* 2020;36:400–10.

50 Haikal L, Ferraz Dos Santos B, Vu DD, Braniste M, Dabbagh B. Biodentine pulpotomies on permanent traumatized teeth with complicated crown fractures. *J Endod.* 2020;46:1204–9.

51 Yang YT, Xia B, Xu Z, Dou G, Lei Y, Yong W. The effect of partial pulpotomy with iRoot BP Plus in traumatized immature permanent teeth: a randomized prospective controlled trial. *Dent Traumatol.* 2020;36:518–25.

52 Bissinger R, Müller DD, Reymus M, Khazaei Y, Hickel R, Bücher K, et al. Treatment outcomes after uncomplicated and complicated crown fractures in permanent teeth. *Clin Oral Investig.* 2021;25:133–43.

53 Wu J, Li X, Xu L, Tang Z, Zhao J, Xiang Y, et al. Radiographic evaluation of immature traumatized incisors following different endodontic treatments. *Dent Traumatol.* 2021;37:330–7.

54 Viduskalne I, Care R. Analysis of the crown fractures and factors affecting pulp survival due to dental trauma. *Stomatologija.* 2010;12:109–15.

55 Bücher K, Neumann C, Thiering E, Hickel R, Kühnisch J. Complications and survival rates of teeth after dental trauma over a 5-year period. *Clin Oral Investig.* 2013;17:1311–8.

56 Fuks AB, Cosack A, Klein H, Eidelman E. Partial pulpotomy as a treatment alternative for exposed pulps in crown-fractured permanent incisors. *Endod Dent Traumatol.* 1987;3:100–2.

57 Bogen G, Dammaschke T, Chandler N. Vital pulp therapy. In: Berman LH, Hargreaves KM (eds.) Cohen's Pathways of the Pulp, 12th Ed., Elsevier, St Louis, Missouri, USA, 2020, 902–38.

58 Kang MK, Bogen G. Regenerative approaches in endodontic therapies of immature teeth. In: Chugal N, Lin LM (eds.) Endodontic Prognosis. Clinical Guide for Optimal treatment outcome, Springer, Switzerland, 2017, 65–86.

59 Cox CF, Bergenholtz G, Fitzgerald M, et al. Capping of the dental pulp mechanically exposed to the oral microflora – a 5 week observation of wound healing in the monkey. *J Oral Path.* 1982;11:327–39.

60 Andreasen JO, Andreasen FM, Mejàre I, Cvek M. Healing of 400 intra-alveolar root fractures. 2. Effect of treatment factors such as treatment delay, repositioning, splinting type and period and antibiotics. *Dental Traumatol.* 2004;20:203–11.

61 Aguilar P, Linsuwanont P. Vital pulp therapy in vital permanent teeth with cariously exposed pulp: a systematic review. *J Endod.* 2011;37:581–7.

62 Mohammadi Z, Dummer PMH. Properties and applications of calcium hydroxide in endodontics and dental traumatology. *Int Endod J.* 2011;44:697–730.

63 Cox CF, Bergenholtz G, Heys DR, Syed SA, Fitzgerald M, Heys RJ. Pulp capping of dental pulp mechanically exposed to oral microflora: a 1–2 year observation of wound healing in the monkey. *J Oral Pathol.* 1985;14:156–68.

64 Parirokh M, Torabinejad M, Dummer PMH. Mineral trioxide aggregate and other bioactive endodontic cements: an updated overview. Part I. Vital pulp therapy. *Int Endod J.* 2018;51:177–205.

65 Parirokh M, Torabinejad M. Mineral trioxide aggregate: a comprehensive literature review. Part III. Clinical applications, drawbacks, and mechanism of action. *J Endod.* 2010;36:400–13.

66 Kaur M, Singh H, Dhillon JS, Batra M, Saini M. MTA versus Biodentine: review of literature with a comparative analysis. *J Clin Diagn Res.* 2017;11:ZG01–5.

67 Hirschman WR, Wheater MA, Bringas JS, Hoen MM. Cytotoxicity comparison of three current direct pulp-capping agents with a new bioceramic root repair putty. *J Endod.* 2012;38:385–8.

68 Vu TT, Nguyen MT, Sangvanich P, Nguyen QN, Thunyakitpisal P. Acemannan used as an implantable biomaterial for vital pulp therapy of immature permanent teeth induced continued root formation. *Pharmaceutics.* 2020;12:644.

69 Matsuo T, Nakanishi T, Shimizu H, Ebisu S. A clinical study of direct pulp capping applied to carious-exposed pulps. *J Endod.* 1996;22:551–6.

70 Cvek M, Cleaton-Jones PE, Austin JC, Andreasen JO. Pulp reactions to exposure after experimental crown fractures or grinding in adult monkeys. *J Endod*. 1982;8:391–7.

71 Gungor HC. Management of crown-related fractures in children: an update review. *Dent Traumatol*. 2014;30:88–99.

72 Shahmohammadi R, Sheikhnezami M, Moradi S, Jafarzadeh H, Azarpazhooh A. Treatment outcomes of permanent immature teeth with crown fracture: a retrospective cohort study. *J Endod*. 2021;47:1715–23.

73 Robertson A. A retrospective evaluation of patients with uncomplicated crown fractures and luxation injuries. *Endod Dent Traumatol*. 1998;14:245–56.

74 Jacobsen I, Kerekes K. Long-term prognosis of traumatized permanent anterior teeth showing calcifying processes in the pulp cavity. *Scand J Dent Res*. 1977;85:588–98.

75 Belobrov I, Parashos P. Treatment of tooth discoloration after the use of white mineral trioxide aggregate. *J Endod*. 2011;37:1017–20.

76 Laux M, Abbott PV, Pajarola G, Nair PN. Apical inflammatory root resorption: a correlative radiographic and histological assessment. *Int Endod J*. 2000;33:483–93.

77 Bendo CB, Paiva SM, Varni JW, Vale MP. Oral health-related quality of life and traumatic dental injuries in Brazilian adolescents. *Community Dent Oral Epidemiol*. 2014;42:216–23.

78 Damé-Teixeira N, Alves LS, Ardenghi TM, Susin C, Maltz M. Traumatic dental injury with treatment needs negatively affects the quality of life of Brazilian schoolchildren. *Int J Paediatr Dent*. 2013;23:266–73.

79 Silva-Oliveira F, Goursand D, Ferreira RC, Paiva PCP, Paiva HN, Ferreira EF, et al. Traumatic dental injuries in Brazilian children and oral health-related quality of life. *Dent Traumatol*. 2018;34:28–35.

80 Antunes LA, Luiz RR, Leão AT, Maia LC. Initial assessment of responsiveness of the P-CPQ (Brazilian Version) to describe the changes in quality of life after treatment for traumatic dental injury. *Dent Traumatol*. 2012;28:256–62.

81 Nagendrababu V, Vinothkumar TS, Rossi-Fedele G, Doğramacı EJ, Duncan HF, Abbott PV, et al. Dental patient-reported outcomes following traumatic dental injuries and treatment: a narrative review. *Dent Traumatol.* 2023. https://doi.org/10.1111/edt.12827.

82 Santini AH. Intraoral comparison of calcium hydroxide (Calnex) alone and in combination with Ledermix in first permanent mandibular molars using two direct inspection criteria. *J Dent*. 1985;13:52–9.

83 Calişkan MK. Success of pulpotomy in the management of hyperplastic pulpitis. *Int Endod J*. 1993;26:142–8.

84 Calişkan MK. Pulpotomy of carious vital teeth with periapical involvement. *Int Endod J*. 1995;28:172–6.

85 Da Rosa TA. A retrospective evaluation of pulpotomy as an alternative to extraction. *Am J Dent*. 2006;54:37–40.

86 Asgary S, Ehsani S. Permanent molar pulpotomy with a new endodontic cement: a case series. *J Cons Dent*. 2009;12:31–6.

87 Asgary S, Eghbal MJ, Ghoddusi J, Yazdani S. One-year results of vital pulp therapy in permanent molars with irreversible pulpitis: an ongoing multicenter, randomized, non-inferiority clinical trial. *Clin Oral Investig*. 2013;17:431–9.

88 Barngkgei IH, Haiboub ES, Alboni RS. Pulpotomy of symptomatic permanent teeth with carious exposure using mineral trioxide aggregate. *Iran Endod J*. 2013;8:65–8.

89 Alqaderi HE, Al-Mutawa SA, Qudeimat MA. MTA pulpotomy as an alternative to root canal treatment in children's permanent teeth in a dental public health setting. *J Dent*. 2014;42:1390–5.

90 Asgary S, Eghbal MJ, Fazlyab M, Baghban AA, Ghoddusi J. Five-year results of vital pulp therapy in permanent molars with irreversible pulpitis: a non-inferiority multicenter randomized clinical trial. *Clin Oral Investig.* 2015;19:335–41.

91 Asgary S, Eghbal MJ, Bagheban AA. Long-term outcomes of pulpotomy in permanent teeth with irreversible pulpitis: a multi-center randomized controlled trial. *Am J Dent.* 2017;30:151–5.

92 Taha NA, Ahmad MB, Ghanim A. Assessment of mineral trioxide aggregate pulpotomy in mature permanent teeth with carious exposures. *Int Endod J.* 2017;50:117–25.

93 Galani M, Tewari S, Sangwan P, Mittal S, Kumar V, Duban J. Comparative evaluation of postoperative pain and success rate after pulpotomy and root canal treatment in cariously exposed mature permanent molars: a randomized controlled trail. *J Endod.* 2017;43:1953–62.

94 Taha NA, Abdulkhader SZ. Full pulpotomy with Biodentine in symptomatic young permanent teeth with carious exposure. *J Endod.* 2018;44:932–7.

95 Taha NA, Abdulkhader SZ. Outcome of full pulpotomy using Biodentine in adult patients with symptoms indicative of irreversible pulpitis. *Int Endod J.* 2018;51:819–28.

96 Asgary S, Hassanizadeb R, Torabzadeb H, Eghbal MJ. Treatment outcomes of 4 vital pulp therapies in mature molars. *J Endod.* 2018;44:529–35.

97 Awawdeh L, Al-Qudah A, Hamouri H, Chakra RJ. Outcomes of vital pulp therapy using mineral trioxide aggregate or Biodentine: a prospective randomized clinical trial. *J Endod.* 2018;44: 1603–9.

98 Ricucci D, Rôças IN, Alves FRF, Cabello PH, Siqueira JF Jr. Outcome of direct pulp capping using calcium hydroxide: a long-term retrospective study. *J Endod.* 2023;49:45–54.

99 Lin LM, Ricucci D, Saoud TM, Sigurdsson A, Kahler B. Vital pulp therapy of mature permanent teeth with irreversible pulpitis from the perspective of pulp biology. *Aus Endod J.* 2020;46:154–66.

100 Schwendicke F, Stolpe M. Direct pulp capping after a carious exposure versus root canal treatment: a cost-effectiveness analysis. *J Endod.* 2014;40:1764–70.

101 Li Y, Sui B, Dahl C, et al. Pulpotomy for carious pulp exposures in permanent teeth: a systematic review and meta-analysis. *J Dent.* 2019;84:1–8.

102 Cushley S, Duncan HF, Lappin MJ, et al. Pulpotomy for mature carious teeth with symptoms of irreversible pulpitis: a systematic review. *J Dent.* 2019;88:103158.

103 Mjör IA, Tronstad L. The healing of experimentally induced pulpitis. *Oral Surg Oral Med Oral Pathol.* 1974;38:115–21.

104 Warfvinge J, Bergenholtz G. Healing capacity of human and monkey dental pulps following experimentally-induced pulpitis. *Endod Dent Traumatol.* 1986;2:256–62.

105 Chueh LH, Chiang CP. Histology of irreversible pulpitis premolars treated with mineral trioxide aggregate pulpotomy. *Oper Dent.* 2010;35:370–4.

106 Dominguez MS, Witherspoon DE, Gutmann JL, Opperman LA. Histologic and scanning electron microscopic assessment of various vital pulp-therapy materials. *J Endod.* 2003;29:324–33.

107 Chacko V, Kurikose S. Human pulp response to mineral trioxide aggregate (MTA): a histologic study. *J Clin Pediat Dent.* 2006;30:203–9.

108 Cvek M, Lundberg M. Histological appearance of pulps after exposure by a crown fracture, partial pulpotomy and clinical diagnosis of healing. *J Endod.* 1983;98:8–11.

109 Cvek M, Granath L, Cleaton-Jones P, Austin J. Hard tissue barrier formation in pulpotomized monkey teeth capped with cyanoacrylate or calcium hydroxide for 10 and 60 minutes. *J Dent Res.* 1987;66:1166–74.

110 Robertson A, Andreasen FM, Andresen JO, Noren JG. Long-term prognosis of crown-fractured permanent incisors. The effect of stage of root development and associated luxation injury. *Int J Paediatr Dent.* 2000;10:191–9.

111 Garcia-Godoy F, Murray P. Systemic evaluation of various haemostatic agents following local application prior to direct pulp capping. *Braz Oral Sci*. 2005;4:791–7.

112 Yilmaz Y, Guler C, Sahin H, Eyuboglu O. Evaluation of tooth-fragment reattachment: a clinical and laboratory study. *Dent Traumatol*. 2010;26:308–14.

113 Garcia FCP, Proubel DLN, Almeida JCF, Dias Ribeiro AP, Toledo IP, Poi WR, et al. Tooth fragment reattachment techniques – a systematic review. *Dent Traumatol*. 2018;34:135–43.

114 Khandelwal P, Srinivasan S, Arul B, Natanasabapathy V. Fragment reattachment after complicated crown-root fractures of anterior teeth: a systematic review. *Dent Traumatol*. 2021;37:37–52.

115 Alonso V, Caserio M. A clinical study of direct composite full-coverage crowns: long-term results. *Oper Dent*. 2012;37:432–41.

9

Regenerative Endodontics

Matthias Widbiller[1] *and Kerstin M. Galler*[2]

[1] *Department of Conservative Dentistry and Periodontology, University Hospital Regensburg, Regensburg, Germany*
[2] *Department of Operative Dentistry and Periodontology, Friedrich-Alexander-University, Erlangen, Germany*

Introduction

Pulp necrosis can be the result of deep caries, trauma or dental anomalies. As a consequence, bacterial colonization of the root canal triggers apical periodontitis, which may be initially asymptomatic (asymptomatic apical periodontitis) or associated with pain or other clinical signs of infection (symptomatic apical periodontitis). Classically, the goal of endodontic treatment is to cure apical periodontitis and resolve the associated clinical symptoms by thorough disinfection and filling of the root canal system.

In this context, root canal treatment of immature teeth poses a particular challenge for clinicians because these teeth typically have short roots with thin dentine walls and a wide apical foramen (Figure 9.1a,b). Various treatment options are available, such as apexification with repeated intracanal dressings with calcium hydroxide or the placement of an apical barrier with a hydraulic calcium silicate cement (HCSC). Traditional apexification involves multiple visits and alternating intracanal applications of calcium hydroxide to induce the formation of a calcified barrier at the root apex (1). Once this barrier is formed, the canal can be obturated with gutta-percha and the tooth can be restored. However, several disadvantages come with this treatment that make it no longer the preferred option. Multiple visits are required, therefore the total treatment time is long, and the prolonged contact of root dentine with calcium hydroxide in combination with the lack of a definitive restoration increases the risk of tooth fracture (2, 3). Given these disadvantages, the current recommendation for immature teeth is to place an apical plug with HCSC and seal the rest of the canal with gutta-percha (Figure 9.1b). This allows the treatment to be completed quickly and with few appointments (4). However, this will still leave short roots with thin root walls, which means an increased risk of fracture (5, 6).

The vision of endodontic regeneration is based on the restoration of the dentine–pulp complex, where a regenerated pulp tissue will take over all the biological functions of the original pulp, leading to the completion of physiological tooth development.

Vital Pulp Treatment, First Edition. Edited by Henry F. Duncan and Ikhlas A. El-Karim.

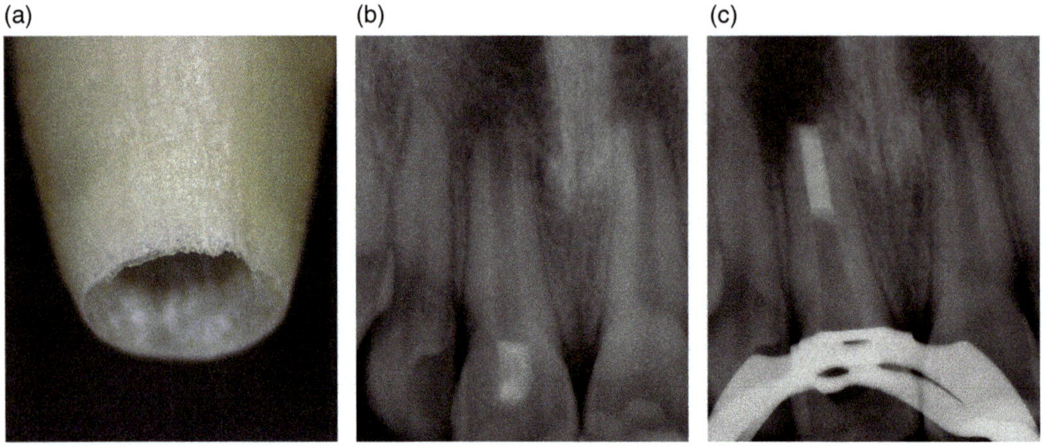

Figure 9.1 (a) The apex of a juvenile tooth without completed root growth is very wide, depending on the stage of development, and has thinly tapering root walls. (b) Root growth is only complete in the first few years after the tooth erupts. When the pulp is lost, the root walls remain thin and the apical foramen wide. (c) The conventional treatment for an immature tooth is to place an apical barrier with HCSC.

Biological and Mechanical Goals of Pulp Regeneration

From a biological perspective, regeneration is the process by which tissue is replaced or restored both in form and function (7, 8). Irreversible inflammation or necrosis of the pulp causes clinical and/or radiological symptoms and entails the removal of damaged tissues (9). With the loss of the dental pulp, its various biological abilities are gone (Figure 9.2).

One of the most important biological tasks of the dental pulp is root formation and the secretion of dentine during and after tooth development. In addition, the pulp tissue can resist invading microorganisms through mineral deposition and defend itself through specific and non-specific

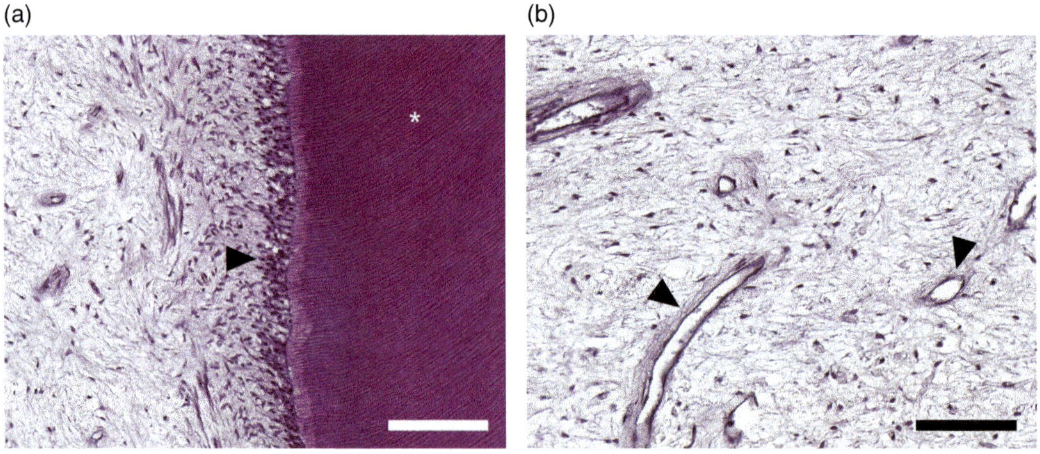

Figure 9.2 Histological representation of the dentine–pulp complex. (a) An odontoblast layer (arrowhead) can be seen at the interface to the dentine (asterisk). (b) The core of the pulp shows a collagenous extracellular matrix. Primarily fibroblasts and blood vessels with erythrocytes are visible (arrowheads) (H&E staining; scale bars: 100 μm).

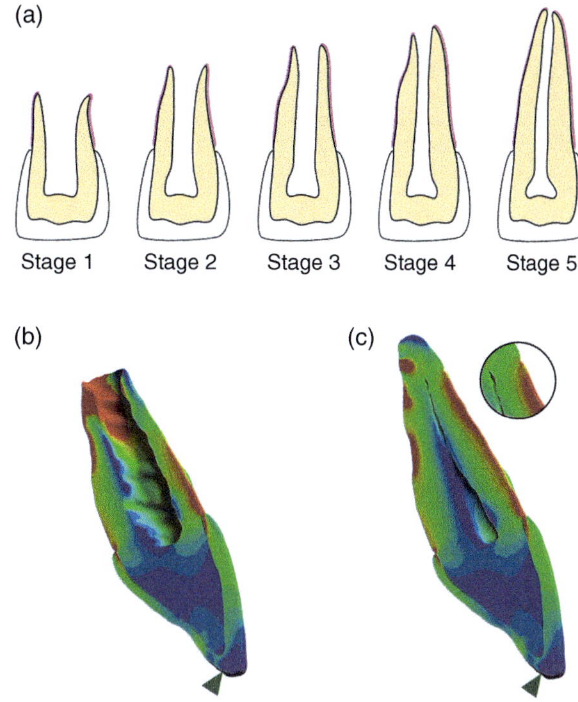

Figure 9.3 (a) Stages 1–5 of root development according to Cvek et al. (3). Stages 1–4 describe tooth roots during maturation, stage 5 the completed root growth. *Source:* Adapted from Cvek et al. (3)/ John Wiley & Sons. (b) Stress distribution pattern of an immature tooth during biting shows concentration of mechanical force in the fragile apical area. *Source:* Adapted from Bucchi et al. (16). (c) A mature tooth with a fully developed root can absorb more force and distribute it better. *Source:* Adapted from Bucchi et al. (16).

immune reactions (10, 11). An additional defence mechanism of the dentine–pulp complex is to ensure an outward flow of dentinal fluid through the tubules (12). Consequently, loss of pulp vitality may allow bacteria to migrate more easily through tubular dentine due to the lack of fluid pressure, which is particularly evident in the significant bacterial invasion of dentine in non-vital teeth (13). Furthermore, the dental pulp is also a sensitive organ that can detect not only thermal, mechanical or chemical stimuli, but also pathogenic irritants. The loss of the pulp inevitably leads to the destruction of neuronal perception, which may play a role in persistent pain conditions and functional changes of the trigeminal nerve (10, 14).

Besides all the biological implications of pulp loss, the long-term survival of the tooth may be compromised by the lack of mechanical strength due to possibly incomplete root maturation. (3, 15). The consequences are particularly severe for immature teeth in an early stage of root development (Figure 9.3a). Because of their short roots and thin dentine walls, these teeth are predisposed to fracture (3, 6). Pulp regeneration could facilitate the completion of root development, resulting in increased mechanical strength (Figure 9.3b) and, thus, long-term survival of affected teeth (16, 17). Due to the thin and fragile root walls of teeth with pulp necrosis in stages 1–3, endodontic regeneration can offer decisive advantages as growth progresses (Figure 9.3c). From stage 4, the root has sufficient stability for both regenerative endodontic approaches and an apical barrier with an HCSC to be suitable for treatment.

Historical Development of Regenerative Endodontics

The field of regenerative endodontics has developed rapidly in recent years and has attracted considerable interest. New biology-based and minimally invasive concepts are increasingly finding their way into everyday clinical practice and are changing the way of thinking in endodontics and

(a) (b) (c)

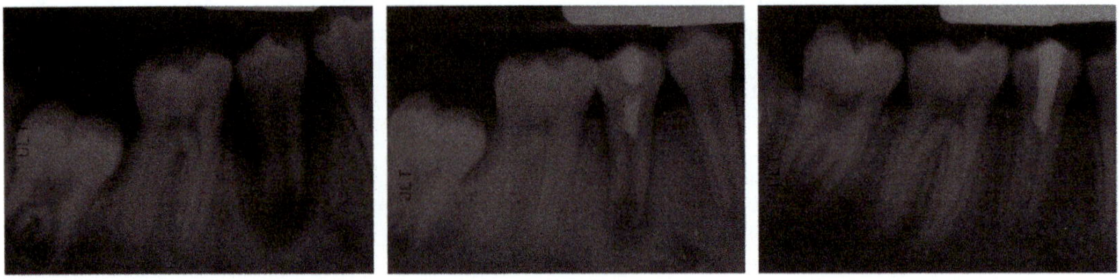

Figure 9.4 (a) Preoperative radiograph of a lower second premolar with an open apex and apical periodontitis. (b) Radiograph confirming the correct placement of MTA over the blood clot. (c) Follow-up radiograph after 18 months showing continued root development and resolution of apical radiolucency. *Source:* Banchs and Trope (20)/Reproduced with permission from Elsevier.

conservative dentistry. However, the idea of regenerating tissue inside the root canal system is not new and dates back to the 1960s. In the paper 'The role of blood clot in endodontic therapy', researcher Birger Nygaard-Østby studied provoked bleeding in the apical third of root canals obturated with gutta-percha in the coronal two-thirds (18). He observed partial or complete replacement of the blood clot, mainly by fibrous connective tissue. These findings were forgotten, and attempts to regenerate the pulp were abandoned for several decades before Iwaya et al. made an interesting observation in 2001 (19). In a case report, the authors described the treatment of a lower premolar with incomplete root formation, chronic apical periodontitis and a sinus tract. After disinfection and intracanal medication, the authors still demonstrated vital tissue inside the root canal and applied calcium hydroxide only to the area of the canal entrance. Thirty months after treatment, the completion of root formation was radiographically evident and the tooth responded again to electrical pulp testing (19). A landmark clinical report was finally published in 2004 by Banchs and Trope, translating this observation into a potential treatment approach (20). Similar to the case of Iwaya et al., the tooth involved was a lower premolar with an apical radiolucency and a sinus tract. The root canal was disinfected and treated with an intracanal medication. After the signs of inflammation had subsided, bleeding into the canal was induced by mechanical irritation of the vital apical tissue (Figure 9.4). The resulting blood clot was covered with mineral trioxide aggregate (MTA) at the level of the enamel-cementum junction. After 24 months, the osseous lesion had healed, root lengthening and thickening as well as apical closure were clearly visible radiographically (20).

This publication was followed by numerous case reports, case series and clinical studies on this biologically based treatment approach known today as revitalization (21, 22). Increasing scientific evidence and experience with revitalization led to official recommendations from the major endodontic societies, the European Society of Endodontology (ESE) and the American Association of Endodontists (AAE), on indications, case selection, procedural details, irrigation, materials and recall (23, 24).

Revitalization

Revitalization has become a well-established treatment alternative to the apical plug after pulpectomy or pulp necrosis in immature teeth and is now an integral part of the endodontic treatment spectrum. The aim is to create new tissue inside the root canal so that, if successful, the tooth root

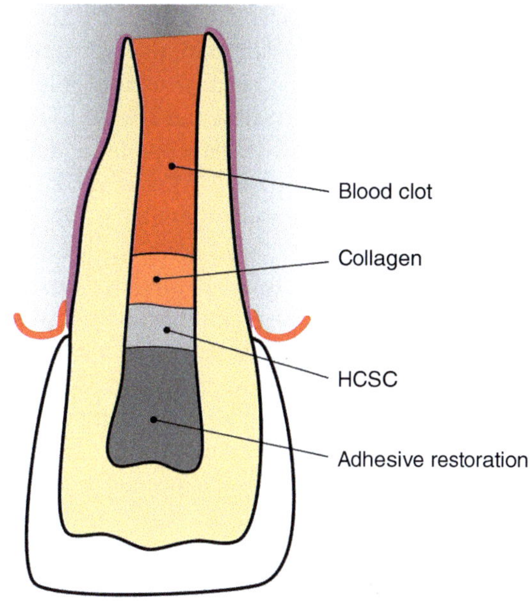

Figure 9.5 During revitalization, bleeding into the root canal is induced by over-instrumentation. A blood clot is formed and covered with a collagen matrix. The root canal is sealed with a bioactive HCSC and the cavity is sealed with an adhesive restoration.

can continue to grow and increase in length and thickness (24). Generally, the revitalization procedure is based on the induction of bleeding into the root canal, whereby mesenchymal stem cells from the periapical tissue are flushed in (Figure 9.5). A stable blood clot is formed, which acts as a biological matrix and contains blood-derived growth factors and multipotent stem cells (25). A key to successful revitalization is optimal infection control and sufficient restoration of the tooth. This allows for the development of a structured connective tissue inside the root canal, which is innervated, supplied by blood vessels and has the ability to form new hard tissue (25).

Indications and Contraindications

Revitalization can now be considered a valid treatment option for immature teeth with pulp necrosis (24). Particularly in the early stages of root development (stages 1–3) (Figure 9.3), when root walls appear thin and fragile, revitalization can offer benefits by continuing root growth. With or without the presence of apical periodontitis, this procedure can allow complete bony healing and progression of root formation. However, revitalization of teeth is not advisable if a dental dam cannot be applied or if extensive coronal hard substance loss would require insertion of an intracanal post. The indication should be given very cautiously, especially in immature replanted teeth after avulsion, as autonomous revascularization is possible due to the wide-open apical foramen and can be expected in about one-third of cases (26). Recommendations for revitalization of luxated teeth cannot be made due to a lack of clinical evidence. Patients with severe general medical impairment (ASA 3 or higher) are also recommended to be treated by conventional approaches (24).

Clinical Protocol

Revitalization usually takes place in two sessions. During the first session, a local anaesthetic is administered, and the tooth is isolated with a dental dam. The necrotic tissue is removed from the root canal, avoiding mechanical debridement of the canal walls. The length of the immature root is determined visually or radiographically, and the canal is disinfected with sodium hypochlorite (NaOCl) just before the apical foramen. A concentration of 1.5–3% is recommended for disinfection and removal of the residual tissue while sparing the local cells (23, 24). The canal is then rinsed with 0.9% normal saline and 17% EDTA to neutralize the cytotoxic NaOCl (27). Subsequently, excel liquid is removed with paper points and the canal is filled with a calcium hydroxide preparation or triple antibiotic paste (TAP: metronidazole, ciprofloxacin and minocycline) and adhesively sealed until the second appointment (23, 24).

After 2–4 weeks, the clinical situation is assessed and, if the tooth is asymptomatic, revitalization may be performed (Figure 9.6). After local anaesthesia, the tooth is isolated again with dental dam and intracanal medication is removed by rinsing with 17% EDTA. This agent has several effects, and it exposes collagen fibres as well as bioactive proteins on the dentine surface (28). After another rinse with saline, the root canal is dried and bleeding is induced by irritation of periapical tissues with an endodontic file, e.g. a pre-bent ISO 30 Hedström file (Figure 9.7a). The blood should reach approximately 2 mm below the cemento-enamel junction and be left to coagulate (Figure 9.6). The coagulum is then covered with a collagen matrix for stabilization, followed by application of an HCSC in direct contact (Figure 9.7b). At this point, a radiographic control is indicated and the tooth is sealed with an adhesive restoration (23, 24).

When selecting bioactive materials to cover the collagen matrix, they should not contain additives that cause crown discolouration, e.g. barium sulphate, which is often added to MTA as a radiopacifier. Synthetic HCSCs are particularly suitable for this purpose as they may not contain

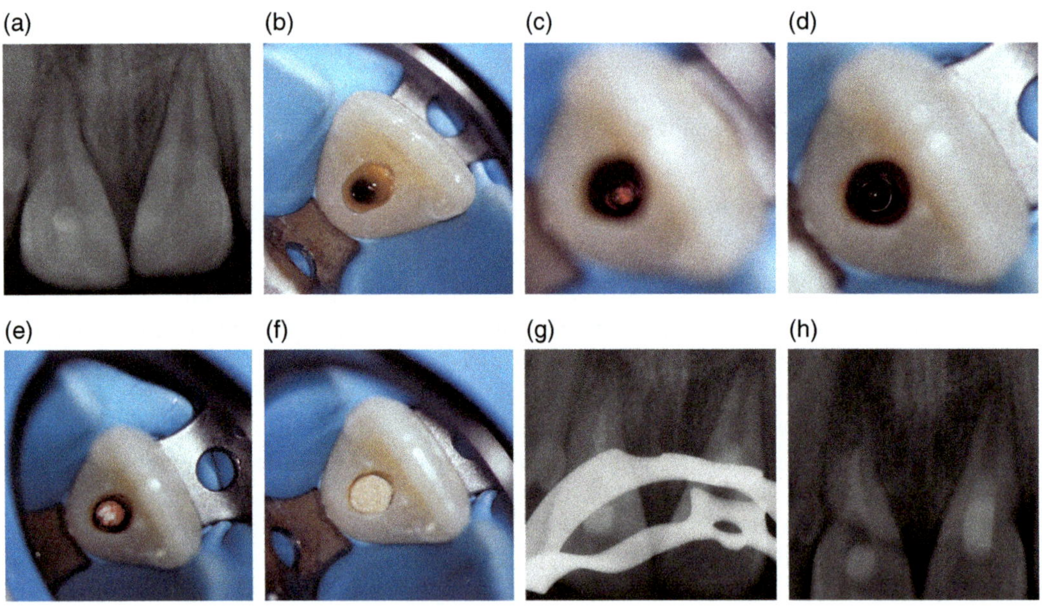

Figure 9.6 (a) The young patient suffered an avulsion of tooth 11, which was replanted, and subluxation of tooth 21, which was diagnosed with necrosis during recall. (b) The root canal was accessed and disinfected. (c) In the second session, the intracanal dressing was removed, the canal was finally rinsed with 17% EDTA and saline, and dried. (d) By over-instrumenting with a file, bleeding was induced into the canal. (e) The blood clot was covered with a collagen matrix and (f) covered with a hydraulic calcium silicate cement (Biodentine, Septodont, Niederkassel, Germany). (g) A radiograph was taken to verify this step. (h) The control radiograph after six months showed no pathological findings.

(a) (b)

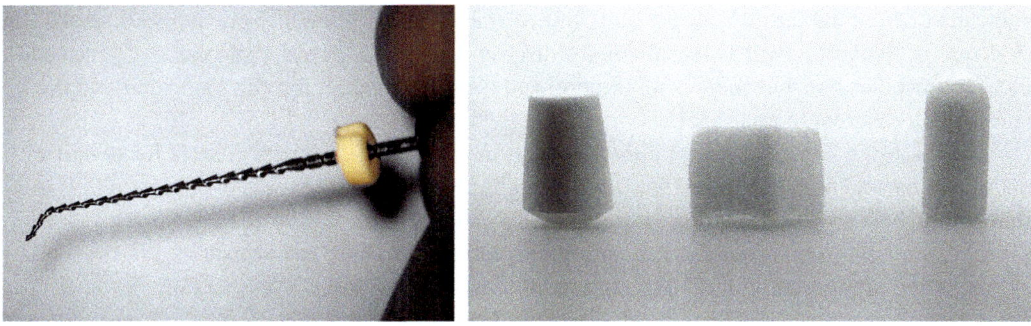

Figure 9.7 (a) A Hedström file may be bent at the tip to cause bleeding when rotated carefully in the periapical tissue. (b) Different collagen preparations for covering the blood clot: PARASORB HD Cone (left; RESORBA Medical, Nuremberg, Germany), Hémocollagène (centre; Septodont, Niederkassel, Germany) and RCP Resorbable Collagen Plug (right; ACE Surgical Supply Company, Brockton, USA).

these additives and also have advantages in terms of workability and mechanical properties (e.g. Biodentine, Septodont, Niederkassel, Germany).

To avoid problems with patient compliance, care should be taken to ensure adequate anaesthesia and a positive treatment atmosphere (24, 29). However, it should be noted that the induction of bleeding into the root canal is often slow in clinical practice and may be compromised by the use of a local anaesthetic containing a vasoconstrictor. Accordingly, it is important to use a local anaesthetic without additional vasoconstrictors to create optimal conditions for the induction of bleeding into the canal. Furthermore, intracanal medications, especially calcium hydroxide, should not be left in place for too long, as this may induce the formation of an calcified barrier and thus alter the conditions for bleeding and revitalization.

Follow-Up

Follow-up visits are recommended after 6, 12, 18 and 24 months and then annually for five years. An additional visit after only three months is particularly useful in cases where the revitalization was preceded by persistent signs of infection, resorptive processes or other risk factors such as reimplantation or transplantation after dental trauma. All clinical and radiological parameters should be reviewed and included in the assessment of treatment outcome.

If, as is often the case, further orthodontic therapy is necessary, it should be borne in mind that revitalized teeth are more susceptible to inflammation and resorptive processes if the aetiology of pulp necrosis was a traumatic dental injury (30, 31). Therefore, in the case of revitalized teeth, bony healing should be observed before tooth movement is started and shorter follow-up intervals should be chosen. If this cannot be guaranteed, revitalized teeth should be excluded from orthodontic movement.

Outcome Measures

Determining the success of a revitalization treatment is a major challenge, especially in young patients, for a number of reasons. The results are often inconclusive due to low patient compliance, poor reliability of sensitivity testing and the almost impossible standardization of two-dimensional radiographs in children and adolescents.

Of critical importance is the distinction between different clinical and radiological outcome parameters (22), as the terms 'success' and 'failure' may not be sufficiently precise with regard to revitalization. Accordingly, it is reasonable to discuss whether a case is a success if a periapical lesion is reduced in size, but there is no mineralized tissue formed within the root canal and thus, no increase in root length and thickness is evident.

For this reason, it is important for clinicians to establish specific success criteria for revitalization. A practical and patient-centred way to describe success is by the absence of pain, swelling and sinus tract (primary goal) and by a response to pulp vitality tests (tertiary goal). Radiological success is defined as the reduction of apical radiolucencies (primary goal) as a result of treatment and the progression of root growth in length and thickness (secondary goal). A clear failure is the failure to achieve the primary goal clinically or radiographically (32).

A comprehensive core outcome set as a checklist for standardized diagnosis and determination of success or failure in clinical practice may include the following aspects (24, 33):

- clinical signs and symptoms of inflammation (e.g. pain, tenderness to percussion, swelling, sinus tract)
- periodontal probing depths and mobility
- tooth discolouration
- response to sensitivity tests (electric, thermal)
- healing of periapical lesion
- root thickening and lengthening

Clinical Outcome

In recent years, a large number of prospective and retrospective clinical studies have been published demonstrating the clinical success of revitalization (21, 34). Due to the initially high survival rates, healing of periapical inflammation and increased growth in immature roots, it has been postulated as an alternative therapy to the apical barrier technique with HCSCs (23, 24).

Despite the growing body of evidence, there is currently a lack of long-term observations, which are essential for a comprehensive assessment of potential complications (21, 35). Although the high survival rate of revitalized teeth motivates the use of the procedure, it must be said that the predictability of the outcome of individual cases in terms of root growth (secondary goal) and restoration of tooth sensitivity (tertiary goal) is poor (34). Considering the available treatment alternatives for immature teeth, there is no significant difference between apexification, apical plug and revitalization in terms of periapical healing and tooth survival (35–38).

Of the many factors that can influence the clinical success of revitalization, root canal infection is considered to be one of the most important. Persistent bacteria are a major cause of treatment failure, as shown by animal studies (39) and a systematic review of failed cases (31). The presence of an apical lesion due to root canal infection can therefore be considered an important prognostic factor. However, incomplete elimination of bacteria in the root canal is not only responsible for failure but may also be responsible for the qualitative outcome of supposedly successful treatments (39, 40). Animal studies have shown that persisting bacteria are clearly associated with reduced or absent hard tissue apposition in the root canal, even in the absence of radiographically visible periapical lesions (39). In fact, a systematic review of existing controlled clinical trials showed that the evidence for revitalization as a treatment for apical periodontitis is limited and that more high-quality studies are needed (35).

In addition to root canal infection, the aetiology of pulp necrosis may also play a role in the success of revitalization. For example, the traumatic impact can damage Hertwig's epithelial root sheath (HERS) and the apical papilla, both structures essential for root growth (41). Especially luxation injuries such as intrusive luxations severely damage the periodontium (42). When the cause of pulp necrosis is caries or infection due to a developmental abnormality, e.g. dens evaginatus, the outcome appears to be different from those following dental trauma (21, 31, 36).

Revitalization of Mature Teeth

The basic indication for revitalization, according to the recommendations of endodontic societies, is the treatment of immature permanent teeth with pulp necrosis (23, 24). Since then, however, there has been increasing interest in applying this regenerative endodontic protocol to mature permanent teeth (43, 44). At the present time, these approaches must be considered experimental, as there are only a few studies, and the long-term prognosis of these teeth is unknown (45, 46). When permanent teeth with mature roots are treated by revitalization, there is currently no evidence of an advantage over established conventional endodontic treatment. Even in teeth with an open apex at an older age, it is biologically unlikely that further root development will occur, as the supply of mesenchymal stem cells decreases with age and HERS degrades. Whereas revitalization of mature teeth may be promising in terms of periapical healing and re-establishment of a response to sensibility testing, clinical studies are needed to assess the clinical relevance of regenerative endodontic procedures in permanent teeth.

Biological Result

The vision of revitalization was originally to regenerate the dentine–pulp complex (9, 47). Over time, the blood clot that has formed inside the root canal is transformed into a vascularized and innervated tissue that exerts at least part of the functions of the original pulp (22, 25). Thus, revitalized teeth may develop sensitivity to cold, periapical inflammation may subside and root development may progress (48, 49).

Histologically, however, this tissue may be different from the original pulp. Typically, the structured odontoblast layer is absent and ectopic components such as cementum or bone can be found (50–52). Accordingly, the biological outcome of revitalization does not represent pulp regeneration but must be considered a classic tissue repair in the biological sense (Figure 9.8) (9). The nomenclature of regenerative endodontics takes this into account, with Diogenes et al. introducing the term 'guided endodontic repair' (53).

Despite the biological limitations, the clinical results of revitalization are promising, and the procedure already represents an important component of clinical endodontic practice. However, due to dissatisfaction with the histological results and the low predictability of outcome, researchers have made great efforts to develop new procedures based on tissue engineering and regenerative medicine strategies to achieve cellular regeneration and biologically restore the dentine–pulp complex in a reproducible manner.

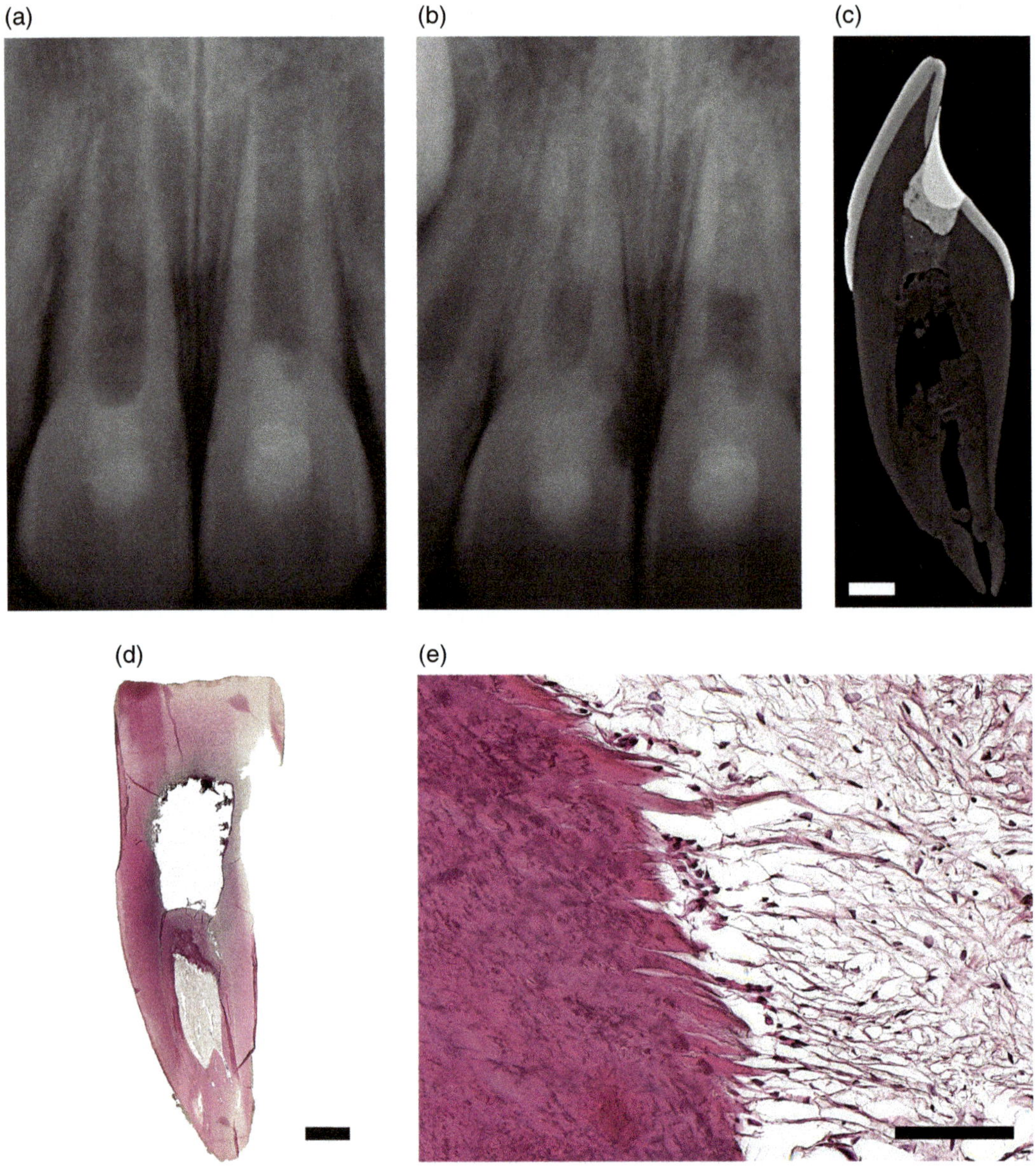

Figure 9.8 (a) Control radiograph after revitalization treatment of teeth 11 and 21, which had pulpal necrosis due to avulsion. (b) Unfortunately, external cervical resorption was noted in tooth 11 after 24 months and the tooth was removed. (c) Sagittal sections after micro-CT-imaging show the new hard tissue on root canal walls and the newly developed root apex. (d) Histological view of the whole tooth shows connective tissue within the canal and hard tissue on the canal walls, which appears structurally different from normal dentine. (e) The magnified view shows that the newly formed tissue does not have a tubular structure and no odontoblast layer has developed (H&E staining; scale bars: 1 mm in c and d; 100 μm in e).

Endodontic Tissue Engineering

Classification

The translational field of regenerative medicine encompasses diverse topics such as gene therapy, stem cell transplantation, the use of soluble molecules, cell reprogramming and tissue engineering (54). However, tissue engineering can be seen as a distinct direction based on the use of stem cells, scaffold materials and signalling molecules to restore tissues (55). Looking at the field of regenerative endodontics and the application of tissue engineering in the root canal, several endodontic tissue engineering (ETE) approaches are conceivable.

In principle, a technical subdivision can be made between cell-based approaches (CB-ETE) and primarily cell-free methods (CF-ETE) (9, 56). Characteristic of cell-based methods is that specific cells are processed *ex vivo* and introduced into the root canal encapsulated in customized scaffolds with added growth factors (Figure 9.9a). Despite the fact that initial clinical studies show promising results (57–59), the practical implementation of cell transplantation is associated with considerable challenges and costs, and its use in everyday practice does not currently seem realistic. The cells needed must first be harvested from donor tissue or pre-stored in a cell bank, expanded in the laboratory and transferred back into the patient under strict regulatory conditions (60). In contrast, the primarily cell-free idea is based on the principle of cell homing (Figure 9.9b). Endogenous stem or progenitor cells that are locally available at the root tip are used as the cell source, thus avoiding *ex vivo* cell manipulation (9, 61). Another advantage of CF-ETE approaches is that they are painless unless blood products are used and easy to administer by injection into the root canal. Following this approach, only scaffold materials are injected into the root canal together with signalling molecules, so that cells from the periapical tissue are attracted and migrate into the root canal (61, 62). In addition, blood vessels and nerve fibres invade the canal lumen, setting the stage for new tissue formation.

In principle, the central goal of ETE is to overcome the limits of repair and enable reproducible pulp regeneration. At present, although preclinical and experimental studies report promising results (58, 63, 64), sufficient evidence of biological pulp regeneration in clinical studies is seen controversial (52, 65).

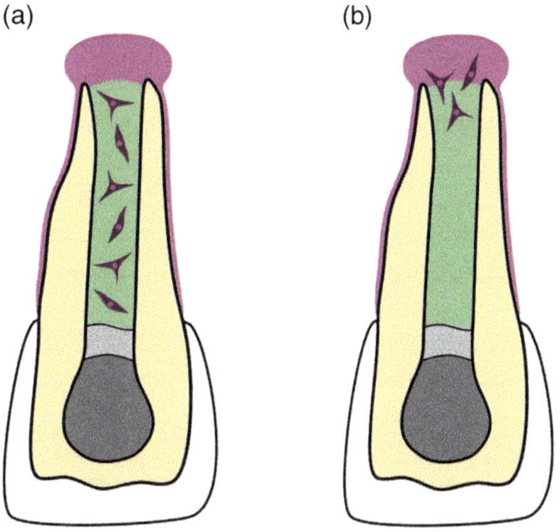

Figure 9.9 (a) Cell-based endodontic tissue engineering involves the expansion of cells *ex vivo* and transplantation into the root canal together with a scaffold and signalling molecules. (b) Cell homing, on the other hand, is a primarily cell-free approach that utilizes locally available cell sources. A customized scaffold containing signalling molecules is placed inside the canal, and cells can migrate from the periapical tissue.

Autologous Platelet Products

During revitalization treatment, the blood clot formed by retrograde bleeding into the root canal serves as a three-dimensional matrix for new tissue formation. On the other hand, autologous platelet products such as platelet-rich fibrin (PRF), plasma rich in growth factors (PRGF) or platelet-rich plasma (PRP) can also be introduced into the root canal through the access cavity from an orthograde direction. Here, the fibrin matrix forms a three-dimensional scaffold and contains blood components as well as platelets, which, according to the CF-ETE concept, provide the opportunity for cells to colonize the root canal. Autologous platelet products appear to improve bone healing and support root growth in clinical studies, however, there is currently a lack of good-quality trials in this field (65–67). It should be noted that the use of blood products involves venepuncture, which is particularly unsettling for young patients. Despite promising clinical outcomes (68–71), platelet-based techniques are, in analogy to revitalization, also emerging as biological repair rather than regeneration (56).

Conclusion

Regenerative endodontics is an exciting field that seeks to regenerate dental pulp and promote root development. Although the conventional apical barrier technique with HCSCs has shown promise, revitalization is a viable option for immature teeth with necrotic pulp, allowing root maturation and restoration of sensibility. However, long-term observations are needed to fully understand its potential and possible complications.

At the same time, researchers are exploring new approaches to achieve cellular regeneration and restore the dentine–pulp complex. Although cell-based methods are promising, their practical implementation is challenging and expensive. On the other hand, primarily cell-free methods based on cell-homing principles have shown to be effective in supporting new tissue formation in the root canal. Despite encouraging preclinical and experimental results, clinical evidence for biological pulp regeneration is lacking. Nevertheless, endodontic tissue engineering and other regenerative approaches have the potential to overcome the limitations of repair and enable reproducible pulp regeneration, offering exciting possibilities for the future of endodontics.

References

1 Mohammadi Z, Dummer PMH. Properties and applications of calcium hydroxide in endodontics and dental traumatology. *Int Endod J.* 2011;44(8):697–730.

2 Andreasen JO, Farik B, Munksgaard EC. Long-term calcium hydroxide as a root canal dressing may increase risk of root fracture. *Dent Traumatol.* 2002;18(3):134–7.

3 Cvek M. Prognosis of luxated non-vital maxillary incisors treated with calcium hydroxide and filled with gutta-percha. A retrospective clinical study. *Dent Traumatol.* 1992;8(2):45–55.

4 Lin JC, Lu JX, Zeng Q, Zhao W, Li WQ, Ling JQ. Comparison of mineral trioxide aggregate and calcium hydroxide for apexification of immature permanent teeth: a systematic review and meta-analysis. *J Formos Med Assoc.* 2016;115(7):523–30.

5 Jamshidi D, Homayouni H, Majd NM, Shahabi S, Arvin A, Omidi BR. Impact and fracture strength of simulated immature teeth treated with mineral trioxide aggregate apical plug and fiber post versus revascularization. *J Endod.* 2018;44(12):1878–82.

6 Talati A, Disfani R, Afshar A, Rastegar AF. Finite element evaluation of stress distribution in mature and immature teeth. *Iran Endod J*. 2007;2(2):47–53.
7 Goss RJ. *Regeneration*, Encyclopaedia Britannica, 2023. Accessed 28 February 2023. https://www.britannica.com/science/regeneration-biology.
8 Gilbert SF. *Developmental Biology*, 6th Ed., Sinauer Associates, Sunderland, 2000.
9 Widbiller M, Schmalz G. Endodontic regeneration: hard shell, soft core. *Odontology*. 2021;109(2):303–12.
10 Schmalz G, Widbiller M, Galler KM. Clinical perspectives of pulp regeneration. *J Endod*. 2020;46(9S):S161–74.
11 Galler KM, Weber M, Korkmaz Y, Widbiller M, Feuerer M. Inflammatory response mechanisms of the dentine–pulp complex and the periapical tissues. *Int J Mol Sci*. 2021;22(3):1480.
12 Maita E, Simpson MD, Tao L, Pashley DH. Fluid and protein flux across the pulpodentine complex of the dog in vivo. *Arch Oral Biol*. 1991;36(2):103–10.
13 Nagaoka S, Miyazaki Y, Liu HJ, Iwamoto Y, Kitano M, Kawagoe M. Bacterial invasion into dentinal tubules of human vital and nonvital teeth. *J Endod*. 1995;21(2):70–3.
14 Lee C, Ramsey A, Brito-Gariepy HD, Michot B, Podborits E, Melnyk J, et al. Molecular, cellular and behavioral changes associated with pathological pain signaling occur after dental pulp injury. *Mol Pain*. 2017;13:1744806917715173.
15 Caplan DJ, Cai J, Yin G, White BA. Root canal filled versus non-root canal filled teeth: a retrospective comparison of survival times. *J Public Health Dent*. 2005;65(2):90–6.
16 Bucchi C, Marcé-Nogué J, Galler KM, Widbiller M. Biomechanical performance of an immature maxillary central incisor after revitalization: a finite element analysis. *Int Endod J*. 2019;52(10):1508–18.
17 Zhou R, Wang Y, Chen Y, Chen S, Lyu H, Cai Z, et al. Radiographic, histologic, and biomechanical evaluation of combined application of platelet-rich fibrin with blood clot in regenerative endodontics. *J Endod*. 2017;43(12):2034–40.
18 Nygaard-Østby B. The role of the blood clot in endodontic therapy. An experimental histologic study. *Acta Odontol Scand*. 1961;19:324–53.
19 Iwaya SI, Ikawa M, Kubota M. Revascularization of an immature permanent tooth with apical periodontitis and sinus tract. *Dent Traumatol*. 2001;17(4):185–7.
20 Banchs F, Trope M. Revascularization of immature permanent teeth with apical periodontitis: new treatment protocol? *J Endod*. 2004;30(4):196–200.
21 Galler KM, Akamp T, Knüttel H, Widbiller M. A critical analysis of clinical research methods to study regenerative endodontics. *Int Endod J*. 2022;55(S2):456–70.
22 Diogenes AR, Ruparel NB. Regenerative endodontic procedures: clinical outcomes. *Dent Clin N Am*. 2017;61(1):111–25.
23 American Association of Endodontists. Clinical Considerations for a Regenerative Procedure. 2023. Accessed 28 February 2023. https://www.aae.org/specialty/wp-content/uploads/sites/2/2017/06/currentregenerativeendodonticconsiderations.pdf.
24 Galler KM, Krastl G, Simon S, Gorp GV, Meschi N, Vahedi B, et al. European Society of Endodontology position statement: revitalization procedures. *Int Endod J*. 2016;49(8):717–23.
25 Kim SG, Malek M, Sigurdsson A, Lin LM, Kahler B. Regenerative endodontics: a comprehensive review. *Int Endod J*. 2018;51(12):1367–88.
26 Andreasen JO, Borum MK, Jacobsen HL, Andreasen FM. Replantation of 400 avulsed permanent incisors. 2. Factors related to pulpal healing. *Dent Traumatol*. 1995;11(2):59–68.
27 Widbiller M, Rosendahl A, Wölflick M, Linnebank M, Welzenbach B, Hiller KA, et al. Isolation of endogenous TGF-β1 from root canals for pulp tissue engineering: a translational study. *Biology*. 2022;11(2):227.

28 Galler KM, Buchalla W, Hiller KA, Federlin M, Eidt A, Schiefersteiner M, et al. Influence of root canal disinfectants on growth factor release from dentin. *J Endod*. 2015;41(3):363–8.

29 Petrino JA, Boda KK, Shambarger S, Bowles WR, McClanahan SB. Challenges in regenerative endodontics: a case series. *J Endod*. 2010;36(3):536–41.

30 Kindelan SA, Day PF, Kindelan JD, Spencer JR, Duggal MS. Dental trauma: an overview of its influence on the management of orthodontic treatment. Part 1. *J Orthod*. 2008;35(2):68–78.

31 Almutairi W, Yassen GH, Aminoshariae A, Williams KA, Mickel A. Regenerative endodontics: a systematic analysis of the failed cases. *J Endod*. 2019;5(45):567–77.

32 Chugal N, Mallya SM, Kahler B, Lin LM. Endodontic treatment outcomes. *Dent Clin N Am*. 2017;61(1):59–80.

33 Cushley S, McLister C, Lappin MJ, Harrington M, Nagendrababu V, Duncan HF, et al. Outcomes reporting in systematic reviews on revitalization: a scoping review for the development of a core outcome set. *Int Endod J*. 2022;55(12):1317–34.

34 Torabinejad M, Nosrat A, Verma P, Udochukwu O. Regenerative endodontic treatment or mineral trioxide aggregate apical plug in teeth with necrotic pulps and open apices: a systematic review and meta-analysis. *J Endod*. 2017;43(11):1806–20.

35 Meschi N, Palma PJ, Cabanillas-Balsera D. Effectiveness of revitalization in treating apical periodontitis: a systematic review and meta-analysis. *Int Endod J*. 2023;56(Suppl 3):510–32.

36 Lin J, Zeng Q, Wei X, Zhao W, Cui M, Gu J, et al. Regenerative endodontics versus apexification in immature permanent teeth with apical periodontitis: a prospective randomized controlled study. *J Endod*. 2017;43(11):1821–7.

37 Nicoloso GF, Goldenfum GM, Pizzol TDSD, Scarparo RK, Montagner F, et al. Pulp revascularization or apexification for the treatment of immature necrotic permanent teeth: systematic review and meta-analysis. *J Clin Pediatr Dent*. 2019;43(5):305–13.

38 Pereira AC, Oliveira ML, Cerqueira-Neto ACCL, Vargas-Neto J, Nagata JY, Gomes BPFA, et al. Outcomes of traumatised immature teeth treated with apexification or regenerative endodontic procedure: a retrospective study. *Aust Endod J*. 2021;47(2):178–87.

39 Verma P, Nosrat A, Kim JR, Price JB, Wang P, Bair E, et al. Effect of residual bacteria on the outcome of pulp regeneration in vivo. *J Dent Res*. 2017;96(1):100–6.

40 Fouad AF. Contemporary microbial and antimicrobial considerations in regenerative endodontic therapy. *J Endod*. 2020;46(9):S105–14.

41 Huang GTJ, Sonoyama W, Liu Y, Liu H, Wang S, Shi S. The hidden treasure in apical papilla: the potential role in pulp/dentin regeneration and bioroot engineering. *J Endod*. 2008; 34(6):645–51.

42 Tsilingaridis G, Malmgren B, Andreasen JO, Malmgren O. Intrusive luxation of 60 permanent incisors: a retrospective study of treatment and outcome. *Dent Traumatol*. 2012;28(6):416–22.

43 He L, Kim SG, Gong Q, Zhong J, Wang S, Zhou X, et al. Regenerative endodontics for adult patients. *J Endod*. 2017;43(9):S57–64.

44 Scelza P, Gonçalves F, Caldas I, Nunes F, Lourenço ES, Tavares S, et al. Prognosis of regenerative endodontic procedures in mature teeth: a systematic review and meta-analysis of clinical and radiographic parameters. *Materials*. 2021;14(16):4418.

45 Arslan H, Ahmed HMA, Şahin Y, Yıldız ED, Gündoğdu EC, Güven Y, et al. Regenerative endodontic procedures in necrotic mature teeth with periapical radiolucencies: a preliminary randomized clinical study. *J Endod*. 2019;45(7):863–72.

46 El-Kateb NM, El-Backly RN, Amin WM, Abdalla AM. Quantitative assessment of intracanal regenerated tissues after regenerative endodontic procedures in mature teeth using magnetic resonance imaging: a randomized controlled clinical trial. *J Endod*. 2020;46(5):563–74.

47 Schmalz G, Smith AJ. Pulp development, repair, and regeneration: challenges of the transition from traditional dentistry to biologically based therapies. *J Endod*. 2014;40(4 Suppl):S2–5.

48 Chan EKM, Desmeules M, Cielecki M, Dabbagh B, dos Santos BF. Longitudinal cohort study of regenerative endodontic treatment for immature necrotic permanent teeth. *J Endod*. 2017;43(3):395–400.

49 Ong TK, Lim GS, Singh M, Fial AV. Quantitative assessment of root development after regenerative endodontic therapy: a systematic review and meta-analysis. *J Endod*. 2020; 46(12):1856–1866.e2.

50 Meschi N, Hilkens P, Gorp GV, Strijbos O, Mavridou AM, et al. Regenerative endodontic procedures posttrauma: immunohistologic analysis of a retrospective series of failed cases. *J Endod*. 2019;45(4):427–34.

51 Digka A, Sakka D, Lyroudia K. Histological assessment of human regenerative endodontic procedures (REP) of immature permanent teeth with necrotic pulp/apical periodontitis: a systematic review. *Aust Endod J*. 2020;46(1):140–53.

52 Minic S, Vital S, Chaussain C, Boukpessi T, Mangione F. Tissue characteristics in endodontic regeneration: a systematic review. *Int J Mol Sci*. 2022;23(18):10534.

53 Diogenes AR, Ruparel NB, Shiloah Y, Hargreaves KM. Regenerative endodontics: a way forward. *J Am Dent Assoc*. 2016;147(5):372–80.

54 Mason C, Dunnill P. A brief definition of regenerative medicine. *Regen Med*. 2008;3(1):1–5.

55 Langer R, Vacanti JP. Tissue engineering. *Science*. 1993;260(5110):920–6.

56 Lin LM, Huang GT, Sigurdsson A, Kahler B. Clinical cell-based versus cell-free regenerative endodontics: clarification of concept and term. *Int Endod J*. 2021;54(6):887–901.

57 Nakashima M, Iohara K, Murakami M, Nakamura H, Sato Y, Ariji Y, et al. Pulp regeneration by transplantation of dental pulp stem cells in pulpitis: a pilot clinical study. *Stem Cell Res Ther*. 2017;8(1):61.

58 Xuan K, Li B, Guo H, Sun W, Kou X, He X, et al. Deciduous autologous tooth stem cells regenerate dental pulp after implantation into injured teeth. *Sci Transl Med*. 2018;10(455):eaaf3227.

59 Brizuela C, Meza G, Urrejola D, Quezada MA, Concha G, Ramírez V, et al. Cell-based regenerative endodontics for treatment of periapical lesions: a randomized, controlled phase I/II clinical trial. *J Dent Res*. 2020;99(5):523–9.

60 Ohkoshi S, Hirono H, Nakahara T, Ishikawa H. Dental pulp cell bank as a possible future source of individual hepatocytes. *World J Hepatol*. 2018;10(10):702–7.

61 Galler KM, Widbiller M. Cell-free approaches for dental pulp tissue engineering. *J Endod*. 2020;46(9S):S143–9.

62 Galler KM, Widbiller M. Perspectives for cell-homing approaches to engineer dental pulp. *J Endod*. 2017;43(9S):S40–5.

63 Rosa V, Zhang Z, Grande RHM, Nör JE. Dental pulp tissue engineering in full-length human root canals. *J Dent Res*. 2013;92(11):970–5.

64 Widbiller M, Driesen RB, Eidt A, Lambrichts I, Hiller KA, Buchalla W, et al. Cell homing for pulp tissue engineering with endogenous dentin matrix proteins. *J Endod*. 2018;44(6):956–962.e2.

65 Widbiller M, Knüttel H, Meschi N, Terol FD. Effectiveness of endodontic tissue engineering in treatment of apical periodontitis: a systematic review. *Int Endod J*. 2023;56(Suppl 3):533–48.

66 Meschi N, Castro AB, Vandamme K, Quirynen M, Lambrechts P. The impact of autologous platelet concentrates on endodontic healing: a systematic review. *Platelets*. 2016;27(7):613–33.

67 Lolato A, Bucchi C, Taschieri S, Kabbaney AE, Fabbro MD. Platelet concentrates for revitalization of immature necrotic teeth: a systematic review of the clinical studies. *Platelets*. 2016;27(5):1–10.

68 Bezgin T, Yilmaz AD, Celik BN, Kolsuz ME, Sonmez H. Efficacy of platelet-rich plasma as a scaffold in regenerative endodontic treatment. *J Endod*. 2015;41(1):36–44.

69 Rizk HM, AL-Deen MSS, Emam AA. Regenerative endodontic treatment of bilateral necrotic immature permanent maxillary central incisors with platelet-rich plasma versus blood clot: a split mouth double-blinded randomized controlled trial. *Int J Clin Pediatric Dent*. 2019;12(4):332–9.

70 Ulusoy AT, Turedi I, Cimen M, Cehreli ZC. Evaluation of blood clot, platelet-rich plasma, platelet-rich fibrin, and platelet pellet as scaffolds in regenerative endodontic treatment: a prospective randomized trial. *J Endod*. 2019;45(5):560–6.

71 Xie Y, Lu F, Hong Y, He J, Lin Y. Revascularisation versus apexification for treatment of immature teeth based on periapical healing and root development: a systematic review and meta-analysis. *Eur J Paediatr Dent*. 2021;22(3):207–14.

10

Outcome of Vital Pulp Treatment and Regenerative Endodontics

Siobhan Cushley[1], Emi Shimizu[2], Yoshifumi Kobayashi[2], and Venkateshbabu Nagendrababu[3]

[1] *Centre for Dentistry, School of Medicine Dentistry and Biomedical Sciences, Queen's University Belfast, Belfast, Northern Ireland, UK*
[2] *Department of Oral Biology, Rutgers School of Dental Medicine, Newark, NJ, USA*
[3] *Department of Preventive and Restorative Dentistry, College of Dental Medicine, University of Sharjah, Sharjah, UAE*

Introduction

Outcomes are objective or subjective variables that are evaluated during a study to assess the influence of a clinical intervention or exposure on the health of a specified population (1). The clinical outcomes selected should be meaningful to the primary stakeholders, namely patients, healthcare professionals, and policymakers (2). Outcomes are assessed using outcome measures (OMs), which are objective or subjective measurements used to evaluate the effectiveness of an intervention compared with the control (3).

A report of a patient's health status by a trained health-care professional is referred to as a clinician-reported outcome (CRO) (4). A CRO can be assessed from patient records and clinical and radiographic examinations; however, they do not reflect perspectives and values of the patient, nor do they illustrate how well an intervention enhanced the patient's oral health (5). A report of a patient's health status that comes directly from the patient, without interpretation by a clinician, is referred to as a patient-reported outcome (PRO) (6). PROs include disease symptoms or therapeutic side-effects such as pain, as well as functional outcomes such as physical, emotional, or cognitive functioning and multidimensional categories such as health-related quality of life (HRQOL) (7, 8). The utilization of PROs in clinical trials has increased over the years (7, 8). The use of PROs is essential for improving clinical care because it develops relationships between doctors and patients and places the patient's priorities at the centre of the process (9). Patient-reported outcome measures (PROMs) are instruments used to evaluate PROs, typically in the form of self-reported surveys (10).

Endodontology is a specialty which includes the following interventions: vital pulp treatment (VPT), root canal treatment (RCT), root canal retreatment, surgical endodontics and regenerative endodontic therapies (RET) (11). The objectives of VPT and RET are the prevention or resolution of pulp and apical disease, which aims to improve the patient's quality of life (QoL) by retaining the natural tooth. This goal is reflected in the preservation of pulp vitality and function, often expressed as success or failure of treatment.

Vital Pulp Treatment, First Edition. Edited by Henry F. Duncan and Ikhlas A. El-Karim.

Clinicians performing VPT and RET should be focused on the well-being of their patients and be in a position to routinely assess the outcomes using the appropriate tools and measures. The purpose of this chapter is to provide an overview of the outcomes of VPT and RET and how and when these outcomes were measured, which ultimately improve patient care. A diverse range of outcomes have been reported with inconsistency and variability across the VPT and pulp revitalization (PR) studies conducted (12, 13). However, VPT and RET outcomes have historically been assessed using clinician-reported OMs, such as radiographic examination and pulp sensibility tests, with less focus on PROs such as pain and QoL. The longitudinal value of VPT and PR for the management of damaged tissue can only be determined if clinicians report agreed key outcomes in such a way as to facilitate their comparison over an appropriate timescale.

The assessment and reporting of endodontic treatment outcomes plays an essential role in treatment decisions, improving care and driving dental health policy.

Outcomes Reporting in VPT

Success

The terminology 'success' merits discussion. From a biological perspective, success demands evidence of pulp preservation and the absence of developing pulpitis or apical periodontitis (14). One challenge in interpreting the success outcome is that it is a subjective term whose meaning has been applied inconsistently across studies. Traditionally, the measure of treatment success used by VPT researchers has been based on the interpretation of the dental history combined with measurement of several different clinical and radiographic outcomes. These outcomes include responses to sensibility testing, absence of pain or other symptoms indicative of pulpal disease, need for the use of medication (analgesia), evidence of hard tissue bridge formation or continued root development in immature teeth and absence of clinical and radiographic signs of internal resorption and apical periodontitis. The lack of standardization of the term success prohibits accurate comparisons of results from studies already completed. The European Society of Endodontology (ESE) 2019 defined the success of VPT as an asymptomatic tooth with maintenance of vitality after at least one year. There should be an absence of apical periodontitis and root resorption and, in the case of immature teeth, continued root development (15). They stipulated that alongside history taking, both clinical and radiographic findings were required to report outcomes (15).

Pain

The asymptomatic tooth can be considered a tooth that is neither painful nor tender to bite on. Whilst both symptoms are frequently reported, reporting of pain differs across VPT studies. The characteristics of pain suggestive of irreversible pulpal changes are sometimes described (16), but equally, studies may simply report on the presence or absence of pain without further comment on the characteristics which could inform a diagnosis (17). Again, the nuances of pain outcomes can introduce an element of uncertainty in results interpretation. Proxy indicators of pain experience reported in VPT studies include the use of medication such as analgesics in the postoperative period (18) and the incidence of flare-ups requiring additional intervention (19). Although the use of analgesics links directly to pain, the other indicator does not and so should be interpreted cautiously. Measurement of pain intensity prior to and in response to treatment demands an accurate tool representing a self-report of the patient's experience (20). It should, however, be remembered that pain is a subjective sensation subject to individual influences, and so it is difficult to make meaningful comparisons between patients (21–23). Several tools have been proposed for routine use in dentistry including multidimensional tools like the McGill questionnaire (MPQ), through to unidimensional tools including visual analogue scale (VAS), numeric rating scale (NRS) and verbal rating scales (VRS). Multidimensional tools assess the impact of complex or persistent acute and chronic pain on a patient's activity or mood and as such are rarely used in VPT pain assessment. The unidimensional VAS, NRS and VRS are often used to report pain intensity in VPT studies.

The VAS is a 100 mm line on which a patient indicates a single point on the line representing their pain intensity, from one extreme representing no pain to 100 mm representing the worst pain imaginable (24). The score is awarded based on the distance between 0 (no pain) and the mark on the line placed by the respondent. The VAS is reliable and sensitive to changes in experience of pain so is useful in representing changes in pain pre and post-VPT. The VAS, however, is not self-explanatory and is open to interpretation by participants and cannot be administered verbally or on the telephone.

The NRS developed by Downie almost 50 years ago is the numeric representation of the VAS. The line is divided into equal segments, 0–10 (NRS-11) or 1–10 (NRS-10), with a verbal descriptor anchor at the two extremes. The respondent selects a whole number that best reflects the intensity of pain they are experiencing (25). NRS is a quick, simple-to-use scale that is reliable across most patients and cultures and can be administered verbally or on the telephone. There is good consistency in results between the NRS and VAS (26) (Figure 10.1).

The VRS, also known as the verbal pain scale (VPS), verbal descriptor scale (VDS) or simple descriptor scale (SDS), is both easy to administer and interpret and involves a patient being given adjectives to assess and describe their experience of pain. This may involve the choice of a single adjective through to a short statement. Each adjective is awarded a score providing an ordered categorical scale assessment of pain (Figure 10.2).

Currently, there are no valid tools to measure the proxy measures of pain described earlier including the use of analgesics in the postoperative period, so typically, this data is collected using a self-administered pain diary or simply having the clinician question the patient at a subsequent visit.

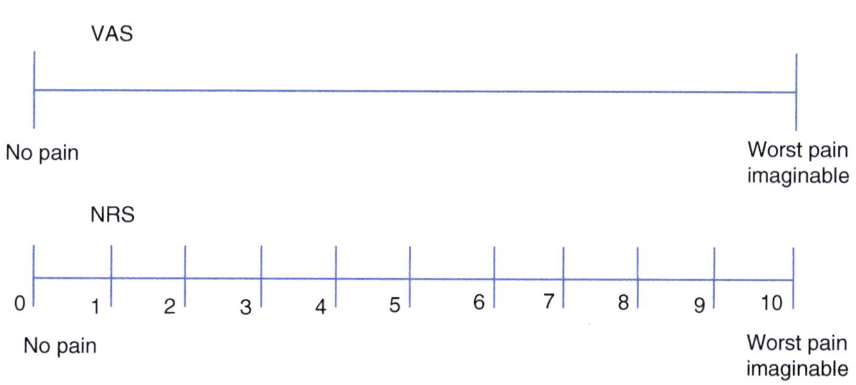

Figure 10.1 Sample visual analogue and numeric rating scales for pain intensity.

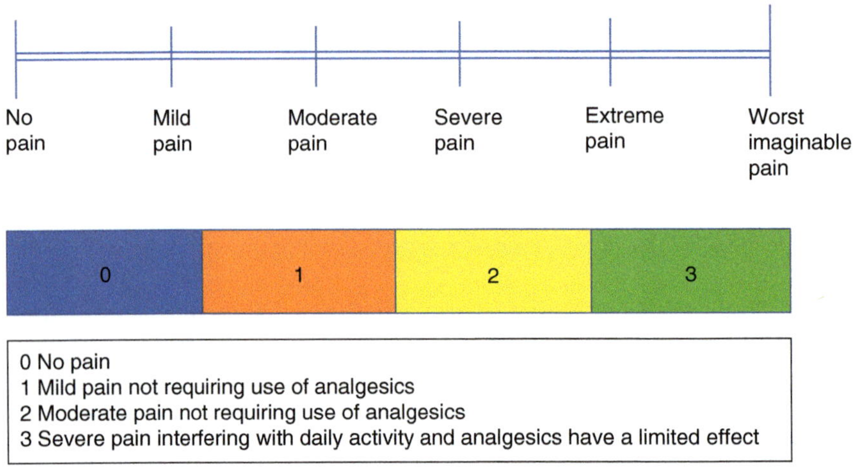

Figure 10.2 Sample verbal rating scales for pain intensity.

Timing of Measurement of Pain

The outcome of VPT must be measured at a consistent time point after treatment has been completed. This optimizes the likelihood that the effect intended for measurement is what is being measured and the true value of treatment can be assessed. Pain and the use of analgesics in the postoperative period should be measured as a minimum at seven days and for a maximum of three months post-treatment (27).

Sensibility/Vitality of Pulp

A key indicator of VPT success is pulpal health status. The gold standard in assessing pulpal health is histological assessment (28); however, as the pulp is encased in a rigid structure, histological assessment can only be carried out after commencing endodontic treatment or extraction of the tooth. In the absence of direct observation of tissue, proxy measures of pulpal status are frequently made based on neural responses to stimuli, the sensibility tests. Sensibility testing includes thermal, both cold and heat and electric pulp tests. The movement of dentinal fluid in response to temperature changes leads to odontoblast movement, which in turn mechanically stimulates the nerves within the pulp or direct electrical stimulation of pulp nerve tissue (29). A positive measure of sensibility is a tooth which responds to testing without an exaggerated response. Whilst these tests can be used singularly or in combination, the ESE 2019 recommends both cold and electric pulp sensibility testing are conducted to monitor outcomes of VPT (15). Owing to the nature of the intervention, teeth that have under-gone VPT may respond differently to sensibility testing and in fact teeth that have under-gone complete pulpotomy may be unresponsive. A recent study explored the reliability of cold and electric sensibility testing in pulpotomized mature permanent teeth. 95% of the teeth treated by complete pulpotomy responded to electric pulp testing, whereas only 13.5% of the same teeth responded to cold testing (30). This lends weight to the ESE's recommendation that both thermal and electric tests should be carried out in sensibility measurement.

Whilst routinely used, sensibility testing measures only sensory response without considering that neural tissue is highly resistant to inflammatory changes and can continue to respond after the pulp tissue has degenerated (31). A better measure of pulp health would be the presence of an intact vascular supply in the pulp tissue and tooth vitality. Such tests include laser Doppler and pulse oximetry; however, owing to the more complex nature of measurement and a lack of commercially available machines, vitality outcome is rarely reported in VPT studies.

Timing of Sensibility Testing

Based on the current ESE guidelines, pulp sensibility testing should be conducted at 6- and 12-months post-treatment, continuing at regular intervals if symptoms persist or when there is doubt about healing (15). The consensus group, however, have suggested that this follow-up reporting should continue for as long as possible beyond one year in all cases (27).

Absence of Apical Periodontitis, Root Resorption and, in the Case of Immature Teeth, Continued Root Development

Radiographic assessment of the principal endpoint of VPT, pulp preservation in the absence of periapical disease and internal root resorption, with continued root development in immature teeth, demands an assessment of the entire root morphology and surrounding bony tissue. There is acceptance that the quality of digital films is superior to that of traditional films (32), which could improve post-op evaluation accuracy; however, currently, there is no recommendation regarding the nature of the imaging technique required from the ESE. Several radiographic assessment criteria have been applied to measure VPT outcomes including modified Strindberg (33), and Periapical index (PAI) criteria (16, 34). Strindberg criteria is an established tool in the reporting of endodontic outcomes; however, its rigidity and failure to acknowledge the continuum of the healing process limits its role. Modification of this tool, however, enables its continued and valid use in the reporting of radiographic outcomes in VPT studies. Alternatively, the PAI is a simple, reproducible 5-point scale used in the reporting of VPT outcomes. The index standardizes the categorization of the radiographic features of apical periodontitis. Conventional radiography, whilst offering cost-effective imaging with good diagnostic performance and accuracy, is subject to geometric distortion and anatomical noise. Periapical lesions may not be visible until demineralization has reached levels of 30–50% leading to difficulties in assessing early disease (35, 36) and two-dimensional radiographs may under-estimate the clinical situation (37). Secondly, root anatomy and any associated pathology may be obscured by neighbouring structures including the maxillary sinus and apical foramen. Cone beam computed tomography (CBCT) has the capacity to overcome these short comings and there has been an increased use of CBCT in endodontics. The PAI scale has been further adapted to allow for this (CBCT-PAI) and its use has been observed in some VPT studies (38). Despite CBCT offering higher detection rate of periapical and associated pathology, (39) its routine use is not yet recommended in endodontics owing to its higher radiation dosage, cost and the need for additional space and operator training (40).

Timing of Radiographic Assessment

Early periapical changes cannot be visualized on radiographs and so sufficient time must elapse before a radiographic assessment can provide the information necessary to make a valid judgement about treatment outcome. The current recommendation is for radiographic assessment at one year, continuing annually if required for up to four years (15).

Other Outcomes Reported in VPT Studies

Whilst the ESE has defined success under strict outcome criteria, a plethora of outcomes have been reported in VPT studies. As a result of all VPTs sharing a common aim of pulp preservation, there is considerable overlap in the reporting of outcomes across studies (Tables 10.1 and 10.2) (12, 13).

Clinician-reported clinical outcomes include the absence of tooth mobility, loss of periodontal attachment, tertiary dentine formation, histological reports including biomarker analysis, definitive restoration integrity/quality, time to complete the procedure, cost-effectiveness, caries progression and pulp, tooth or restoration survival. Additional radiographic outcomes include lamina dura uniformity, canal calcification, hard tissue formation/remineralization and carious lesion progression.

Table 10.1 Clinician-reported outcomes (CROs) in VPT and PR studies (12, 13).

Outcome measure	Selective caries removal	Pulp capping	Pulpotomy	PR
Signs and symptoms disease	X	X	X	X
Sensibility testing	X	X	X	X
Pulp or restoration survival	X	X	X	—
Loss of periodontal attachment	—	X	X	X
Tooth mobility	X	X	X	X
Swelling/sinus	X	X	X	X
Need for further intervention	X	X	X	X
Formation of hard tissue barrier	X	X	X	X
Integrity/quality of restoration	X	X	X	—
Exposure during caries removal	X	—	—	—
Success	X	X	X	X
Time to complete procedure	X	X	X	X
Root resorption	X	X	X	X
Development secondary caries	X	X	X	—
Evidence of apical/furcal radiolucency	X	X	X	X
Periodontal ligament/lamina dura changes,	X	X	X	—
Continued root development/apexogenesis	X	X	X	X
Bacterial activity	X	—	—	—
Biomarker measurement	—	X	X	—
Inflammatory cell activity	X	X	X	—
Pulpal calcification	—	X	X	X
Cost-effectiveness	—	—	X	—
Reinfection	—	—	—	X
Tissue regeneration	—	—	—	X
Unpredictable pattern in root morphology	—	—	—	X
Thickening dentine walls	—	—	—	X
Tooth fracture	—	—	—	X

X, reported; —, not reported.

Table 10.2 Dental patient-reported outcomes (PROs) in VPT and PR studies (12, 13).

Outcome measure	Selective caries removal	Pulp capping	Pulpotomy	PR
Tooth survival	X	X	X	X
Pain	X	X	X	X
TTP/palpation	X	X	X	X
Use of analgesics post-op period	X	X	X	—
Tooth function	—	X	X	X
Satisfaction with treatment	—	X	—	—
Patient comfort	—	X	—	—
Discoloration/aesthetics	X	X	X	X

X, reported; —, not reported.

Quality of the Definitive Restoration

The quality/integrity of the definitive restoration across all VPTs links to how treatment may fail in the future. Elimination and exclusion of bacteria from the pulpal space and surrounding areas are critical to long-term treatment success (41, 42). A defective or deteriorating restoration provides free access for bacterial penetration, and with the hard tissue barrier formed at the pulp wound potentially porous or lacking in structural uniformity, adequacy of the coronal restoration is essential to maintain an environment conducive to maintaining pulpal health. Without factoring this dimension into reporting, it could be that the overall outcome reported may indeed not truly reflect the impact of the intervention but rather the result of other influencing factors. Restoration integrity and quality can be assessed radiographically and clinically by direct observation utilizing the modified US Public Health Service/Ryge criteria or indirectly utilizing digital photography.

Survival

Survival is often reported as an outcome of VPT. Whilst studies may report survival, some are reporting survival of the restoration, others pulp survival or possibly tooth survival. All three outcomes are legitimate, but the lack of consistency prohibits comparison and again reinforces the need for outcome terminology to be clearly defined.

Histopathological Outcomes

Histopathological outcomes include measures of bacterial activity, biomarkers, hard tissue deposition/remineralization and pulpal inflammatory response. Whilst histopathological assessment is the gold standard in understanding the biological impact of the treatment, these findings are infrequently reported in clinical studies in VPT because of the inaccessible nature of the pulp without commencing endodontic treatment. Biomarker quantification is increasingly reported in more recent studies (25), where it seeks to address the short comings with the current diagnostic tools and may offer an objective tool to accurately evaluate pulpal health status.

Formation of Hard Tissue Barrier

Formation of a mineralized hard tissue bridge is often reported as an outcome in VPT studies. The methods of identification/measurement of this barrier in VPT studies include histological assessment, visual inspection and probing of the tissue, and radiographic assessment (43–45). Whilst histological assessment represents the gold standard, in a treatment designed to be conservative it would not be appropriate to reopen the tooth to simply assess hard tissue deposition and mineralization. In clinical studies radiographic assessment is frequently used to measure this outcome but simple intra-oral imaging is subject to several limitations including restricted detection of early mineralization processes and a subjective assessment of the quality of the bridge. CBCT imaging has been used in a small number of VPT studies and offers the advantage of better visualization of the bridge but with its associated limitations, consideration must be given to whether the benefits outweigh the risks. As such CBCT is not currently recommended by the ESE as a measurement tool for hard tissue bridge formation in VPT.

Oral Health-Related Quality of Life

Additional PROs include the subjective assessment of the functional and psychosocial impact of pulpal disease and its management, a measure of QoL. More specifically, the oral health related quality of life (OHRQoL) arguably represents one of the most important PROs. Outcomes that inform OHRQoL include pain and analgesic use in the postoperative period, flare-up, chewing ability and tooth function, swelling and sinus, tenderness to percussion and palpation, aesthetics/tooth discoloration, need for further intervention, impact on daily activities both in receiving the intervention and its effect and patient comfort. Stand-alone scores of individual outcomes such as pain measurement or patient satisfaction which may contribute to an overall assessment of QoL, cannot be interpreted as a measure of improved OHRQoL. Additionally, often, these outcomes have been based on ad hoc questioning of a patient without the use of a validated instrument. Several tools are available to measure QoL, including HRQoL, OHRQoL and oral health impact profile (OHIP), but this outcome is not often reported in VPT. There is a recommendation that QoL outcomes should be measured at a minimum time-point of six months and for as long as possible (27).

Composite Outcomes

Frequently in VPT studies, in lieu of a single outcome measure, a composite endpoint is reported. The composite endpoint comprises two or more single-component outcomes combined to give an overall outcome of treatment effect (46). This methodology increases the incidence of the endpoint being observed, and as a result, the statistical precision of the result is increased, and the study can achieve its aim with fewer patients in a shorter time frame, at less cost. An example of a composite endpoint in VPT is success. With different studies often including diverse single-component measures it should be remembered that composites must be interpreted cautiously to ensure that the measures being reported are equivalent. Adoption of the ESE 2019 description of success should resolve inconsistency in reporting success.

With such a diverse range of reportable outcomes, there needs to be clarity regarding which outcomes are the most important and should be reported as a minimum in all cases. Early work in this field has resulted in a consensus group identifying and ranking outcomes that should be reported in the treatment of pulpitis and agreeing appropriate follow-up periods (27) (Table 10.3).

The consensus group determined that the duration of follow-up for all outcomes should be 'a minimum of one year and a maximum of as long as possible' except for pain, tenderness, swelling

Table 10.3 Outcome consensus for the treatment of pulpitis.

Critical outcome	Important outcome
Tooth survival (PRO)	Tooth function (fracture, restoration longevity) (PRO)
Pain, tenderness, swelling and need for medication (analgesics) (PRO)	Need for further intervention (PRO)
Evidence of emerging apical radiolucency (CRO)	Adverse effects (exacerbation, restoration integrity, allergy) (PRO)
Response to sensibility test (not complete pulpotomy or pulpectomy) (CRO)	Sinus (CRO)
	OHRQoL (PRO)
	Radiographic evidence of continued root formation (CRO)

and need for medication, which was determined as 'a minimum of seven days and a maximum of three months' and OHRQoL with 'a minimum of six months and maximum of as long as possible'.

Stakeholder Considerations in Outcome Reporting

The importance of PROs has already been outlined, but now consider the choice of outcomes from the viewpoint of different stakeholders in the measure of the composite success. A clinician may define success as an asymptomatic tooth which responds to sensibility testing with evidence of normal or healing apical tissues and an absence of root resorption. A patient may simply require survival of a functional tooth within their budgetary limitations. Let us consider a scenario reporting the success of VPT. At 12 months, there is an absence of clinical and radiographic signs and symptoms indicative of treatment failure. However, what if the patient reported that they were dissatisfied with the cost of the treatment? Would this scenario be seen as an overall treatment failure? Typically, with composite outcomes, failure of any variable within the composite would equate to overall failure of the measure. Montori et al. (47) stated that for composite outcomes to be reliably applied, three prerequisites must be met: the component endpoints must be of equal importance to patients as they are to clinicians, the more and less important endpoints should occur with similar frequency and the endpoints should share similar relative risk reductions. If these prerequisites are not met, a composite endpoint may not be appropriate and single primary outcomes should perhaps be reported. So, in our scenario, it may have been more appropriate to include only clinical and radiographic outcomes within the composite of success and report satisfaction with the cost as a stand-alone measure.

Pulp Revitalization as a Regenerative Endodontic Therapy

Outcomes and Outcome Measures

Success/Survival

In PR, the outcome 'success' is defined as the absence of periapical disease or clinical symptoms throughout the observation period, whilst 'survival' is defined as the presence of treated teeth regardless of biological and/or clinical symptoms. The meta-analysis of seven clinical trial studies indicated no significant differences in the success rate between PR (83%) and apexification (86%)(48).

Compared with the implant-based study, the observation periods for PR reported in the literature are relatively shorter, with no patients being followed for more than 10 years (49–52). Therefore, a longer observation period may be required to define the success and survival in RET in the future.

Radiographic Measurement of Outcomes

The good prognosis in PR consists of asymptomatic functional teeth, no periapical radiolucency and increased root development including elongation of root length and increased root wall width. Failure to achieve these objectives is considered an unfavourable outcome.

1) The following points must be considered when performing radiographic measurements: The use of CBCT for radiographic evaluation allows for a more detailed assessment of the outcome after PR (53–56).
2) It is recommended to use the standardized paralleling technique with the Rinn XCP alignment system to measure root length and root wall width before and after the procedure (57).
3) The radiograph images need to be adjusted or modified by SIDEXIS XG (Dentsplay Sirona) (58), TurboReg plug-in application of Image J (National Institutes of Health) (59) or Photoshop (Adobe) (60).
4) Root length should be measured from the cementoenamel junction (CEJ) to the radiographic apex of the tooth (57–59).
5) To measure the root thickness and pulp space, Mittmann et al. (58) used the point at the half of the root length line and a right-angle straight line on the point (Figure 10.3 ½ l). After the line was generated with 90 degrees from the point (Figure 10.3 ½ l), the root thickness (Figure 10.3 r) and pulp space (Figure 10.3 p) were measured.
6) The diameter of apical foramen should be measured by dragging a straight line across the apical foramen (58).

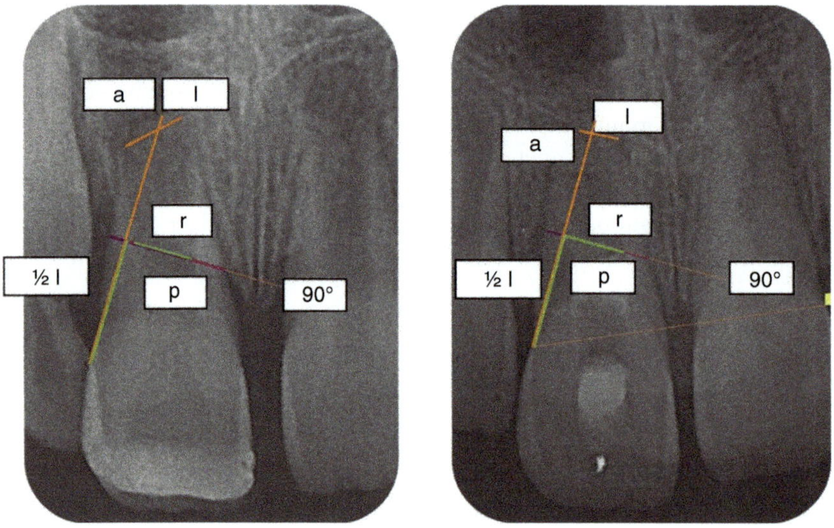

Figure 10.3 Radiographic measurement. l: root length, it was measured from the cemento-enamel junction (CEJ) to the radiographic apex of the tooth. r: root thickness, p: pulp space, a: diameter of apical foramen. *Source:* Mittmann et.al. (58)/Reproduced from Springer Nature/CC BY 4.0.

Pain

Several studies reported postoperative pain within 24 hours after PR (61–63). According to these reports, there was no statistically significant difference regarding the time-point and incidence of postoperative pain between the PR group and the conventional RCT group (61, 63). Therefore, PR practitioners need to follow up on their patients' postoperative pain for 24 hours, as they do for RCT patients. As postoperative pain should be decreased until 72 hours after the procedure (62), if patients have severe symptoms such as continuous pain, swelling (flare-up), or fever even after 72 hours, the treated tooth needs to be re-evaluated. In case of mild pain after PR, non-steroidal anti-inflammatory drugs (NSAIDs) such as Ibuprofen (Advil, Motrin) or alternatively Acetaminophen (Tylenol) have been used for the management (64).

To measure the intensity in postoperative pain of PR, several pain tools (MPQ, VAS, NRS, VRS) are available (described in VPT section). From the clinical trial, PR with platelet-rich plasma (PRP) reduced the intensity of postoperative pain assessed by NRS after 12 hours compared with the RCT group (63), indicating that PRP can be useful for RET. To improve outcome data of PR, it is important to measure pain intensity using these tools during the follow-up period.

Tooth Function

To evaluate tooth function after RET, tooth sensitivity is one of the pulpal functionality to be checked. Indeed, some case series and clinical trials reported the regain of tooth sensitivity after RET including PR and stem cell-based therapy (58, 65–69) in cold test or electric pulp tests. The meta-analysis of the clinical trials showed the positive vitality response is significantly higher in PR with platelet concentrate including PRP and platelet-rich fibrin (PRF) compared to blood clot only (48), indicating that PRP or PRF has a benefit to use for PR.

Seek Emergency Treatment

A few studies of clinical trials indicated the incidence of flare-ups after PR procedure (63, 70). According to the reports, there is no significant difference in the incidence of flare-ups between PR and conventional RCT (63). The causative factors of flare-ups are microbial infection, injured periradicular tissues by mechanical or chemical factors, apical extrusion of debris and host defences (71). Although flare-ups happen in a similar frequency compared to RCT, there are limited reports regarding flare-ups in clinical trials and case series of RET. Thus, it is recommended all information including flare-ups should be reported in clinical trials of RET in the future.

Adverse Effects

The main adverse effect of PR procedure is crown discoloration, as mentioned in many clinical trials and case series (69, 70, 72–74). Discolouration is caused by minocycline of triple antibiotic paste (TAP), calcium silicate cement as well as reactions of calcium silicate cement with irrigation solutions or blood (73). Currently, bleaching (internal bleaching) is the standard treatment of discoloration teeth caused by PR procedure.

Vertical or horizontal fractures have been reported after PR procedure (75–77); however, the reason for facture was not related to the adverse effect of the procedure in all of those reports. One of the fractured teeth had pre-existing large crown restorations with thinner root dentin, and two other fractured teeth had untreated trauma or cracked roots.

Follow-Up and Optimal Timing for Reporting Outcomes

American Association of Endodontists (78) and ESE released the recommendation of follow-up (6-, 12-, 24-months) of a regenerative procedure (79, 80). Additionally, most case series and clinical trials show the period of the follow-up is less than three years for RET (48, 69). These time spans for follow-up should be recognized as a minimum requirement because those periods are considerably shorter than the follow-up period of implant studies (49), which exceeds 10 years in many cases. The follow-up period for RET can be extended to the same span of implant studies in the future.

Improvement of Current RET by Assessing OHRQoL

OHRQoL is a component of HRQoL associated with the patient's impact of oral disease and dental treatment. As the goal of oral health care is to reduce and eliminate oral disease in patients, the concept of OHRQoL that captures these effects is the primary target of dental treatment in a patient-centred approach. OHRQoL is not only important for individual patients but also a major indicator of dental public health (13, 81, 82). Unfortunately, there are no studies regarding OHRQoL on RET including PR and stem cell-based regenerative endodontic study (13). OHRQoL of each patient receiving RET needs to be evaluated, whilst every clinical study or case report containing RET operation should document patients' OHRQoL in the future.

The OHIP-14 is commonly used for assessment of OHRQoL in the dental field (83). The OHIP-14 includes 14 questions over 7 domains (physical functioning, physical pain, physiological disability, physical disability, psychological disability, social disability and handicap) based on the World Health Organization's theoretic model of disease-impairment-disability-handicap (84, 85) (Table 10.4).

Table 10.4 OHIP-14 questionnaire.

Dimension	Question	Weight
Functional limitation	Have you had trouble *pronouncing* any words because of problems with your teeth, mouth or dentures?	0.51
	Have you felt that your *sense of taste* has worsened because of problems with your teeth, mouth or dentures?	0.49
Physical pain	Have you had *painful aching* in your mouth?	0.34
	Have you found it *uncomfortable to eat any foods* because of problems with your teeth, mouth or dentures?	0.66
Psychological discomfort	Have you been *self-conscious* of your teeth, mouth or dentures?	0.45
	Have you *felt tense* because of problems with your teeth, mouth or dentures?	0.55
Physical disability	Has your *diet been unsatisfactory* because of problems with your teeth, mouth or dentures?	0.52
	Have you had to *interrupt meals* because of problems with your teeth, mouth or dentures?	0.48
Psychological disability	Have you found it *difficult to relax* because of problems with your teeth, mouth or dentures	0.60
	Have you been a bit *embarrassed* because of problems with your teeth, mouth or dentures?	0.40
Social disability	Have you been a bit *irritable with other people* because of problems with your teeth, mouth or dentures?	0.62
	Have you had *difficulty doing your usual jobs* because of problems with your teeth, mouth or dentures?	0.38
Handicap	Have you felt that life in general was *less satisfying* because of problems with your teeth, mouth or dentures?	0.59
	Have you been *totally unable to function* because of problems with your teeth, mouth or dentures?	0.41

References

1 Ferreira JC, Patino CM. Types of outcomes in clinical research. *J Bras Pneumol.* 2017;43(1):5.
2 Lamont TJ, Clarkson JE. Core outcome sets and dental patient reported outcomes. *J Evid-Based Dent Pract.* 2022;22(1, Supplement):101659.
3 Smith PG, Morrow RH, Ross DA (eds.). *Outcome Measures and Case Definition*, OUP Oxford, Oxford, UK, 2015.
4 Powers JH 3rd, Patrick DL, Walton MK, Marquis P, Cano S, Hobart J, et al. Clinician-reported outcome assessments of treatment benefit: report of the ISPOR clinical outcome assessment emerging good practices task force. *Value Health.* 2017;20(1):2–14.
5 Hua F. Increasing the value of orthodontic research through the use of dental patient-reported outcomes. *J Evid Based Dent Pract.* 2019;19(2):99–105.
6 Guidance for industry: patient-reported outcome measures: use in medical product development to support labeling claims: draft guidance. *Health Qual Life Outcomes.* 2006;4:79.
7 Mercieca-Bebber R, King MT, Calvert MJ, Stockler MR, Friedlander M. The importance of patient-reported outcomes in clinical trials and strategies for future optimization. *Patient Relat Outcome Meas.* 2018;9:353–67.
8 Mercieca-Bebber R, Williams D, Tait MA, Roydhouse J, Busija L, Sundaram CS, et al. Trials with patient-reported outcomes registered on the Australian New Zealand Clinical Trials Registry (ANZCTR). *Qual Life Res.* 2018;27(10):2581–91.
9 Pantaleon L. Why measuring outcomes is important in health care. *J Vet Intern Med.* 2019;33(2):356–62.
10 Johnston BC, Patrick DL, Devji T, Maxwell LJ, Bingham CO III, Beaton DE, et al. Patient-reported outcomes. In: Cochrane Handbook for Systematic Reviews of Interventions Version 63 (updated February 2022), 2019, 479–92.
11 Torabinejad M, Bahjri K. Essential elements of evidenced-based endodontics: steps involved in conducting clinical research. *J Endod.* 2005;31(8):563–9.
12 Cushley S, Duncan HF, Lundy FT, Nagendrababu V, Clarke M, El Karim I. Outcomes reporting in systematic reviews on vital pulp treatment: a scoping review for the development of a core outcome set. *Int Endod Jo.* 2022;55(9):891–909.
13 Cushley S, McLister C, Lappin MJ, Harrington M, Nagendrababu V, Duncan HF, et al. Outcomes reporting in systematic reviews on revitalization: a scoping review for the development of a core outcome set. *Int Endod J.* 2022;55(12):1317–34.
14 Asgary S, Hassanizadeh R, Torabzadeh H, Eghbal MJ. Treatment outcomes of 4 vital pulp therapies in mature molars. *J Endod.* 2018;44(4):529–35.
15 Duncan HF, Galler KM, Tomson PL, Simon S, El-Karim I, Kundzina R, et al. European Society of Endodontology position statement: management of deep caries and the exposed pulp. *Int Endod J.* 2019;52(7):923–34.
16 Taha NA, Ahmad MB, Ghanim A. Assessment of mineral trioxide aggregate pulpotomy in mature permanent teeth with carious exposures. *Int Endod J.* 2017;50(2):117–25.
17 Witherspoon DE, Small JC, Harris GZ. Mineral trioxide aggregate pulpotomies: a case series outcomes assessment. *J Am Dent Assoc.* 2006;137(5):610–8.
18 Simon S, Perard M, Zanini M, Smith AJ, Charpentier E, Djole SX, et al. Should pulp chamber pulpotomy be seen as a permanent treatment? Some preliminary thoughts. *Int Endod J.* 2013;46(1):79–87.
19 Casagrande L, Seminario AT, Correa MB, Werle SB, Maltz M, Demarco FF, et al. Longevity and associated risk factors in adhesive restorations of young permanent teeth after complete and selective caries removal: a retrospective study. *Clin Oral Investig.* 2017;21(3):847–55.

20 Hjermstad MJ, Fayers PM, Haugen DF, Caraceni A, Hanks GW, Loge JH, et al. Studies comparing numerical rating scales, verbal rating scales, and visual analogue scales for assessment of pain intensity in adults: a systematic literature review. *J Pain Symptom Manage.* 2011;41(6):1073–93.

21 Cascella M, Thompson NS, Muzio MR, Forte CA, Cuomo A. The underestimated role of psychological and rehabilitation approaches for management of cancer pain. A brief commentary. *Rec Prog Med.* 2016;107(8):418–21.

22 Friedman S, Abitbol S, Lawrence HP. Treatment outcome in endodontics: the Toronto Study. Phase 1: initial treatment. *J Endod.* 2003;29(12):787–93.

23 Farzaneh M, Abitbol S, Lawrence HP, Friedman S. Treatment outcome in endodontics-the Toronto Study. Phase II: initial treatment. *J Endod.* 2004;30(5):302–9.

24 Atav Ates A, Dumani A, Yoldas O, Unal I. Post-obturation pain following the use of carrier-based system with AH Plus or iRoot SP sealers: a randomized controlled clinical trial. *Clin Oral Investig.* 2019;23(7):3053–61.

25 Ballal NV, Duncan HF, Rai N, Jalan P, Zehnder M. Sodium hypochlorite reduces postoperative discomfort and painful early failure after carious exposure and direct pulp capping-initial findings of a randomized controlled trial. *J Clin Med.* 2020;9(8).

26 Rosas S, Paço M, Lemos C, Pinho T. Comparison between the visual analog scale and the numerical rating scale in the perception of esthetics and pain. *Int Orthod.* 2017;15(4):543–60.

27 Duncan HF, Nagendrababu V, El-Karim I, Dummer PMH. Outcome measures to assess the effectiveness of endodontic treatment for pulpitis and apical periodontitis for use in the development of European Society of Endodontology S3-level clinical practice guidelines: a consensus-based development. *Int Endod J.* 2021;54(12):2184–94.

28 Patro S, Meto A, Mohanty A, Chopra V, Miglani S, Das A, et al. Diagnostic accuracy of pulp vitality tests and pulp sensibility tests for assessing pulpal health in permanent teeth: a systematic review and meta-analysis. *Int J Environ Res Public Health.* 2022;19(15):9599.

29 Matthews B, Hughes SHS. Chapter 9 The ultrastructure and receptor transduction mechanisms of dentine. In: Hamann W, Iggo A (eds.) Progress in Brain Research, vol. 74, Elsevier, 1988, 69–76.

30 Aravind A, Rechithra R, Sharma R, Rana A, Sharma S, Kumar V, et al. Response to pulp sensibility tests after full pulpotomy in permanent mandibular teeth with symptomatic irreversible pulpitis: a retrospective data analysis. *J Endod.* 2022;48(1):80–6.

31 Jafarzadeh H, Abbott PV. Review of pulp sensibility tests. Part I: general information and thermal tests. *Int Endod J.* 2010;43(9):738–62.

32 Kanagasingam S, Hussaini HM, Soo I, Baharin S, Ashar A, Patel S. Accuracy of single and parallax film and digital periapical radiographs in diagnosing apical periodontitis – a cadaver study. *Int Endod J.* 2017;50(5):427–36.

33 Kumar V, Juneja R, Duhan J, Sangwan P, Tewari S. Comparative evaluation of platelet-rich fibrin, mineral trioxide aggregate, and calcium hydroxide as pulpotomy agents in permanent molars with irreversible pulpitis: a randomized controlled trial. *Contemp Clin Dent.* 2016;7(4):512–8.

34 Galani M, Tewari S, Sangwan P, Mittal S, Kumar V, Duhan J. Comparative evaluation of postoperative pain and success rate after pulpotomy and root canal treatment in cariously exposed mature permanent molars: a randomized controlled trial. *J Endod.* 2017;43(12):1953–62.

35 Bender IB, Seltzer S. Roentgenographic and direct observation of experimental lesions in bone: II. 1961. *J Endod.* 2003;29(11):707–12. discussion 1.

36 Bender IB, Seltzer S. Roentgenographic and direct observation of experimental lesions in bone: I. 1961. *J Endod.* 2003;29(11):702–6. discussion 1.

37 Rechenberg DK, Munir A, Zehnder M. Correlation between the clinically diagnosed inflammatory process and periapical index scores in severely painful endodontically involved teeth. *Int Endod J.* 2021;54(2):172–80.

38 Hashem D, Mannocci F, Patel S, Manoharan A, Brown JE, Watson TF, et al. Clinical and radiographic assessment of the efficacy of calcium silicate indirect pulp capping: a randomized controlled clinical trial. *J Dent Res.* 2015;94(4):562–8.

39 Estrela C, Bueno MR, Leles CR, Azevedo B, Azevedo JR. Accuracy of cone beam computed tomography and panoramic and periapical radiography for detection of apical periodontitis. *J Endod.* 2008;34(3):273–9.

40 Patel S, Brown J, Semper M, Abella F, Mannocci F. European Society of Endodontology position statement: use of cone beam computed tomography in Endodontics: European Society of Endodontology (ESE) developed by. *Int Endod J.* 2019;52(12):1675–8.

41 Mjör IA, Tronstad L. Experimentally induced pulpitis. *Oral Surg Oral Med Oral Pathol.* 1972;34(1):102–8.

42 Goldberg M. *The Dental Pulp: Biology, Pathology, and Regenerative Therapies*, Springer, 2014.

43 Eghbal MJ, Asgary S, Baglue RA, Parirokh M, Ghoddusi J. MTA pulpotomy of human permanent molars with irreversible pulpitis. *Aust Endod J.* 2009;35(1):4–8.

44 Negm M, Grant A, Combe E. Clinical and histologic study of human pulpal response to new cements containing calcium hydroxide. *Oral Surg Oral Med Oral Pathol.* 1980;50(5):462–71.

45 Nosrat IV, Nosrat CA. Reparative hard tissue formation following calcium hydroxide application after partial pulpotomy in cariously exposed pulps of permanent teeth. *Int Endod J.* 1998;31(3):221–6.

46 Cordoba G, Schwartz L, Woloshin S, Bae H, Gøtzsche PC. Definition, reporting, and interpretation of composite outcomes in clinical trials: systematic review. *Bmj.* 2010;341:c3920.

47 Montori VM, Permanyer-Miralda G, Ferreira-González I, Busse JW, Pacheco-Huergo V, Bryant D, et al. Validity of composite end points in clinical trials. *Bmj.* 2005;330(7491):594–6.

48 Panda P, Mishra L, Govind S, Panda S, Lapinska B. Clinical outcome and comparison of regenerative and apexification intervention in young immature necrotic teeth-a systematic review and meta-analysis. *J Clin Med.* 2022;11(13):3909.

49 Simonis P, Dufour T, Tenenbaum H. Long-term implant survival and success: a 10-16-year follow-up of non-submerged dental implants. *Clin Oral Implants Res.* 2010;21(7):772–7.

50 Abu Zeid ST, Alamoudi RA, Alothmani OS, Mokeem Saleh AA, Siddiqui AY. A prospective study of long-term regenerative endodontics outcomes of necrotic immature permanent teeth: an 8-year follow-up. *Healthcare (Basel).* 2021;9(12):1670.

51 Casey SM, Fox D, Duong W, Bui N, Latifi N, Ramesh V, et al. Patient centered outcomes among a cohort receiving regenerative endodontic procedures or apexification treatments. *J Endod.* 2022;48(3):345–54.

52 Aksel H, Serper A. Recent considerations in regenerative endodontic treatment approaches. *J Dent Sci.* 2014;9(3):207–13.

53 Law AS. Outcomes of regenerative endodontic procedures. *Dent Clin N Am.* 2012;56(3):627–37.

54 Markandey S, Das Adhikari H. Evaluation of blood clot, platelet-rich plasma, and platelet-rich fibrin-mediated regenerative endodontic procedures in teeth with periapical pathology: a CBCT study. *Restor Dent Endod.* 2022;47(4):e41.

55 Arango-Gómez E, Nino-Barrera JL, Nino G, Jordan F, Sossa-Rojas H. Pulp revascularization with and without platelet-rich plasma in two anterior teeth with horizontal radicular fractures: a case report. *Restor Dent Endod.* 2019;44(4):e35.

56 Linsuwanont P, Sinpitaksakul P, Lertsakchai T. Evaluation of root maturation after revitalization in immature permanent teeth with nonvital pulps by cone beam computed tomography and conventional radiographs. *Int Endod J.* 2017;50(9):836–46.

57 Caleza-Jiménez C, Ribas-Pérez D, Biedma-Perea M, Solano-Mendoza B, Mendoza-Mendoza A. Radiographic differences observed following apexification vs revascularization in necrotic immature molars and incisors: a follow-up study of 18 teeth. *Eur Arch Paediatr Dent.* 2022;23(3):381–9.

58 Mittmann CW, Kostka E, Ballout H, Preus M, Preissner R, Karaman M, et al. Outcome of revascularization therapy in traumatized immature incisors. *BMC Oral Health.* 2020;20(1):207.

59 Bose R, Nummikoski P, Hargreaves K. A retrospective evaluation of radiographic outcomes in immature teeth with necrotic root canal systems treated with regenerative endodontic procedures. *J Endod.* 2009;35(10):1343–9.

60 Waheed A, Van Etten RL, Koob R, Drenckhahn D. Targeting of phosphomannosyl-deficient arylsulfatase A to lysosomes of I-cell fibroblasts. *Eur J Cell Biol.* 1988;45(2):262–7.

61 Tawfik M, Morsi M, Ibrahim A. A comparative study to assess the post operative pain intensity following non-surgical root canal treatment and pulp revascularization in mature necrotic teeth. *Egypt Dent J.* 2019;65(4):3899–905.

62 Omaia M, Negm M, Nashaat Y, Nehal Nabil N, Othman A. The effect of triple antibiotic paste as an intracanal medication with an anti-inflammatory drug on post-operative pain of asymptomatic uniradicular necrotic teeth: a double blind randomized clinical trial. *F1000 Res.* 2019;8(1687):1–16.

63 Ahmed YE, Ahmed GM, Ghoneim AG. Evaluation of postoperative pain and healing following regenerative endodontics using platelet-rich plasma versus conventional endodontic treatment in necrotic mature mandibular molars with chronic periapical periodontitis. A randomized clinical trial. *Int Endod J.* 2022;56:404–18.

64 Schuh C, Benso B, Aguayo S. Potential novel strategies for the treatment of dental pulp-derived pain: pharmacological approaches and beyond. *Front Pharmacol.* 2019;10:1068.

65 Cehreli ZC, Isbitiren B, Sara S, Erbas G. Regenerative endodontic treatment (revascularization) of immature necrotic molars medicated with calcium hydroxide: a case series. *J Endod.* 2011;37(9):1327–30.

66 Keswani D, Pandey RK. Revascularization of an immature tooth with a necrotic pulp using platelet-rich fibrin: a case report. *Int Endod J.* 2013;46(11):1096–104.

67 Nakashima M, Iohara K, Murakami M, Nakamura H, Sato Y, Ariji Y, et al. Pulp regeneration by transplantation of dental pulp stem cells in pulpitis: a pilot clinical study. *Stem Cell Res Ther.* 2017;8(1):61.

68 Nageh M, Ahmed GM, El-Baz AA. Assessment of regaining pulp sensibility in mature necrotic teeth using a modified revascularization technique with platelet-rich fibrin: a clinical study. *J Endod.* 2018;44(10):1526–33.

69 Yan H, De Deus G, Kristoffersen IM, Wiig E, Reseland JE, Johnsen GF, et al. Regenerative endodontics by cell homing: a review of recent clinical trials. *J Endod.* 2023;49(1):4–17.

70 Meschi N, EzEldeen M, Garcia AET, Lahoud P, Van Gorp G, Coucke W, et al. Regenerative endodontic procedure of immature permanent teeth with leukocyte and platelet-rich fibrin: a multicenter controlled clinical trial. *J Endod.* 2021;47(11):1729–50.

71 Jayakodi H, Kailasam S, Kumaravadivel K, Thangavelu B, Mathew S. Clinical and pharmacological management of endodontic flare-up. *J Pharm Bioallied Sci.* 2012;4(Suppl 2):S294–8.

72 Wei X, Yang M, Yue L, Huang D, Zhou X, Wang X, et al. Expert consensus on regenerative endodontic procedures. *Int J Oral Sci.* 2022;14(1):55.

73 Žižka R, Šedý J, Gregor L, Voborná I. Discoloration after regenerative endodontic procedures: a critical review. *Iran Endod J.* 2018;13(3):278–84.

74 Pereira AC, Oliveira ML, Cerqueira-Neto A, Gomes B, Ferraz CCR, Almeida JFA, et al. Treatment outcomes of pulp revascularization in traumatized immature teeth using calcium hydroxide and 2% chlorhexidine gel as intracanal medication. *J Appl Oral Sci.* 2020;28:e20200217.

75 Martin G, Ricucci D, Gibbs JL, Lin LM. Histological findings of revascularized/revitalized immature permanent molar with apical periodontitis using platelet-rich plasma. *J Endod.* 2013;39(1):138–44.

76 Shimizu E, Jong G, Partridge N, Rosenberg PA, Lin LM. Histologic observation of a human immature permanent tooth with irreversible pulpitis after revascularization/regeneration procedure. *J Endod.* 2012;38(9):1293–7.

77 Shimizu E, Ricucci D, Albert J, Alobaid AS, Gibbs JL, Huang GT, et al. Clinical, radiographic, and histological observation of a human immature permanent tooth with chronic apical abscess after revitalization treatment. *J Endod.* 2013;39(8):1078–83.

78 AAE Special Committee to Develop a Microscope Position Paper. AAE Position Statement. Use of microscopes and other magnification techniques. *Journal of endodontics.* 2012;38(8):1153–5.

79 Endodontists AAo. AAE Clinical Considerations for a Regenerative Procedure. 2021.

80 Galler KM, Krastl G, Simon S, Van Gorp G, Meschi N, Vahedi B, et al. European Society of Endodontology position statement: revitalization procedures. *Int Endod J.* 2016;49(8):717–23.

81 John MT. Foundations of oral health-related quality of life. *J Oral Rehabil.* 2020;48:355–9.

82 Liu P, McGrath C, Cheung GS. Improvement in oral health-related quality of life after endodontic treatment: a prospective longitudinal study. *J Endod.* 2014;40(6):805–10.

83 Slade GD, Spencer AJ, Locker D, Hunt RJ, Strauss RP, Beck JD. Variations in the social impact of oral conditions among older adults in South Australia, Ontario, and North Carolina. *J Dent Res.* 1996;75(7):1439–50.

84 Locker D. Measuring oral health: a conceptual framework. *Community Dent Health.* 1988;5(1):3–18.

85 Slade GD. Derivation and validation of a short-form oral health impact profile. *Commun Dent Oral Epidemiol.* 1997;25(4):284–90.

Index

t

u

v